P9-DCV-808

Also by Harlan Lane

AS AUTHOR

The Wild Boy of Aveyron

When the Mind Hears: A History of the Deaf

The Mask of Benevolence: Disabling the Deaf Community

AS EDITOR

Recent Perspectives on American Sign Language
(François Grosjean, co-editor)

The Deaf Experience: Classics in Language and Education
(translated from the French by Franklin Philip)

Parallel Views: Education and Access for Deaf People in France and the United States

Looking Back: A Reader on the History of Deaf Communities and Their Sign Languages
(Renate Fischer, co-editor)

Also by Robert Hoffmeister

Discourse Processes in American Sign Language
(James Gee, co-editor)

Also by Ben Bahan

American Sign Language Literature Series: Bird of a Different Feather
(with Sam Supalla)

Signs for Me
Basic Sign Vocabulary for Children, Parents & Teachers
(with Joe Dannis)

My ABC Signs of Animal Friends
(with Joe Dannis)

A Journey into the Deaf-World

Cover art:

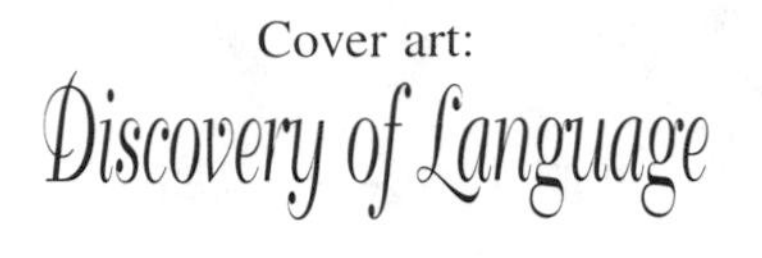

by Harry R. Williams

As a Deaf boy, the artist struggled to understand the connections between words and images. His discovery of language came when he grasped that the fingerspelled word "B-A-L-L" matched the picture of a ball, and the door of enlightenment opened for him. Before, his mind was a desert. After, his vision was transformed by the primary colors—red, blue, yellow—which were to change his life. The flower in full bloom is Williams' rendering of the moment of discovery: "I understand!"

L. K. Elion
My Eyes are My Ears;
Homage to Harry R. Williams

A Journey into the Deaf-World

HARLAN LANE

ROBERT HOFFMEISTER

BEN BAHAN

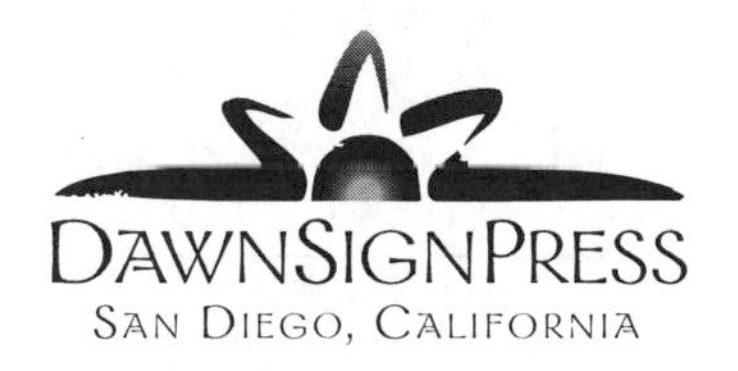

DAWNSIGNPRESS
SAN DIEGO, CALIFORNIA

A Journey into the DEAF–WORLD

Editor: Corona A. Machemer Editorial Services
Producer: Joe Dannis
Sign Illustrator: Paul Setzer
Manufactured in the United States of America.
Published by DawnSignPress.

The paintings of the abbé de l'Epée on his deathbed, by Peyson; of the abbé de l'Epée giving a lesson, by Privat; and of Sicard and Massieu, by Langlois are from the collection of the library of l'Institut National des Jeunes Sourds, 254 rue St Jacques 75005 Paris.

The information contained in this book is intended to be educational and not for diagnosis, prescription, or treatment of health disorders, whatsoever. This information should not replace competent medical care. The Authors and Publisher are in no way liable for any use or misuse of the information.

Library of Congress Cataloging-in-Publication Data
Lane, Harlan L.
A journey into the deaf–world / Harlan Lane, Robert Hoffmeister, Ben Bahan.
p. cm.
Includes bibliographical references and index.
ISBN 0-915035-63-4 (paper: alk. paper). — ISBN 0-915035-62-6 (hardcase: alk. paper)
1. Deaf—Social conditions. 2. Deaf—United States—Social conditions. 3. Deaf—Means of communication—United States. I. Hoffmeister, Robert. II. Bahan, Benjamin J. III. Title.
HV2380.L27 1996
305.9′08162′0973—dc20 96-19522
CIP

10 9 8 7 6

For our parents and the Deaf people who have led us on the journey

Contents

Acknowledgments

MANY of our colleagues have greatly assisted us in preparing this book and it is a pleasure to acknowledge their help: Thomas Allen, Yerker Andersson, Elliot Aheroni, Douglas Bahl, Charlotte Baker-Shenk, Donald Bangs, Sue Burnes, John Campton, Kathee Christensen, Oscar Cohen, Dennis Cokely, Janis Cole, Betty Colonomos, Jay Croft, Amy Czisk, Kristin Diperri, Lindsay Dunn, Gilbert Eastman, L.K. Elion, Karen Emmorey, Kathy Girod, Neil Glickman, Debra Guthmann, Michael Harvey, David Hays, William Isham, Trudy Schafer-Jeffers, Jerald Jordan, Debbie Kneisell, Michel Lamothe, Jessica Lee, Ruben Leon, Ella Mae Lentz, Ceil Lucas, Alan Marcus, Marina McIntire, Paula Menyuk, Betty G. Miller, Ilene Miner, Elizabeth Monaco, William Moody, Elissa Newport, Carol Padden, Peter Paul, Hal Rosenblatt, Susan Rutherford, Al Santoro, Carol Santoro, Jerome Schein, Brenda Schertz, Michael Schwartz, Ginger Smith, Theresa Smith, Jim Tourangeau, and Clayton Valli.

We want to record particular gratitude to our gifted editor, Corona Machemer, who has been an invaluable advisor, collaborator and critical reader; to Lynn Stafford, our copyeditor; and to the skilled and dedicated team at DawnSignPress.

Authors' Note

YOU are about to begin an intellectual journey that will introduce you to the language, culture, community and daily lives of the members of the DEAF–WORLD. Our focus is on the DEAF–WORLD in the United States, for it has been the most thoroughly investigated. We do, however, discuss the "worlds" of culturally Deaf people elsewhere around the globe.

We thought it appropriate to designate the minority language group that is the focus of our study using the term with which they designate themselves in American Sign Language: the *DEAF–WORLD*. We follow the convention of identifying signs from signed languages with English glosses (approximate translation equivalents) in small capital letters. The dash in DEAF–WORLD indicates that this is a compound sign; as in English, the initial letters of this proper noun are capitalized.

When we refer to the DEAF–WORLD in the U.S., we are concerned with a group (an estimated million people) possessing a unique language and culture. This language and culture have only become recognized and accepted of late. "Deaf: The New Ethnicity," was the cover line for a 1993 lead story in the *Atlantic Monthly*. In truth, however, this linguistic minority is not so new; it traces its roots in America to pre-revolutionary times. What is new is the avalanche of scientific evidence concerning Deaf language and culture and the growing social acceptance of DEAF–WORLDS in many lands.

The rapidly growing body of linguistic and cultural knowledge about Deaf people has lacked a coherent and comprehensive presentation to the many interested parties: professionals in diverse fields (including audiology; speech-language pathology; medicine; education; school, rehabilitation and mental health counseling; psychology; interpreting; American

Sign Language and Deaf studies), as well as concerned lay people, such as parents of Deaf children, and Deaf people themselves. *A Journey into the DEAF–WORLD* seeks to fill this need and, in so doing, to contribute to reducing the gap between professional perceptions of Deaf people and Deaf people's perception of themselves.

The terms *deaf, hearing-impaired,* and *deaf community* are commonly used to designate a much larger and more heterogeneous group than the members of the DEAF–WORLD. Most of the estimated 20 million U.S. citizens in this larger group communicate primarily in English or one of the spoken minority languages, such as Spanish. Some lost their hearing as adults, some in childhood, and some were born with a hearing loss. The DEAF–WORLD has traditionally forged ties with groups of people with hearing-impairments who do not identify with the DEAF–WORLD but rather with the mainstream national language and culture, and it continues to do so. However, in order to tell the story of a culture that remains too little known and poorly understood, we have abstained from exploring the lives and concerns of people with hearing-impairments who do not use the language and have not internalized the culture of the DEAF–WORLD. Readers with an interest in people with hearing impairments can call on a very large clinical literature, summarized in many textbooks, as well as compelling and illuminating first-person accounts, such as Henry Kisor's *What's That Pig Outdoors?*; Kay Thomsett and Eve Nickerson's *Missing Words*; and the David Wright classic, *Deafness*.

As a constant reminder that this book is about the "new ethnicity," we follow the growing practice of capitalizing Deaf to designate the members and institutions of the DEAF–WORLD. We take it that a child who has not acquired spoken language and culture because of limited hearing is a culturally Deaf child, even if that child has not yet had the opportunity to learn DEAF–WORLD language and culture. This issue is examined in chapter 5, on Deaf culture.

Harlan Lane
Northeastern University

Robert Hoffmeister
Boston University

Ben Bahan
Gallaudet University

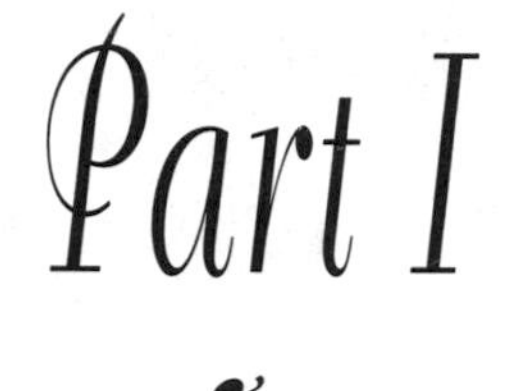

Part I

In the Center of the DEAF-WORLD

Chapter 1

Welcome to the DEAF-WORLD

HELLO, my name is Ben Bahan, and I am from New Jersey. I went to the Marie Katzenbach School for the Deaf, a residential school in West Trenton. I have Deaf parents. My mother went to the same school I went to; my father went to different schools but graduated from the New York School for the Deaf in White Plains. I grew up in the DEAF–WORLD. My parents were active in Deaf clubs and associations and took me and my hearing sister to those places when we were young. After I graduated from the Katzenbach School, I went to Gallaudet University in Washington, DC. Then I moved to California to do research in American Sign Language (ASL) linguistics at the Salk Institute for Biological Studies in La Jolla. In 1980, with Joe Dannis, I became a founding partner of DawnSignPress, and have been vice-president ever since. I also taught ASL at several community colleges and worked at the California School for the Deaf at Fremont for two years as a dormitory counselor. Then, in 1985, I decided to advance my education, so I entered Boston University. While pursuing my doctorate in applied linguistics there, I helped direct the Deaf Studies Program in the School of Education. Meanwhile, at Boston University I met my wife, Sue Burnes, who is also a Deaf child of Deaf parents. There are a lot of stories to tell about what has happened since then, but let us jump now to where I am today—back at Gallaudet University as an assistant professor in the newly formed Deaf Studies Department.

Let me also introduce my colleagues and co-authors, Harlan Lane and Bob Hoffmeister. Harlan is hearing, but I first met him through his book about the history of the DEAF–WORLD, *When the Mind Hears*. I recall that when I read it I felt an overwhelming sense of pride in the accomplishments of the past and in the DEAF–WORLD, which has survived despite attempts to eradicate it. In Harlan's book, Deaf people at last had a document, similar to a monument, to which we could point, making sure that succeeding generations would not forget how we were treated by many of those in the hearing world who claimed to want to help us, and how our language was suppressed. A specialist in the psychology of language, Harlan received his B.A. and M.A. from Columbia University and his Ph.D. from Harvard, where he was a student of renowned psychologist B.F Skinner, who chaired his thesis work. Harlan has taught at the University of Michigan; at the Sorbonne in Paris, where he earned a state doctorate in linguistics; and at the University of California at San Diego. A man with many titles, he is University Distinguished Professor at Northeastern University, Research Affiliate at M.I.T., and Research Associate at the Massachusetts Eye and Ear Infirmary. Harlan's background makes for important contributions to this book. But to the DEAF–WORLD his contribution is much more important, because in the world of hearing intellectuals, we Deaf people are often looked upon as deficient, in need of intervention. Harlan, by contrast, believes, as we do, that we are a language minority, and he takes up our point of view and champions it in the hearing world.

While Harlan looks at the DEAF–WORLD from his perspective, which is that of an intellectual, Bob Hoffmeister faces the issues from the trenches, because he is a *coda*, the hearing **c**hild **o**f **D**eaf **a**dults. I first got to know Bob the same way many Deaf people first learn about each other, not through books so much, but rather face-to-face. Bob grew up on the campus of the American School for the Deaf in West Hartford, Connecticut, where his parents were teachers. As a child, he was exposed to every nook and cranny of the DEAF–WORLD. Like many codas, as a young adult he decided to stay away from the Deaf community, but was eventually drawn back into it and went on to become a specialist in ASL language acquisition and bilingual education for Deaf children. The themes of psychology, language, and Deaf education run through Bob's academic training: B.S. at the University of Connecticut; M.A. from the University of Arizona; and Ph.D. from the University of Minnesota. Bob is currently a professor at Boston University and director of the Programs in Deaf Studies. In 1980, at Boston University, he created the first university major and specialization in Deaf Studies in the U.S.

The paragraphs above may strike you as odd ones to be the opening passage of a book about Deaf culture (or any book, for that matter), but they are here for a purpose: to give you a taste of that culture at the very outset of the journey upon which we are now embarked, into the world Deaf people call the DEAF–WORLD.[1] When members of the DEAF–WORLD meet, they introduce themselves and their companions as Ben has here introduced the three of us who will be your guides on this journey. They give capsule life-histories so that each can see how the others are connected to the DEAF–WORLD network. For unlike other cultures, Deaf culture is not associated with a single place, a "native land"; rather, it is a culture based on relationships among people for whom a number of places and associations may provide common ground.

Deaf people in the U.S. use the sign DEAF–WORLD to refer to these relationships among themselves, to the social network they have set up, and not to any notion of geographical location. Instead of a spot marked X on a map, the term is used to account for many places, from the clubs where Deaf people meet to socialize or to play competitive sports, to associations where they exchange ideas and through which they engage in political action, to religious organizations. In other words, the meaning of the ASL sign *WORLD* in the compound DEAF–WORLD corresponds to one of the meanings of the English word *world*, as stated in the American Heritage Dictionary: "A class or group of people with common characteristics or pursuits and a particular way of life."

One way to understand what we mean by DEAF–WORLD is to examine how one gets to be a member of that world, and who its members are. Generally, we can say that the inhabitants of the DEAF–WORLD are people who possess *DEAF–WORLD Knowledge* (more on that below) and who share the experience of what it is like to be Deaf. But within that overall definition, there are distinctions to be made. For one thing—and perhaps this will surprise you—the extent of a person's hearing is not the central issue in deciding membership in the DEAF–WORLD. There are people who have very limited hearing or none at all but choose not to be part of the DEAF–WORLD. Conversely, there are many Deaf people who hear well enough to use a telephone and speak well enough to be understood, but choose to live in the DEAF–WORLD.

Like other language minorities, most people in the DEAF–WORLD were born into it. However, unlike other minorities, children born into this one gain access to the language and culture at various ages. Some start that acquisition at birth, some later in life—for example, on arriving at a preschool for Deaf children, or even as late as adolescence. And not all members of the DEAF–WORLD are born into it. A small percentage lose their hearing after learning spoken language and mainstream culture, and then undertake to acquire DEAF–WORLD language and culture.

Signed language is the most important instrument for communicating in the DEAF–WORLD. The language competency of the members varies, depending on whether signed language is their native language (true only of the children of members of the DEAF–WORLD) or whether they learned the language as small children or later in life. (As we shall see, very few Deaf children of hearing parents learn signed language from infancy, when learning languages is easiest and mastery greatest.) But regardless of when they learn it, from the day Deaf Americans enter the DEAF–WORLD, ASL becomes their primary language, and is, in itself, a big chunk of DEAF–WORLD Knowledge. Using it, Deaf people can join the networks, local and national, which link the members of the DEAF–WORLD. They can learn the accumulated wisdom of generations of Deaf people, master the subtleties of relating appropriately in that world, and become familiar with the culture, history, traditions, values and signed-language literature of the Deaf society.

Sometimes hearing people who are genuinely interested in the DEAF–WORLD and desire to participate in it feel that they are not accepted. In the same way, for example, American expatriates might feel they are not totally accepted in France. But it is not true that hearing people are unwelcome among the Deaf. It's just that Deaf people, like all people, have a need for being, at least part of the time, with others who share the same language and culture, values and concerns. In this regard, the DEAF–WORLD might be likened to a revolving door that spins at its own rate. If you are able to walk in and keep up the pace and, more importantly, are committed to staying the course, then you are more than welcome. Most hearing people, however, only want to go around once or twice and then exit, back to their own circle of friends. The impression that hearing people have—that the door is spinning too fast for them to join in—is partially accurate, for when Deaf people use their own language among themselves, they use it at their own pace. When they behave differently from hearing people, they are following customs of the DEAF–WORLD. The DEAF–WORLD has its own rate of spinning; it may slow down now and then, here and there, for some "outsiders," but when it returns to speed, it is the newcomer's responsibility to keep up. In this respect, is it really any different from any other culture?

The goal of this book is to slow the spin enough so that those of you who wish to do so may enter and join us for a while. As we thought about how best to do this, it occurred to us that, because a vital part of Deaf culture is stories and the telling of stories (as in any culture where knowledge and tradition are passed down face-to-face), and because Ben is known as a storyteller in the DEAF–WORLD, we might start off with a story. This story will illuminate some of the themes to be discussed, and more importantly, give you some notion of the ways members of the community differ from one another, as well as what they have in common. For in considering the culture of any community, it is essential to keep in mind the diversity of those who belong to it, even as one focuses on what binds them together and makes their group distinct from others.

You will discover more about storytelling as a vital part of Deaf culture in subsequent chapters. Here, suffice it to say that in order to become a storyteller, there is a path you must follow; along the way, you are given opportunities to demonstrate your talent in front of an audience. Eventually you may be acclaimed and recognized. Storytellers like Ben are more than entertainers; they are the culture's oral historians and teachers, and their stories have messages embedded in them about DEAF–WORLD values.

Oral historians in any culture without a written language have several ways they can go about telling their stories; they choose among them depending on the audience, the story, and their resources. They can tell their stories live in front of an audience; record them on film or videotape;

translate them into a language of broader communication that has a writing system (most often English or French); or compose them in that written language in the first place. Ben composed the story you are about to read in English. Sometimes DEAF-WORLD stories have to do with the relationship between the DEAF-WORLD and hearing people. The story to be told here is one of those. It is divided into three parts, one in each part of this book. Its setting is a place that is a constant in the DEAF-WORLD, a Deaf club. It concerns a hearing reporter who has been assigned to write a series of articles on Deaf people. To do this, the reporter visits a Deaf club and interviews four members.

The lives of the four Deaf characters in this story are based on the lives of real Deaf people; however, the names of the characters and the schools they attended (except for their universities) are fictional and the characters are to some extent composites, so that we may bring up many issues succinctly without introducing you to too many people.

At the Metro Silent Club I

*Gloria Cosgrove was getting worried. She had been waiting to meet Jake Cohan, with her yellow-lined pad of paper and ballpoint pen, for over twenty minutes. She'd begun to wonder if she'd come to the right place until she saw two people speaking signed language go in the door beside which she was standing. Now she thought maybe she'd gotten the time wrong or that something else had happened. She and Jake had set up this interview a few days before through a TTY relay operator, and she didn't have much confidence that the operator had gotten it right.**

With Jake typing what he wanted to say and the operator reading it to her and then typing her replies for Jake to read . . . well, she just didn't trust it. Besides, Jake had been reluctant to set up this meeting, and had only agreed after double-checking with the director of the Deaf education

* A TTY relay operator uses a TTY (the acronym comes from teletypewriter) to relay calls between hearing and Deaf clients. A TTY resembles a typewriter with an electronic display. As each key is struck, the device emits a distinctive tone that is transmitted over the telephone line and causes the corresponding letter to appear on both users' TTY screens. See chapters 12 and 15.

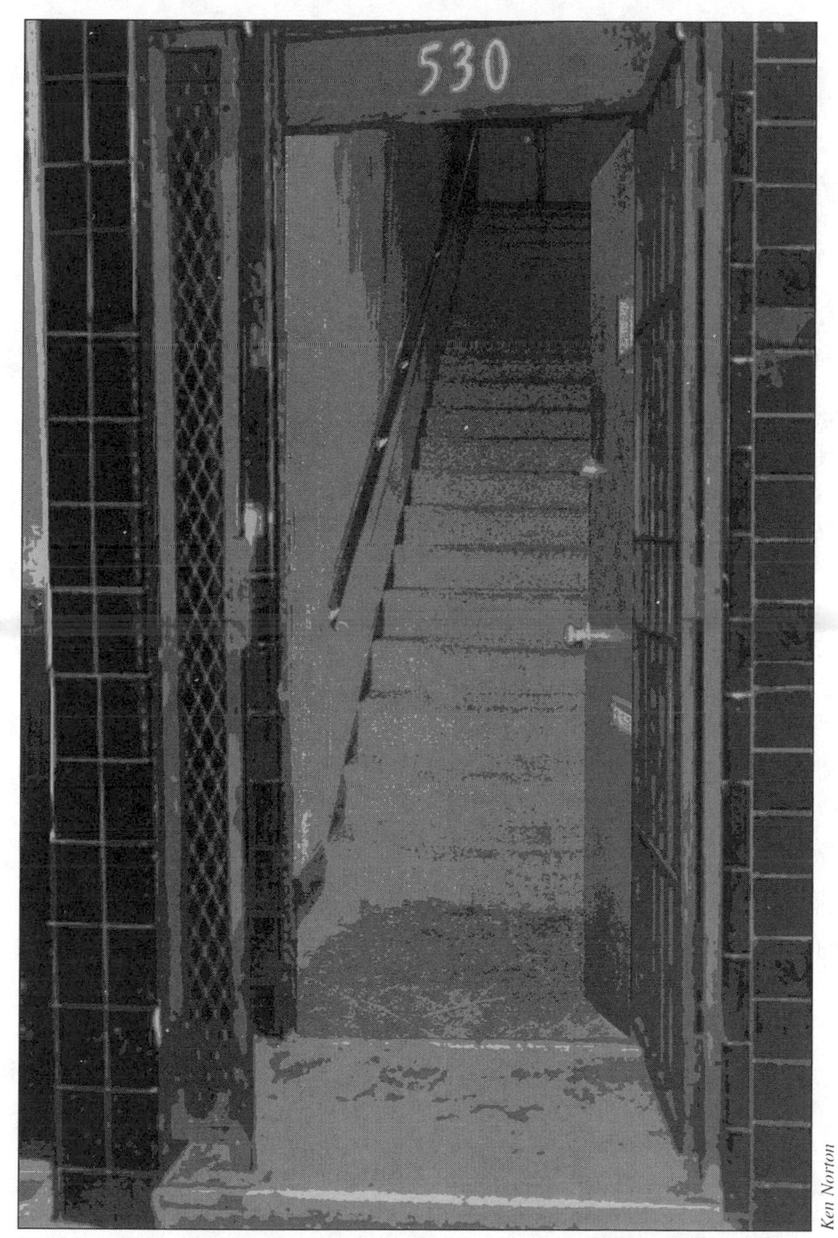

Ken Norton

Fig. 1-1. **Entering the San Francisco Club for the Deaf. Stairs to the second floor are a hallmark of Deaf clubs in the United States.**

program at the state university, whom Gloria had interviewed first and who had recommended Jake to her. He'd been "burned before," Jake said, but he didn't elaborate.

She glanced once more down the street, where the streetcar was just pulling out, and spotted a dark-haired man who appeared to be in his mid-forties heading in her direction. He glanced to the right and left twice before stepping off the curb, and again when he was halfway across the street. This must be Jake, she thought, as he hurried up to her. Gloria held out her pad and pen, but instead of taking them, he extended his hand and said, "Hello, I am Jake, are you Gloria Cosgrove?"

For a moment she was too astonished to respond. She hadn't been sure how she was going to communicate with Jake, but the last thing she'd expected was that he could speak, and she felt silly standing there with her pad and pen. She recovered quickly, however, and, relieved that the communication problem was solved, returned his greeting and explained that she had been looking forward to meeting him and his friends and was worried that something might have happened. But instead of responding to her implied question about his late arrival, he said, "There are interpreters inside," and took her arm. She flushed with embarrassment. Obviously he hadn't understood a word she'd said, and once again she wondered what she'd let herself in for.

After entering the building, they climbed a long steep stairway and proceeded down a dimly lit corridor to an open doorway with a sign beside it announcing the Metro Silent Club. Gloria's heart was beating rapidly—from the climb or nervousness, she wasn't sure which—as they walked through the door. Before her was a big room with a bar at one end and a small makeshift stage at the other. Scattered about the edges were a few round tables and chairs. There were some twenty-five people present, with concentrations at strategic locations: a dozen or so at the bar, signing madly; a couple over by a telephone with a machine attached to it, on which one of them was typing, and which she supposed was a TTY; two sets of four at tables, playing cards; and two people by the stage who looked as out of place as she felt. But what struck her most was the eerie silence. Despite all the activity, there was very little noise.

She was still taking in the scene when she felt a hand on her shoulder. She glanced around to see a young man who began signing to her.

When she said she didn't understand, he frowned and shook his head and again signed something. Frantically she looked around for Jake, but he was signing away with the two people over by the stage. She started to call him, then realized the uselessness of that and made a move in his direction, only to find the young man's hand once again on her shoulder. Was she going to get bounced from this place? In her confusion, she had forgotten her pad and pen, but the young man, apparently taking pity, now reached for them and wrote something and handed them back. Who are you? *she read.* What are you doing here? *She flushed, and once again looked toward Jake. How could she explain in a few words what she was there for? Finally she wrote,* I came with Jake Cohan, *and handed the pad back. The doorkeeper nodded, left her standing there and went to consult with Jake, who returned with the people he'd been talking to; they turned out to be interpreters, one of whom now translated for Gloria as Jake explained to the doorkeeper that Gloria was a reporter and that it was okay with the club president for her to enter the club and do an interview.*

As she, Jake, and one of the interpreters seated themselves at a table, Gloria asked Jake, through the interpreter, "Is it always that difficult to get into this club?"

Jake laughed. "Oh no," he signed (while the interpreter spoke), "he knew you weren't a member, and if you're not, there's a cover charge. I'm sorry it was a bit awkward, but you wanted to learn about the DEAF-WORLD. *That kind of thing—being at a loss because you can't understand what people are saying, or because you can't make yourself understood—is the sort of experience Deaf people have every day on the job or when they go shopping or wander into a strange neighborhood."*

While Gloria was digesting this, he went on, explaining that the Metro Silent Club was one of the oldest in the region, founded in 1933, and that people had been coming there ever since to socialize, and "because the drinks were cheaper," though nowadays it was only open on weekends. He'd arranged for her to meet several of the members for a group interview. Was that all right with her?

Before she could answer, he was waving his hands to summon three people from across the room, who pulled up chairs and joined them.

"This is Laurel Case, Roberto Rivera, and Henry Byrnes," Jake said. "I asked them to join us in the interview because they all come from dif-

ferent backgrounds, so they can give you an idea about the varied backgrounds of the people in this club. Also, they can show you how different their lives are in other respects as well. That way maybe you'll be able to tell your readers how strongly we're bound together in the DEAF–WORLD. *Despite major differences, we do all belong to this club."*

Clearly Jake had taken charge of the interview, and Gloria wasn't sure she liked the idea. It was almost as if he were challenging her. But she'd come here to get a story. Shrugging, she pulled out her tape recorder. At least she wouldn't have to worry about background noise obscuring the interpreters' voices.

"Okay," Jake said, "we'll start by introducing ourselves. Who wants to go first?"

When the others glanced at each other, clearly at a loss, Jake announced that he'd get the ball rolling. "My parents and brother are Deaf," he said. "I grew up in Peabody, Massachusetts, and my brother and I went to the Cogswell School, a residential school for the Deaf. After that came Gallaudet University. Now I'm an independent-living counselor at a rehabilitation center run by Deaf people. I'm forty-five years old, divorced, and live in a townhouse in the city. Roberto?"

Roberto nodded to Gloria and his hands started moving. "Everybody in my family but me is hearing. I was born in Puerto Rico, and we moved to Lowell when I was about eighteen months old. I became Deaf a few months later from spinal meningitis. I went to public school in Lowell where I was in a self-contained class."

"What does self-contained *mean?" Gloria asked. She had to keep reminding herself to look at Roberto, as she had been told, and not at the interpreter. Roberto and the others, on the other hand, watched the interpreter; it was disconcerting.*

"We'll explain later," said Jake. "Go on, Roberto."

Roberto nodded. "I work as an assembler at a plant that makes household appliances. I am twenty-seven years old and not married, but I have a girlfriend."

Laurel went next. "I grew up in Fairfield, Connecticut, outside New York City. Everyone in my family is hearing. I was educated at the Hubbard School, a residential school for the Deaf that had a strict oral program. I was first exposed to signed language six years ago when I entered Gallaudet. Now I can't stop signing. I work in the post office."

"She's twenty-five," Roberto said. "She just broke up with her boyfriend."

This remark elicited a slap on the arm from Laurel.

"Okay, you're next, Henry," said Jake, taking command again.

"I am thirty-six years old and was born and brought up in Philadelphia. My family are all hearing. I graduated from the Frank Booth Day School for the Deaf. I am married and have two beautiful Deaf children. I was recently laid off from my job as a graphic artist."

"Well, that's us in a nutshell," said Jake. "Now it's time to change interpreters. They like to change off every twenty minutes or so. Then you can tell us what you're up to, Gloria."

The interpreter, who had been sitting beside Gloria and facing the others, got up and the other took his place. Meanwhile, Gloria tried to collect her thoughts. She wasn't used to being quizzed by her interviewees. Again, she had the unsettling feeling that she was being challenged.

"I am writing about the Deaf community and how, recently, the Deaf seem to be defining themselves and seeing themselves in new ways. I interviewed the director of the Deaf education program at the university, who put me onto Jake. The professor suggested that I meet Jake at the independent-living center where he works, but Jake suggested this place, so here I am."

"Have you ever met a Deaf person before?" asked Laurel.

"Not really, except for my great aunt, who became pretty hard-of-hearing in her old age. I've seen people signing to each other, but except for her, you're the first hearing-impaired people I've actually met."

As soon as the words were out, Gloria wished them back. She'd used the term hearing impaired *in her TTY conversation with Jake and he'd set her straight then. Deaf people didn't consider themselves hearing impaired, he'd said, and didn't want to be called hearing impaired. It was like calling a Black person a Negro.*

"I'm sorry," she said, looking at Jake. "I didn't mean to say that. You'll have to be patient with me."

Their eyes met, and for a moment Jake held her gaze, as if trying to see into her mind. Then, apparently satisfied, he nodded. "Apology accepted," he said. "At least you didn't say aurally challenged."

As the others laughed, Gloria relaxed. This is going to be all right, she thought, and said, "That's why I need your help. There are a great many people out there like me who don't know how Deaf people really feel. We read about Deaf students protesting at Gallaudet University, shutting the place down until a Deaf president was appointed. We read that, when Heather Whitestone became Miss America, Deaf people weren't happy because she chooses not to sign. We wonder what is really going on. I want you to tell me so I can share it with others. The straight dope."

Again Jake nodded, and this time he smiled. "Okay, shoot," he said. "Where do you want to start?"

"Why don't we begin at the beginning," Gloria said. "How and when did you and your parents learn you were Deaf and what was their reaction?"

And so, with periodic interruptions to switch interpreters, the four began telling her their stories, responding to Gloria's occasional questions, but mostly just talking, giving her—she hoped—what she'd asked for: the unvarnished truth, as they saw it.

Once more Jake went first. "Remember, I have Deaf parents, and that makes my situation different from theirs," he said, glancing at the other three. "Unlike their parents, my parents knew when my mother was pregnant that there was a possibility their child might be Deaf. They weren't really expecting it, though, because it was generally believed in the DEAF-WORLD *that if a Deaf couple didn't themselves have Deaf parents it was unlikely that they would have Deaf children. All my grandparents were hearing and my aunts and uncles, too. So my folks weren't expecting a Deaf child. Shortly after I was born, my mother said that she and my father ran a few homemade hearing tests, screaming and banging on the pots to see if I would respond to the sound. Those tests, according to my mother, were inconclusive in her eyes, but my father was sure I was Deaf. She explained that she wasn't sure because sometimes I reacted to the sounds and sometimes I didn't. But they had decided in any case to raise me to be the way they are. So, from day one, I was exposed to ASL and was treated as one of them. My mother did tell me that after the doctors confirmed that I couldn't hear, she and my father felt a sense of loss, but nothing like what hearing parents go through. What my parents faced was the reality that their child was Deaf and they were concerned about the kind of life I would have and the hardships I'd face, and vowed to make my life better than theirs had been."*

Laurel went next: "My parents' reaction was entirely different. My mother told me that when she was pregnant, she and my father had great expectations. I would be like them—college graduates with high-powered careers. About two years after I was born, my mother started to suspect 'something wasn't right,' because I wasn't talking. My father and the rest of the family thought she was being over-anxious. My mother said her suspicion was confirmed one day when my aunt came over for lunch. After she fed me, I fell asleep in the highchair. While they were washing dishes, my aunt dropped a glass. She glanced at me to make sure I was okay, and I was still sound asleep. My parents took me to a specialist who confirmed that I was Deaf. They were devastated by the news, and soon after they were arguing a lot. My father plunged deeper and deeper into his work, while my mother decided to make a new career out of raising me."

"I was two and a half when I became Deaf," Roberto said. "Most of what I know of my situation I got much later from my younger hearing sister, who knows how to sign. My parents experienced the same kind of emotions as Laurel's. The difference is that my parents spoke very little English. So they were extremely confused about what was going on and had little understanding of what should be done to raise a Deaf child. The doctors and audiologists recommended that they contact a Spanish-speaking specialist affiliated with the hospital, who ran an early intervention program for Deaf children at a local school, and that's what they did."

Finally, Henry spoke. "From what my mother has said, my parents went through the same thing Laurel's and Roberto's did. My mother suspected something wasn't right when I was around two years old, but she thought I was just a bit slow in my development and would pick up when I got older. That assumption originated from my grandmother's recollection that my father had begun talking and crawling relatively late. And, like Jake, at certain times I appeared to react to noise, while at other times I didn't. But when I was three, and my situation still hadn't improved, they took me to a doctor, and the fact that I was Deaf was confirmed.

Many years later my mother told me that, after hearing the news, she cried for days. My father withdrew into a shell like a turtle and just wanted to be left alone. After a while, they decided to seek another opinion, and then another. They went to five different doctors and audiologists within a span of six months. They kept hoping they'd find someone who could help. They just couldn't stop. When I was five or six years old, my mother took me to a faith healer, although I didn't understand that at the time. I remember there was a big audience and I was standing in front of a guy in a dark suit beside an altar. He stuck his fingers into my ears and pulled them out as fast as he could to create a sucking effect. I remember that it hurt."

Nobody said anything for a moment after this, and Gloria took the opportunity to turn the tape over in her recorder while the interpreters changed shift. When everyone was settled again she said, "You've all told me about your parents' reactions to the news of your being Deaf. How about your reactions? How did you feel about it when you were old enough to understand?"

There was no immediate response, and Gloria was beginning to think she'd put her foot in it again, when finally Jake touched her shoulder to get her attention. He pointed to a woman sitting at the bar. "See that blonde girl in the blue dress?" he said. "She's what we call a coda, which is an acronym for child of deaf adults. Everyone in her family is Deaf—her grandparents, aunts, uncles, cousins—everybody. She grew up with them on a farm, where everyone signed. She just grew up signing to everyone, not knowing until she first attended school, at the age of five, that the rest of the world used speech to communicate. At school she had to go through speech therapy and learn how to talk.

"You see," Jake went on, "my situation was exactly like hers, only I didn't realize until even later that most of the people in the world communicated differently from my family. The point is, both Rhoda—that's her name—and I grew up thinking that signed language was normal as a way of communicating. We had no idea that other people might make a fuss about it and try to prevent us from using it."

"You're not answering the question," said Laurel.

"I know it," said Jake. "That's because there isn't an answer, not really. You see, none of us knows what we're, quote-unquote, 'missing,' from the hearing point of view."

"And once we made it into the DEAF-WORLD, that became the important thing," Henry added. "I mean, the important thing is what we have, not what we don't have."

"Even late-deafened people sometimes feel that way," Laurel put in. "The treasurer of this club, a woman named Alice, lost her hearing when she was sixteen. I asked her once how she felt about becoming Deaf after hearing for sixteen years. She said the experience of suddenly being plunged into a life of soundlessness had been humbling, but the ones who suffered most were her hearing parents and relatives. I thought that Alice's response was somewhat strange, that someone older going Deaf would be traumatized. But Alice wasn't, not really.

"Her family was another matter, though. They thought they were being punished by God for something they or she had done. So Alice ended up feeling guilty. She spent a lot of time trying to figure out what sins she'd committed: sneaking out at night to meet a boyfriend? smoking? kissing before she was fifteen? She said a lot of Hail Marys in hopes of changing things, so her parents could stop grieving. Nothing came of it. And in fact, she says now that when she became Deaf, it was a turning point in her life for the better."

"I. King Jordan says the same thing," Henry said. "He says that losing his hearing at the age of twenty-one from a motorcycle accident was the best thing that ever happened to him. It led him into the DEAF–WORLD *and to becoming a student, then a professor, and finally the president at Gallaudet University, none of which would have occurred if he had remained hearing."*

Gloria glanced down at her notebook and wrote "GU, I. King Jordan," then underlined the name.

"Why'd you do that?" asked Roberto, peering at the book, which Gloria had left open on the table in front of her. She'd had the feeling from the start that to win and keep the trust of these people, she shouldn't appear to be concealing anything.

"It's just a reminder to myself. I wrote about the protest and I want to go back and review my old notes."

"You were there?" asked Laurel.

"No, but I interviewed a local teacher of the Deaf about it for a sidebar to one of the Associated Press articles. As I recall, she was pretty negative about the whole thing, but I can't remember why. I'll need to go look it up."

"Was she Deaf or hearing?" asked Roberto.

"You know, come to think of it, she was Deaf. Funny, but I forgot all about her when you asked me if I'd met any Deaf people."

"It's not so funny," said Henry. "I bet she did the interview without an interpreter and was probably a very good speaker. I bet she called herself hearing-impaired, *too."*

"You know, you're right," said Gloria. "How did you guess?"

"It's easy if you know the Deaf community as well as Henry does," said Jake, taking control again. "But we're getting off the track. Henry, what was it like for you when you learned your kids were Deaf?"

"Yes, Henry," said Gloria. "You used the word beautiful *earlier."*

Henry's hands were in the air to reply when suddenly the lights in the clubroom flashed on and off, stopping him in mid-sign. That does it, Gloria thought, the electricity's going. No one else seemed concerned, however. Instead, as one, everybody in the room looked towards the stage. "What's going on?" Gloria asked. The interpreter touched Jake's shoulder to get his attention as, up on stage, a man started signing.

"It's a fund-raising effort," said Jake. "He's announcing a raffle. Now where were we?"

"We were starting on my kids," said Henry. "Like Jake's folks, my wife and I weren't expecting our children to be Deaf because we both have hearing parents and the rest of our extended families are all hearing. So it was a surprise to us with both kids, but we were thrilled when we found out. It was pretty confusing for the doctors, let me tell you. The audiologist came in after the test looking very apprehensive and said, 'I am so sorry. The test shows that your baby is Deaf, although there may be a chance of residual . . . .' He stopped because my wife and I were hugging each other, we were so happy. He thought we were nuts."

As Henry and the others burst out laughing, Gloria felt totally lost for the first time since she'd been stopped at the club door. It was one thing to accept being Deaf and get on with your life. It was another entirely to relish the thought. "I . . . I don't understand," she said lamely.

"You think we're nuts, too, don't you?" asked Laurel.

Gloria started to shake her head no, then thought better of it. They could read her face like a book. "Well, yes, sort of," she said. "I mean, I just don't get it."

"You will eventually," said Jake. "I hope. That's what we're here for,

isn't it? For now, let's just say that the DEAF–WORLD *places a higher value on Deaf kids than almost anything else. Okay?"*

Still bewildered, Gloria knew she had no choice but to wait. Again she'd detected that wariness, in Jake especially.

"How did your parents react to your son's deafness?" she asked Henry finally. "You said they took you to faith healers. I bet they had a hard time dealing with it."

For several moments no one moved, and when Henry at last lifted his hands, it was, she thought, reluctantly. "When our son was born, my parents came over to visit. Periodically throughout the day my father would go into the nursery. I thought he was going to beam with pride at his grandson, but eventually I learned it was something else. After his fourth or fifth trip, I decided to follow him, and I caught him standing behind the crib clapping. He was testing a two-day-old baby! He never said anything, but his actions said plenty. And it hurt.

"It was like finally seeing how my parents reacted when they found out I *was Deaf, which, of course, I was too young to remember. I thought that by this time my dad would have accepted the fact that I'm a human being who's happily married with a good job—this was before I got laid off—and not some freak of nature. It gave me a chance to see how they really thought of me. I would have liked them to say, 'Oh it's not a big deal,' but it is to them, I guess, and it always will be.*

"My wife's parents were almost worse, because they kept grilling us on how we were going to bring the kid up and recommending speech-and-hearing specialists. They wanted to be sure we raised him to speak. They couldn't accept that we had a pretty good idea of what it was like growing up Deaf and that we were capable of deciding what would be best for our child. They were not pleased when we decided he'd learn ASL first. But we weren't about to put him through what we went through.

"We want our children to have the kind of head start Jake had, growing up just like any hearing kids in the neighborhood, with their parents using their normal daily language. We bring them with us to the Deaf club, the way Jake's parents brought him to the Deaf club—this very one, in fact—where they can find other Deaf kids to play with and Deaf adults too, and storytellers to watch and learn from.

"With me it was so different. Since my parents didn't find out I was

Deaf until I was three, I missed those three years of language and had to wait one more year after that, while my parents tried to pound speech into me and dragged me from one clinic to the next. My mother would accompany me and try to learn different techniques for teaching me how to speak. At home she would make me go through some drills, but I was so stubborn and strong-willed. I threw such tantrums that she would just give up and drive me to the therapist's office and let the therapist teach me. This went on for a while until the last therapist decided I wasn't trying hard enough and recommended that I be enrolled in a day school for the Deaf in the city. There, I finally met other Deaf kids and began acquiring signed language, four years too late. There's no way anything like that's going to happen to my kids. No way."

"Right on," Laurel said. "But if you think you had it tough . . ."

"Actually, I didn't, not the way you did."

"You're so right," Laurel said. "You see, Gloria, after finding out I was Deaf, my parents took me to a specialist in New York City who recommended that they get in touch with a parent-infant program coordinator at his hospital. After the coordinator explained different approaches, it didn't take them long to decide they were going to do their utmost to make me 'normal'—that's the word my mother uses. Signing, they felt, was not normal. It was that simple.

"The first thing that happened was that I was fitted with hearing aids, and from that time on—I was two years old—my mother would take me to a speech therapist in my home town. While I was being drilled, she would devour all the literature she could on how to teach speech and lipreading. Soon she found out about this pre-school home correspondence kit from a clinic in California that specialized in oral instruction. She immediately subscribed. After that, every morning for about an hour, she would sit me down and go over different speech games and drills from that kit. Sometimes it was fun, but mostly it was tedious for both of us.

"My mother tells me now that many times she wanted to give up, but she forced herself to stay with it. In the evenings, my father took his turn drilling me for another half-hour. An hour and a half every day. My mother says there were many times when she had to bribe me with candy or toys. And not only was I corrected during the speech sessions, I was corrected throughout the day. For example, when I asked my mother where

something was, if I pronounced the word wrong, she would correct me and make me say it right before telling me where the thing was. My mother was more a therapist than a mother."

Gloria was saddened by Henry and Laurel's obvious anger with their parents. Of course, it was different for Jake. And Roberto? He seemed to read her mind: "Before today I used to envy Laurel and Henry, because they had a good education," Roberto said. Now I'm not so sure. I said my parents were devastated when they learned I was Deaf, but the fact is, my sister told me that. They never showed me that they felt that way. I was the third child in a family of five children and the only one Deaf.

"The language we used at home and in my neighborhood was, and still is, primarily Spanish, so I grew up around three different languages: Spanish, English and signed language. I am most comfortable using signed language, though, and feel it is most natural for me to communicate my ideas and feelings, so I primarily use ASL, which makes me different from the rest of my family.

"My mother speaks very little English, because most of the time she stayed home raising us children. My father has a little more English because of his work. But even though my father speaks more English, I find him hard to understand. I actually understand my mother better; I guess some basic Spanish has stayed with me all these years and also, she is better than my dad at miming things. Even my Deaf Anglo girlfriend used to understand my mother much better than my father. They could have good conversations using gestures and facial expressions, and my mother knows some basic signs.

"You see, when they found out I was Deaf, and placed me in that early intervention program, I met other Deaf children. Then, later, when I was about four, the program encouraged my parents to learn Signed English so they could communicate with me. My father was unable to go because they scheduled the classes at three in the afternoon, when he was working. But my mother went to a few classes and picked up some rudimentary signs, like* NO, BATH, EAT, FATHER, MOTHER, BED. *Then she stopped going because no one there spoke Spanish and she figured she could learn signs from me, since I was already correcting her. She would come home and*

---

* Signed English is one of the systems designed to represent English manually using some signs, but not grammar, borrowed from ASL and some invented signs. See chapter 9.

sign some signs wrong, and I would shake my head and say WRONG, *and show her the right way. I guess my mother figured I would teach her even better than the teachers. It turned out that we stuck to our own way of communicating, which was a combination of gestures, homemade signs, and signed language.*

"That's what I'm getting to. I mean, I don't recall my mother ever making me sit and try to talk, like Laurel's mother and Henry's. She just brought me up like the other kids in the family."

"You were lucky," said Laurel. "You learned to sign pretty early and didn't have to wear hearing aids. That was the worst, for me and my mother. She'd put them on me in the morning and a few minutes later would find me walking around without them. I would take them off and hide them. She tried using two-sided tape to stick them on my head, but I'd still pull them off. Once my dad found a set—five-hundred-dollars' worth—in the toilet. Two little pink, shrimp-shaped things. He laughs about it now, but then it wasn't so funny. My parents were relentless. I was going to talk, come hell or high water. Signing was absolutely forbidden."

"Yet here you are," said Henry.

"That's right," said Laurel. "Here I am. Even though I speak well and can lip-read well enough to carry on a decent conversation with hearing people, now I am more in favor of signed language. Until I learned it, I had no idea how much I was missing out on. When I did realize it, I became angry with my parents, because I'd learned from them, and from my teachers, that any involvement in the DEAF–WORLD *would isolate me from the world in general and make me a very limited person. Now I know this to be false. I can't believe I actually believed it, because in fact the opposite is true. Being in the* DEAF–WORLD *makes me even more worldly."*

The others nodded their agreement. "So you see," Jake said, "no matter how you raise your Deaf kids, no matter how much speech you try to drill into them, chances are they will end up becoming a member of a club like this one, because signing just comes naturally to you if you're Deaf. You just gravitate towards the DEAF–WORLD. *Learning ASL as a baby, the way I did, gives you a head start, that's all."*

Roberto glanced at his watch and said, "I need to call my friend now, so can we take a quick break?"

"That's a good idea. I'll go buy everybody drinks," Gloria said.

"What would you like?" "Coke." "Coke." "Scotch and soda." "Beer." Grabbing her purse, she got up and went to the bar, only to find that the bartender was taking orders in ASL and she had to go back to the table for her pad and pen. By the time she'd returned to the table with the drinks, the interpreters had gone outside for a smoke. Jake, Henry and Laurel were signing away and laughing uproariously.

Jake wrote on her pad: We're talking about Laurel's experience buying a new car. Hilarious.

Gloria sat there watching the conversation ping-pong back and forth, listening to their laughter. Then suddenly she thought she knew what it must have been like for them growing up—all except Jake. Even though she was among a lot of people in the clubroom, she felt completely alone.

❦

Chapter 2

Families with Deaf Children

THE birth of a child is a momentous and happy occasion in the lives of most parents. Parents expect not only a joyous addition to the family, but also the assured continuation of the family lineage. The belief that children will be able to benefit from the life experiences of their parents contributes to the coalescing of the family unit. Parents look forward with excitement to planning their child's future.

When their child is Deaf, however, these generalizations no longer hold; the response of the parents to the advent of a Deaf child is likely to depend on whether the parents are hearing or Deaf. Hearing parents and their Deaf child commonly act out roles that are socially prescribed and extremely painful. Deaf parents, on the other hand, commonly welcome the birth of a Deaf child.

The Birth of a Deaf Baby to Deaf Parents

The reactions of Deaf parents on learning that their child is Deaf are as diverse as the parents themselves. In general, however, many members of the DEAF–WORLD would prefer having a Deaf child to having a hearing child, and those whose happiness at the advent of a Deaf child is tinged with sadness (after all, that child will face many extra challenges) commonly overcome their reservations quickly.[1] If you belong to a hearing culture, you may find such Deaf preferences hard to understand; yet all cultures have preferences about children: some prefer male babies, others fair-skinned or dark-skinned babies. Of course, Deaf parents' preference for Deaf children does not mean that they love their hearing children less, only that the birth of a Deaf baby in a Deaf household signifies that the Deaf heritage of the family will be secure. Deaf families with many Deaf members are commonly proud of their genealogy.

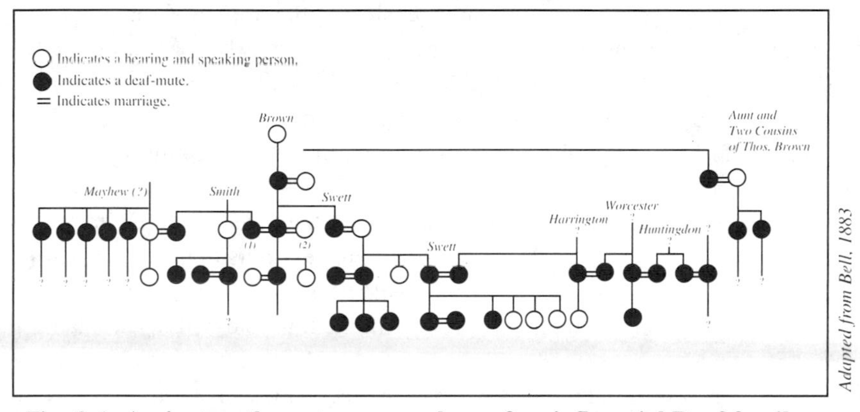

Fig. 2-1. **A nineteenth-century genealogy of an influential Deaf family, the Browns of Henniker, New Hampshire**

In other words, when a Deaf infant of Deaf parents is diagnosed as Deaf, the joy of the parents reflects the fact that most Deaf parents, like parents generally, look forward to having children who are a reflection of themselves. (Recall Henry's remark at the Metro Silent Club that he and his wife were thrilled to discover that their first baby was Deaf, and later that their second was, too.) Deaf parents bring their Deaf baby home to a nurturing environment in which communication is naturally dependent on visual, not aural, cues. Almost all use the signed language of the DEAF–WORLD (American Sign Language in the U.S. and most of Canada) to interact with their child. Their home is already functioning as an environment conducive to using vision as the main means of learning and development. The house is wired to respond to environmental signals with visual ones. For example, doorbells and telephones don't ring. Instead, they flash lights, each with its own pattern. Deaf parents usually have a TTY so they can communicate over the telephone.

Like the hearing child born to a well-functioning hearing family, the Deaf infant in a Deaf family, as Jake explained at the Deaf club, is immediately exposed to a world suited to maximizing his or her social, emotional, psychological, cognitive, and linguistic development. Social development is assured through exposure to adults who function normally as models for the child. Emotional development is encouraged by the positive responses of the family to its new member. Psychologically, Deaf parents treat their Deaf child as an extension of themselves. Cognitively, parental expectations are high: with proper nurturing, there are no Deaf-dependent limits on intellectual development. Finally, and most importantly, as we shall see in subsequent chapters, the child will enjoy a full command of language through exposure to ASL, allowing him or her to grasp the idea of communication, its purpose, and its form.

Deaf parents are able to communicate with their Deaf children immediately. They present a viable model for language acquisition, so the Deaf child is able to reach naturally and easily the milestones of language development essential to effective social interaction. We will discuss language acquisition at some length in chapter 3. Here, suffice it to say that all children pass through stages when they practice vocalizations and play with sounds as precursors to developing the language of their community. The cooing, babbling, and first-word stages of hearing children are paralleled in Deaf babies by their play with variations in handshape and movement, and by their first signs.[2] (Deaf babies also coo and babble orally, but since these sounds are not the building blocks of a language the children will naturally acquire, they eventually stop making them.) Deaf parents are able to communicate with their Deaf child, to respond to their child's developing language appropriately, and thus to show that he or she has been understood, just as the child shows by making appropriate responses that he or she has understood the parents. Deaf parents also naturally present original language forms (words and sentences) that are slightly above the language level of the child, and so they are able to assist their child in the natural acquisition of increasingly complex language.

Incidental, unplanned learning plays a large role in any child's acquisition of knowledge about the world. In hearing families, children observe and overhear conversations and discussions that are not directed at them. The information the children glean in this way helps them learn the mores, values, and behaviors that the family and the culture consider desirable or undesirable. Children of Deaf parents are also able to observe and oversee such interactions, especially if they have Deaf relatives. They become accustomed to interpreting other elements of the visual world, including signals that come from technology. The flashing doorbell, for example, signifies the arrival of new people, both strangers and acquaintances. But the most important visual information comes from the signed language being used all around them.

At the dinner table in a Deaf family, the Deaf child is part of the conversation from the beginning. Interaction proceeds using ASL, and all the family is included. When the doorbell flashes and friends arrive, the conversation will be conducted using ASL. The infant or toddler is able to see and receive the input, and to categorize, store, and make sense of it. An older Deaf child is able to engage in discussions concerning why it's time to go to bed, why there's no school today, how to play fair, and so on—meaningful exchanges that enhance the child's development.

Deaf parents are able to maximize these interactions. When their children are infants, they know how to get their attention by waving a hand in the baby's line of sight or by gently touching the child. They place the baby on their lap with the baby's back touching their chest and read, using signs that, when they touch the body, touch the baby's body rather than their own. This allows the baby to observe and internalize how signs are seen from the signer's perspective. Deaf parents also read to their children the traditional way, with the child sitting beside them. The combination of methods permits a comparison of perspectives, both of which allow parents and children to view the signs and the printed page simultaneously.

The visual environment and language, the enriched interactions and these small accommodations, all result in large payoffs for the development of Deaf children. Most Deaf children of Deaf parents function better than Deaf children of hearing parents in all academic, linguistic, and social areas.[3] Deaf children of Deaf parents develop a sense of identity that is strong and self-governed. At the same time, they feel included in social interactions as members of a tight-knit group. In the past, some Deaf children of Deaf parents did not even realize that there were hearing people in the world until they were of school age. (It is not uncommon for children to discover belatedly that there exist people who are different from them in profound ways.) One Deaf scholar, a member of a distinguished Deaf family in the United States, relates that he did not realize the world had hearing people in it until he was six years old. Before his mother finally explained, he was baffled by the failure of some playmates to understand him and by their habit of moving their lips.[4]

Other things being equal, Deaf children of Deaf parents have as good a chance as any other children of becoming adults with a strong sense of who they are and a highly positive sense of their ability to accomplish what they set out to do. It is no surprise that the Deaf President Now movement, which was able to change the governing structure of the world's only university for the Deaf, Gallaudet University in Washington, DC, from one dominated by hearing people to one controlled and operated by Deaf professionals—see chapter 5—was led by Deaf children of Deaf parents who felt that Deaf people should no longer tolerate the hearing world's modest view of their capabilities. By their highly effective use of the media, they projected nationwide, indeed internationally, a positive image of the DEAF-WORLD. (There is another yardstick by which the functioning of the Deaf home and the role of ASL in child development may be measured. Most of the children born to Deaf parents are hearing. These children of Deaf adults—codas—frequently function bilingually, using ASL and spoken English with ease. Even though many have parents with limited education and blue-collar occupations, a large majority—85 percent in one survey—enter the professions.[5])

As noted earlier, however, not all Deaf parents react in the same way to the birth of a Deaf baby. Some are saddened, at least in part. This is not surprising. Some Deaf parents are influenced by the values and instructions of hearing professional people who see the arrival of a Deaf child as a regrettable event, and one that will require professional intervention. These parents may adopt the hearing professionals' perspective, especially since the specialists' education and status seem to give their views special credibility. Then, too, Deaf parents know that their Deaf child must endure many arduous trials on the way to adulthood in a world dominated by hearing people. Their own experiences may have been so negative at times that they do not wish the same for their child.

Deaf parents face considerable obstacles in raising their children. They are frequently educated below their capacity, employed below their capability, and viewed negatively by the hearing world because they are Deaf. In some cases, that stigma has led social workers to seek to remove children from Deaf families. Because of social opprobrium, and because the system of Deaf education often fosters low self-esteem, some Deaf parents question their ability to function as good parents. Their daily encounters with oppression because they are Deaf may be a constant reminder that they should be something they are not—people who speak and hear. Deaf parents, like all parents, are sometimes baffled about how to manage their children. Unlike hearing parents, however, there are few places they can turn for advice.

The fact that being Deaf is viewed negatively in our society creates complicated interactions between the Deaf parents of a Deaf newborn and the hearing professionals with whom they come in contact. The difficulties begin at the well-baby checkups that are a typical part of medical practice in the United States, when the parents are exposed to what pediatricians, otolaryngologists, and audiologists generally have in mind for their Deaf child. Though the Deaf family may arrive enthusiastic, cohesive, and full of positive thoughts about their Deaf child, they are likely to encounter a perspective that, while caring, is also concerned, and thus implicitly negative. In particular, according to reports of many Deaf parents, professionals who work with the families of Deaf infants commonly give Deaf parents two pieces of strategic advice that are poorly received.

First, many professionals, in accord with accepted practice and the recommendations of books in their field, encourage Deaf parents not to use signed language with their hearing children, because that is reputed to delay the acquisition of English. (As we shall see in subsequent chapters, the opposite is closer to the truth and, in any event, for parents not to communicate with their child in signed language is tantamount to not communicating with the child at all.) This advice frequently makes the parents feel guilty (for not providing "the best" language environment), angry (since they cannot live up to the professionals' ideal), and mistrustful (since the advice is counter to their loving desire to communicate).

Second, professionals commonly encourage Deaf parents to put hearing aids on their Deaf babies, reasoning that some sound and exposure to spoken language is better than none. Since sound plays a marginal role in the lives of the Deaf parents and the family unit, many parents are naturally loath to put a prosthesis on their healthy child. Moreover, hearing aids are expensive, their use must be enforced, and many Deaf children hear no better with them than without them.

If professional people offer such alien advice, viewing the Deaf baby not as a godsend but as a problem, then Deaf parents who are secure in their cultural identity, recognizing that they have more experience and knowledge about growing up Deaf than the professionals advising them, ignore this professional input. Reassured that nothing has been found wrong with their baby, that their child is simply Deaf, they go home and proceed with their lives, drawing on the resources of the DEAF–WORLD, which offers support, encouragement, and a means to function as a self-fulfilled, contributing member of society, in the world at large as well as in the DEAF–WORLD.

A Deaf Child Born to Hearing Parents

Deaf people marry other Deaf people ninety percent of the time, but these marriages rarely produce Deaf children.[6] Of the children in educational programs for the Deaf, only five to ten percent have Deaf parents.[7] So most Deaf children are born to hearing parents, whose response to the birth of a Deaf infant usually contrasts markedly with the response of Deaf parents.

Families in America are influenced by the expectation that their children will live better than their parents. The birth of a Deaf child to hearing parents alters this expectation, less because the child does not hear than because of the way Deaf people are understood and valued in the culture of the larger society. If a child is born Deaf, and especially if there are other Deaf family members, the hearing parents may feel that they have produced a genetically defective child, a weak link in the family lineage. Relatives (and professionals) may contribute to this feeling by insisting that the parents must work very hard to mitigate the child's impairment. Proceeding with only this clinical perspective, hearing parents of a Deaf child may blame themselves for having inflicted a burden on their other children and on society at large.

Deaf parents raise their Deaf children with their personal experience and the DEAF–WORLD as their primary resources, but hearing parents of

Deaf children, who seldom have such resources, may be driven to begin a process of professionally guided identity development for their child that might appropriately be called "the making of a hearing-impaired person."[8] The process begins with professional people, perhaps unwittingly, reinforcing the hearing parents' and hearing society's deficit model of their child—that is, a model founded on the idea of hearing loss. This Deaf-child-as-patient needs otologists to determine the cause of the hearing loss and to consider remedies such as hearing aids and surgery. The child needs audiologists to quantify and characterize the loss in detail. The child will need speech therapy to develop oral communication as far as possible, and special education, provided by teachers trained in managing children with disabilities. If the child is thoroughly socialized into the role of patient-client, child and parents will not only accept these services, they will seek them out. Hearing parents are commonly unaware that other parents, Deaf parents, raise their Deaf children successfully without many of these services; indeed, they raise them more successfully than hearing parents who rely on such services extensively, judging by the results of psychological and academic tests and by the testimony of the DEAF–WORLD.[9]

One reason hearing parents are so vulnerable may be the shock of discovering that their child, whom they had considered normal in every way, is in fact unable to hear. Initially unaware that they have a Deaf child, they experience a time of joy and expectation. Because Deaf babies display the same kind of sensorimotor development, babbling, and gestural behavior as hearing infants, the first few months of the infant's life will follow typical patterns. Mother-child interaction will be reciprocal, because much of it involves touch and vision. Infants, Deaf and hearing, track the movement of their parents' hands, and distinguish their parents from strangers through visual identification of facial features and physical contact. Because these normal interactions lead hearing parents to believe that their child is functioning as expected, the emotional high from the birth and enjoyment of their child goes on for months.

Typically, it is the mother who develops the closest attachment to the child during these first months of life. She notices the nuances of her infant's behavior and is the first to identify and react to the various stages of the infant's development, both physical and social. It is she, then, who usually begins to suspect when her child is a few months old that he or she is not responding "normally." Then, over the next year or two, until a definitive diagnosis is made and accepted, parents commonly experience a series of dizzying highs of hope and lows of fear, an emotional roller coaster.[10]

Because the mother's sense that something is amiss is grounded in her uniquely close relationship with the infant, her initial suspicions are often met with skepticism on the part of extended family members, the baby's pediatrician, and sometimes even the father, all of whom perceive the baby to be "normal." A mother often may air her concerns first at the twelve-week well-baby visit to the pediatrician. We know from parental reports that many pediatricians discount her feelings as over-protectiveness, however, and suggest that "there is nothing to worry about." Some, in an effort to assuage her fears, perform rudimentary tests to assess whether the child actually has some level of hearing loss. In many cases, these tests are no different from those the parents have already performed: walking behind the child and clapping, calling out, or banging objects to make noise. Many Deaf infants appear to respond to the sound in these little tests because they are so attuned to using their vision that they visually track the actions of the pediatrician.[11] The mother leaves the doctor's office with a sense of relief and looks forward to the future with the belief that there are no significant differences between her child's behavior and what might be expected. She redefines her child's observed behaviors as simply minor anomalies in ways of interacting. The infant contributes to her belief by continuing to interact with her using gesture, vocalization, and babbling.[12]

During the period from four to twelve months, however, the parents increasingly struggle to interpret behavior that, while it generally matches their expectations for child development, also includes many "misfires." For example, they may successfully and enjoyably play patty-cake with their child, yet notice that the child does not respond when urged to sing along. At approximately the ninth or tenth month, when children are expected to produce their first words, suspicion and doubt again emerge in the mother and, now, often in the father as well. A return trip to the pediatrician results in further examination and referral to an audiologist. An audiological appointment at a major medical center takes three to four weeks to obtain.

It is during this period that the interactions between parent and child begin to involve a cycle of negativity, in which the child increasingly attempts to manipulate the parents and the parents punish those initiatives in their effort to manipulate their child. The Deaf toddler is now attempting to communicate, but lacks a model that is accessible because communication for the hearing parents is based on spoken language. As a result, the child resorts to physical gestures and other "tricks" in order to express herself or himself and to control the parents' behavior. The techniques available to the child include pulling on clothing ("Let's go out and play!"), pointing to objects or walking over to them ("Give me that"), pounding or stamping of feet, and tantrums ("I am frustrated," or "I am angry"). These moves gain attention or communicate wants, but they are extremely imprecise, and they make the parents feel powerless. Many times it is difficult for the hearing parents not only to understand their child's desires, but also to discipline the child, and to explain even simple things. Frustration builds as communication fails.

The months pass. Finally, after repeated cycles of suspicion that a problem exists, rejection of the suspicion, and its re-emergence, when the Deaf child of hearing parents is about a year old, he or she undergoes extensive audiological testing and the parents are told that their child has "a hearing loss." Many times this information is delivered as though it were exclusively medical, as if the diagnosis were one of diabetes, and little is said about how to cope with the news, or how to find more information.

To determine the actual extent of the hearing loss, as many as four visits to the audiologist may be required. Finally, the diagnosis is confirmed. The child abruptly changes from a toddler with some developmental problems into a gravely impaired child whose language, socialization, and education are imperiled. Thus begins the "stages of trauma" that hearing parents are said to experience, including grief, mourning, denial and anger.[13] (Laurel and Roberto said at the Deaf club that their parents were "devastated"; Henry's parents reacted similarly.)

It is during this difficult time that the hearing parents' understanding of their problem is constructed. The medical and audiological discussions that follow diagnosis can hardly provide an in-depth knowledge of the DEAF–WORLD. Even when clinicians do their best on this count, the novel information and perspective are difficult for most parents to grasp at this tumultuous moment. Alas, the parents do not fully grasp that countless children such as theirs grow up to become successful Deaf adults, members of the DEAF–WORLD who are engaged in the wider society as well, living fulfilled lives and becoming parents in their turn. Since the professionals are hearing and since the premise of their profession is that lack of hearing is a serious impairment, it is only natural for their discussions with the parents to end up by reinforcing the parents' view that something very bad has happened. The residual hearing the child may possess and the professional services he or she will require frequently become the focus of attention. Consultations are concerned with the need for hearing aids, speech therapy, and "language" training, by which is meant training in spoken English (in the U.S.). The idea of impairment becomes central to all the choices relating to the child's future that confront the family. Indeed, the professionals' preferred term for the child is *hearing-impaired.*[14] The professional reasons: a child with a loss of a bodily function has an impairment; the impairment gives rise to a disability, a severe restriction in a normal human activity, namely, communication; and the disability handicaps the child, preventing him or her from fulfilling various social roles.[15]

Hearing parents are recruited unwittingly to this understanding of their child in terms of disability, but they are recruited explicitly to a collaboration with professionals in the effort to provide "saturation services" to the family.[16] Professionals commonly see parental acceptance that their child is Deaf as a reluctant last choice; this may not be so much in what they say as in their vigorous, multi-faceted campaign to mitigate the child's hearing loss and its consequences. The parents naturally conclude that to do anything that would deter their child from functioning like a hearing person would be a disaster of enormous consequences.[17] For example, a priority of the audiology profession has become early detection of hearing loss. The purpose of early detection is to enable early fitting of hearing aids and other remediation. Some textbooks recommend that hearing aids be fitted on children with hearing loss as early as possible, whether they can be shown to benefit the child or not.[18] Parents who choose not to have their child fitted with aids are often viewed as negligent, and deemed to be closing off options for their Deaf child. Indeed, ignorant of the DEAF–WORLD and unable to foresee what life in that world would be like for their child, hearing parents understandably think only in terms of their familiar hearing world and of the importance of hearing.

(There are some professionals—especially, but not only, Deaf professionals—who struggle against this approach. They encourage the parents of the Deaf child to talk to Deaf adults, who can inform them about growing up Deaf, about the mores and values of Deaf culture, and about the ways they have learned to accommodate to a hearing society. Such professionals may remind the parents that someday their child is going to be a Deaf adult.)

A second priority for audiology today (in addition to early detection) is said to be parental empowerment. Professionals are urged to recognize the "suitability of a parent-centered paradigm . . . which requires [parents'] extensive and prolonged involvement in health and educational delivery systems."[19] The announced goal is to give parents information about all the different options with regard to prostheses, therapies, and educational placements. In practice, however, the options exercised by Deaf parents, such as the early use of ASL, and hiring Deaf baby-sitters and day caretakers, are rarely presented to hearing parents. Hearing parents often say that they "just didn't know about" such options.

This, too, is understandable. Much research on the DEAF–WORLD is relatively recent and has not been incorporated into the training of many professionals. Second, what the professional seeks is a collaboration of health-care professional and parent; orienting the family and child toward the DEAF–WORLD is not usually seen as advancing that collaboration. It may even be seen as undermining it. Deaf adults are rarely to be found in the professions consulted by hearing parents.[20] Third, health-care professionals are naturally oriented toward a health-care perspective, one that emphasizes the latest medical and prosthetic technology. It is not necessarily that they exclude the cultural perspective, but rather that their information and their enthusiasm lie preponderantly with the clinical approach.[21]

Associated with the hearing-impaired model of their child, there is, of course, a staggering amount of information. Parents who have the leisure, the means, and the education to inform themselves well are soon bewildered by claims and counter-claims, and by the sheer volume of all that appears to be relevant. Having learned about hearing aids, audiograms, the principles of hearing, the methods of speech therapy and of aural rehabilitation, they are likely to encounter an alphabet soup of invented sign systems for representing English on the hands, which we generically call *manually coded English* (MCE); these include Signed English, SEE 1, and

SEE 2.* ASL and PSE (Pidgin Sign English, see chapter 3) may be mentioned, as may techniques for oral communication, like cued speech. How is the parent to distill all this information and make choices without knowing the consequences of choosing one or another option?[22] After receiving a great deal of information about what to do with their Deaf child, parents feel guilty and fearful. They feel guilty because they are unprepared to make the right decisions, fearful because of what the future may hold.

Each of the professions concerned with assisting hearing parents of a Deaf child has its own history, body of knowledge and techniques. Hence, the wealth of information encountered by the parents is compartmentalized. Parents are commonly not led to an overview of the life-trajectory that is probable for their Deaf child, nor are they led to imagine possible futures. Because of professional compartmentalization, each segment of their child's life will involve a different group of people. There will be the initial medical and audiological group of professionals, then will come the parent-infant group, the preschool group, the elementary school group and the high school group (primarily groups of educational specialists and social workers), and then the rehabilitation group (primarily rehabilitation counselors).

Deaf adults who could present to hearing parents a positive view of their child's prospects are very rarely to be found in any of these groups. Professionals in parent-infant programs and early intervention programs, and most school district special educators, appear not to appreciate adequately the valuable resource that Deaf professionals represent. Indeed, the salient themes of many professional references to Deaf adults concern their limited academic achievement, their inability to speak, the limited utility of ASL, and the DEAF–WORLD as isolated.[23] Some physicians even inform parents and other medical professionals that the opinions and experiences of Deaf adults have no bearing on how to raise and "manage" their Deaf child.[24] The result of all this is to extend the duration of the parents' trauma and exacerbate their fear of the unknown.[25] Having spent months on an emotional roller coaster, some parents, like those of Henry at the Deaf club, are reluctant to accept the diagnosis that their child is Deaf. They engage in a process of denial that may last for years.

---

* MCE systems are discussed in chapter 9.

Some hearing parents continue to shop among professionals, attempting to find either a conflicting diagnosis or a diagnosis more acceptable (for example, that the child has an encouraging amount of residual hearing). Parental denial is buttressed when their Deaf child is placed in programs designed for hearing children. This may occur first in early-intervention programs, where Deaf children are often placed with hearing children who have disabilities. Although the parents may find this reassuring, such a placement delays the start of effective educational programming, and the Deaf child's academic achievement is likely to reflect the delay.[26] Academic placements that reinforce parental denial may continue in elementary and high school, where many Deaf children spend much of the school day isolated in a group of hearing children. In the absence of substantive reciprocal communication between teacher and student, Deaf students may resort to a kind of communication through manipulative behavior such as disrupting the class by acting out. Frequently, the result is estrangement between the Deaf child and his or her parents. Deaf adults who were placed in regular school programs where they were the only Deaf child report their exhilaration when they were first able to congregate with other Deaf people, in school, at work, or at a Deaf club. They then discovered, many say, that they were not imperfect copies of hearing people; rather, they were proud Deaf people. Whom do they blame for their long isolation? Many blame their parents, as well as the professionals who, despite the best of intentions, misled them.

Because so few children are Deaf, many physicians who come into contact with young Deaf children and their families fail to recognize all that a hearing family with a Deaf child must be grappling with, linguistically, psychologically and socially. It has been suggested that not enough training is provided to physicians and other health professionals regarding the diagnosis, prognosis, and treatment of early childhood deafness.[27] Further, some physicians may withdraw from the unpleasantness of facing families who are in pain and may fail to relay necessary factual information, preferring to restrict their comments to medical matters. To guard against this, some professionals (but all too few) work closely with Deaf adults and support groups comprised of parents of Deaf children.[28] Parents have a right to professional advice that provides a balanced view of the possible futures for their Deaf children, including the many positive possible futures for Deaf people in our society.

The effects of all this on the family are problematic. The family constellation can become more solid or, as in Laurel's case, more divided, as family members attempt to come to terms with the diagnosis that one of its members is Deaf. There are not many support systems available that can realistically help hearing families through the trials we have described, and there are even more trials to come. Bills for medical and audiological consultations begin to mount in the months after diagnosis. There are enormous time pressures. Parents need time for visits to the audiologists for the fitting of hearing aids and for hearing tests; they need time to schedule visits with other professionals and to keep the appointments; they need time to gather information, to read that information, and to make life-changing decisions. Parents' inquiries will leave them unsure of what to do, but at the same time they will be convinced that it is urgent to do something, and the right decisions are their responsibility. Faced with these stresses, some parents begin to blame each other.

As the Deaf child in a hearing family approaches his or her eighteenth month, the lack of communication is frequently a growing source of frustration. Parents are unable to explain to their Deaf child why the child cannot have certain objects or do certain things. Frustration builds in both parents and child, increasing parental feelings of inadequacy. Adults who are unable to communicate with their Deaf child may resort to manipulation and overdisciplining.[29] The search for answers is intensified. The stresses created by the highs and lows of the previous eighteen months begin to surface. Husband and wife communicate less. Typically, the mother is left to handle the interactions with the Deaf child. The mother also assumes responsibility for dealing with professionals, visiting the clinic and the parent-infant program, and for collecting information. The mother's investment, both emotionally and in time, is enormous, but her love for her baby drives her to do all that she can do, and eventually to neglect other family members, who may feel shut out. Because the investment in whatever decisions are made is so enormous, expressions of doubt are not long entertained. If the parents decide, with professional guidance, to try to teach their child to speak "so he will be able to cope with the hearing world," they encounter further stress, as this commitment is a vast undertaking. And if there is little progress or outright failure in teaching the child to speak, a common explanation from the professionals is "inadequate parental involvement."[30] Some parents resent this responsibility and burden and become angry with the professionals who counseled them.[31]

Extended family members who become involved sometimes increase the tension. Grandparents tend to support the professionals' encouragement of more speech training. In the face of all this, the mother, trying to develop strategies to cope, often unwittingly becomes more controlling of her child physically, and she becomes overprotective. She begins to fear leaving her child with a sitter, for example, as normal parental separation anxieties become magnified. Many parents worry that their child will be unable to live up to their aspirations, will not be in touch with them as an adult, will not be a productive and happy member of society, and even will not be able to live independently.

The Deaf child in a hearing family also develops strategies for coping. Many young Deaf children cling to their hearing mothers excessively. The child's tremendous fear of separation results in excessive crying, holding, and visual contact. There is almost no meaningful communication, and very few interactions have the result of rewarding the child's positive behaviors. There are times in a young child's life when he or she wants to say, "Mom, I'd rather do it myself."[32] The young Deaf child of hearing parents commonly cannot. The maturation process leading to independence and autonomous behavior thus may be stunted. The limits on the young Deaf child's world, in the areas of language, cognitive explanations of the environment, intellectual reasoning, and encouragement to explore, take their toll.

The interaction between parent and child becomes more the relation of teacher to pupil. Parents are encouraged to function as speech teachers, as Laurel's mother did. Mothers and fathers spend months, sometimes years, in the naming-of-objects period of language acquisition.[33] Some parents incorporate gestural communication, as did Roberto's parents, but it becomes idiosyncratic to the families and the child.[34] The functional use of home gestures can range from simple pointing at objects and acting out messages, to a repertoire of agreed-upon gestures that convey a much more extensive range of information, sometimes even effective information.[35] However, even where such *home sign* is well developed, the restricted communication between hearing parents and their Deaf child is reflected in the child's temper tantrums, which are often the product of frustrated attempts to communicate even simple ideas. There are also often long moments of staring during communicative interactions, and these may exacerbate the parents' fears and self-doubt.

As their Deaf child grows older, hearing parents may resort unwittingly to practices that actually inhibit the child's development.[36] A survey at one school for the Deaf found that only one parent in ten could communicate with his or her Deaf child.[37] Because of this limited ability to communicate, hearing parents tend to control interactions—to dictate the topic of the interaction, for example, and to prevent their child from exploring the physical and social environment. Having difficulty in managing the normal taking of turns in a discussion, they respond to their child's attempts to introduce new topics by hurriedly retreating to the topic they themselves introduced. Most hearing parents talk *to* their Deaf children, not *with* them.[38] Reliance on spoken English as the sole means of communication with a Deaf child restricts parent-child interaction severely and interferes with the natural bonding process. When communication breaks down, the child's cognitive, linguistic, emotional and educational progress suffers.[39]

Because the parents are unable to communicate information, rules of behavior, and values to their Deaf child—the bases for the child's independent decision-making—they find they must devote a disproportionate share of their attention to their Deaf child. Sibling relationships may be jeopardized. An imbalance in the natural hierarchy of the family constellation is created. Unhealthy stress and depression sometimes persist. Coping mechanisms are blunted, causing both the family and the child to become handicapped.[40]

Compare the common differences in approach of Deaf parents and of hearing parents to raising a Deaf child. On the one hand, Deaf parents are likely to have close rapport with their Deaf child, fluent communication, high expectations, and a well-founded positive outlook. On the other, fearful and frustrated hearing parents may not be able to communicate substantively with their Deaf child, who, in turn, is frustrated and tantrum-prone. *Yet it is the same child in both family situations.* So the root of the problem cannot be the Deaf child. Rather it must lie with the parents. It lies indeed with the hearing parents' inability to expose their Deaf child to a natural language without taking special measures.

The central issue in raising a Deaf child is language: the human capacity for language, and the roles that language fulfills in a social existence. We turn now to a consideration of the natural language that is fully accessible to the Deaf child if he or she is merely exposed to it. This language is at the center of the DEAF–WORLD. Once we have examined what the DEAF–WORLD has to offer its members, we will return to our discussion of hearing parents' loving concerns.

❦

Chapter 3

The Language of the DEAF-WORLD

WHAT is the language of the DEAF–WORLD? What is this language that Jake acquired as a matter of course from his Deaf parents without any special provision; that Roberto and Henry belatedly learned from other Deaf children; that Laurel was prohibited from learning until she was an adult? It is the visual-manual language of a visual people, Deaf people. It is the thread that binds the members of the DEAF–WORLD to one another, and to Deaf people across the ages. It is signed language.

The signed language of the DEAF–WORLD in the U.S. is American Sign Language (ASL). ASL is the language of a sizable minority. Estimates range from 500,000 to two million speakers in the U.S. alone; there are also many speakers in Canada.[1] Compared to data from the Census Bureau, which counts other language minorities, ASL is the leading minority language in the U.S. after the "big four": Spanish, Italian, German and French.[2] This large population of ASL speakers, and the several means for the transmission of ASL across the generations (residential schools, Deaf children of Deaf parents, the Deaf club), assure a rich culture for the DEAF–WORLD. Nothing is more central to that culture and dearer to the hearts of Deaf people than their language.

In the past few decades, linguists have uncovered a wealth of information about ASL and other signed languages. That knowledge is just beginning to be incorporated into educational and rehabilitative practices.

Perhaps the most astonishing and fundamental discovery of that research is that ASL *is* a language—a complete natural language, quite independent of English. The now overwhelming evidence that signed languages are among the world's natural languages contradicts what scholars and laymen once believed—that languages were spoken and heard, and thus that signed languages were actually just pantomime or alternate forms of spoken languages. Linguists now recognize that the capacity to acquire a language naturally and to pass it on to one's children is rooted deeply in the brain. Whether the capacity surfaces in a signed language or a spoken language is quite immaterial. The point is, it does surface, one way or another. In our mind, words like *speak* and *say* have a greater scope than we had realized—they apply to language production, whether the sentences be articulated orally or signed. When a child learns how words sound or how signs look, then that child has mastered merely the surface expression of language. The most basic principles of language are actually dictated by the capacities of the human brain.

In the next chapter we will focus on what is special about ASL—its visual and spatial form, and how that form affects language and thought in the DEAF–WORLD. In this chapter, we show that, even though ASL has a form different from that of spoken languages, it is fundamentally like spoken languages in the purposes it serves and in the way in which it is acquired. We further describe how, like other minority languages, ASL has struggled for survival and evolved into its present form, despite hearing efforts to eradicate it. Finally, we discuss the roles of ASL in the culture of the DEAF–WORLD in the United States, roles that mirrors those served by other languages in their respective cultures.

In our experience, people learning about the DEAF–WORLD and its language for the first time make some natural but mistaken assumptions that render their task more difficult. Let's take a moment, therefore, to explain what ASL is not, before examining all that it is. The first fallacy to clear out of the way is that signed language is pictorial. Visual communication is often pictorial, as pantomime testifies. However, pantomime and ASL are very different; to know a pantomime is not to know a grammar, but as we shall see, ASL has a grammar, with rules of word and sentence formation. If signed languages were thoroughly pictorial, they would be immediately understood and easy to learn; they are not.

The mistaken assumption that signs are highly pictorial, or *iconic*, leads many people to expect that signed languages can only be used to discuss concrete matters. Actually, ASL abounds in signs for abstract ideas, such as *soul, privilege, fake* and *abstract.*

People who assume mistakenly that signed language is pictorial and concrete are often led to the erroneous belief that it is universal as well. However, signed languages are not the same all over the world: Deaf communities that evolve independently have independent signed languages. ASL speakers are unintelligible to speakers of signed languages in Great Britain and Thailand, for example.

Finally, those who assume signed language is concrete are led to assume that it is primitive. They are encouraged in this mistaken belief when they read word-for-word transcriptions of ASL (called *glosses*), as in ME MOTHER RESPONSIBLE CHILDREN ME TAKE-CARE-OF FEED CLEAN LIST.* This method of transcription may well leave the reader with the impression that there are only verbs in the present tense and a few nouns in ASL. Such transcriptions record very little of the grammar of the utterance, much as Tonto left out grammar when addressing the Lone Ranger. The glosses may seem to be close to the original utterance, but in fact they can be very far from conveying its meaning. An actual *translation* of the original sentence, which takes into account not only the basic signs but also how they were modified to convey the structure of the sentence, yields: *I'm a mother, which means I have a lot of responsibilities. I must take care of the children, feed them, clean them up—there's a whole list.* Similarly, ASL has been naively criticized for having only one sign where English has several words. But the converse is also true: for example, one linguist enumerated thirteen different meanings of *run* in English for which ASL has thirteen different corresponding signs.[3] These problems of translation arise whenever different languages are compared. They are most striking when the languages are not closely related.

Hearing people naturally assume at first that all languages are spoken, so many start out with the mistaken belief that ASL is spoken English expressed on the hands according to certain conventions. However, as we

* Multi-word glosses connected by hyphens are used when more than one English word is required to translate a single sign, as in TAKE-CARE-OF.

shall show, ASL has developed as a fully autonomous language with a complex grammar not derived from English. Like spoken languages, ASL has rules for constructing words from a small set of combining elements, and rules for binding its words together into sentences and discourses. We noted in chapter 2 that there are also invented systems of manually coded English, but such systems have little to do with the natural language of the DEAF–WORLD, passed on from Deaf parents to their children, and from their Deaf children to those of hearing parents.

ACQUIRING ASL

Each language minority differs from others in significant ways. For example, some language minorities are in the course of dying out, while others are growing in numbers. Minorities that speak signed languages, however, are different from other language minorities in the ways in which they acquire the language. This has profound consequences for the group and its culture. As we saw in chapter 1, some DEAF–WORLD members acquire ASL natively, from birth on; others relatively early, when starting preschool or school; and still others much later in life, as late as adolescence.

In studying native acquisition of signed language, investigators have videotaped Deaf children of Deaf parents in their homes periodically and then analyzed the tapes in order to describe the stages in the Deaf child's acquisition of ASL (or any other signed language). The striking finding of these studies, noted in chapter 2, is that the progression through stages is very similar to that followed by hearing children learning spoken languages. Thus, Deaf children "babble" (manually) before producing their first words in signed language.[4] As with their hearing counterparts, Deaf children's one-word stage consists of individual signs produced one at a time in isolation. A common sign at this stage is POINT. Early two-sign productions may consist of two POINTS: if a child wants to indicate that a particular toy is his, he might show possessor and possessed with a sequence of two POINTS, one to the toy, the other to the child himself. Many other signs at the one-word stage are simple nouns and verbs, such as MOTHER and EAT. Sign productions at this stage frequently contain errors in the way they are produced, comparable to the hearing child's *tum* for *come*, and so on. These are characteristic of "baby-talk."

Some studies indicate that the acquisition of ASL may be faster than that of spoken language. Several studies find that the first sign tends to appear in a Deaf child's language two to three months earlier than a hearing child's first spoken word. (Other studies do not confirm this, however.) The growth of ASL vocabulary also appears to be faster: one Deaf child studied used eighty-five signs at thirteen months. Hearing children at that age are usually just acquiring their first few words.[5] If indeed the manual modality does provide a particularly accessible means of communication for very young children, it may be because its "speech mechanism" is directly visible to both the child and the parents, who can even reach out and mold the sign production. Investigators have also suggested that motor control of the hands may develop earlier than that of the vocal apparatus.

However, two-word utterances in ASL usually emerge at about the same age as two-word utterances in English, and in both cases they consist of basic words without grammatical markings. The range of meanings is also similar: existence statements appear first (POINT MOTHER), then statements about actions (FATHER EAT) and states of being (MOTHER HAPPY). These are followed by statements of location (POINT TRUCK), and finally by characteristics of actions, such as manner (RUN FAST) and indirect object (GIVE MOTHER).[6]

Although there are many more pronouns in ASL than in English, Deaf children's acquisition of ASL pronouns appears around twenty months of age, beginning with the first person pronoun POINT (directed at the speaker), meaning *I, me* or *mine.*[7] This is just the age at which hearing children also start using the analogous set of pronouns. Deaf and hearing children make similar pronoun errors. Psycholinguist Laura Petitto reports a videotaping session in which a 23-month-old Deaf child signed YOU when she clearly meant herself. Her Deaf mother signed, "NO, NO, NO, YOU MEAN YOU." Then she took her child's hand and made the pointing gesture directly on the child. The child, however, continued to point away from herself when referring to herself, much as a young hearing child would echo the mother's *you* in "You're a bad girl." Petitto found that the transition from gesture to sign in Deaf children begins with the pointing gesture, which then drops out for several months, only to return as a pronoun—an element in a grammar, with occasional grammatical mistakes.[8]

By the time Deaf children reach age two, pronouns for all three persons are evident and their acquisition has proceeded through stages and on a time schedule strikingly parallel to that reported for English. As chapter 4 explains, ASL has many more pronouns that refer to things than to people. These begin to appear when the child is around three years of age and are not completely mastered as a set of rules until age eight or nine.

Although ASL does not rely extensively on word order, as English does, to convey meanings, it appears that Deaf children learning ASL favor a particular word order, namely subject-verb-object. When they later master the rules for modifying words to show their roles in the sentence (such as subject and object), the children will relax this S-V-O word order, for example, moving the topic of the signed sentence to the front position (CAR FATHER BUY).

Two forms of negation in ASL develop early: the negative head shake and the sign NO. At the start of the two-word stage, the child forms negation by putting the negative at the beginning of the sentence, prior to the verb and without a subject (NO EAT), as in English acquisition. In later development, NO is used less. NOT emerges next, and then CAN'T. This is the same order of acquisition as observed in English.

The first indication of mastering ASL grammar, which appears around age three, is *verb agreement*, in which the verb moves from its subject location to its object location. For example, the child makes the one-sign utterance, MOTHER-GIVE-ME by starting the sign GIVE where the mother is located and moving the sign to a location close to the child's chest. At this early stage, the movement of verbs is modified in this way only if those locations are present in the room—in the example, only if the mother is actually there. At about this time, the child also masters a more sophisticated use of verbs and their grammatical conventions. In particular, the child performs some of the regular changes in the movements of verbs, called *inflections*, showing how an action is carried out, whether it is, for example, habitual, continuing, or repetitive. English conveys some of these same changes in the manner of an action by adding word-endings like *-ing* and adverbs like *always*. In a later stage of ASL acquisition, the child produces most of the regular changes in the movements of verbs but has not yet figured out how to combine those changes simultaneously according to rule (as in LOOK-REPEATEDLY-OVER-A-LONG-TIME). The Deaf child may go on mastering the system for complex verbs until as late as age seven or eight.

In ASL, the ability to describe the relation of objects in space also follows a developmental sequence. *On* is acquired first, then *in back of* and then *between*; this is the same order reported for children learning several spoken languages.[9]

To summarize, signed and spoken language acquisition follow identical stages of development: babbling (7-10 months), first-word stage (12-18 months), two-word stage (18-22 months), stage of word modification and rules for sentences (22-36 months).[10] What seems to determine the progress of language acquisition is the complexity of the rules the child must master and not the mode of language, spoken or manual, in which they must be mastered. These findings have led some scientists to conclude that the brain is programmed biologically to carry out language acquisition whatever its modality, spoken or signed.

So far we have spoken only about Deaf children of Deaf parents, exposed in the normal way to language models and acquiring ASL as a native language. As we said in chapter 2, such children are a minority in the DEAF–WORLD, which is mostly comprised of Deaf people with hearing parents. The acquisition story is often quite different for Deaf children with hearing parents, who have limited access to signed language because their parents generally do not know ASL. In addition, they have limited access to English because English is a spoken language and they are Deaf. Such children spontaneously gesture to members of their families or each other. Their gestures are idiosyncratic, reflecting salient features of their environment. Thus the gesture signifying *father* may touch the chin if father has a beard.

These Deaf children of hearing parents first produce one gesture at a time, and then combine gestures to produce two-gesture utterances and even longer stretches.[11] The gestures tend to be ordered in a consistent way, which reveals who is doing what to whom. Most utterances follow one of two orders. Here is an example of the first order, which states what is acted upon and then the action: "POINT at cowboy GIVE," meaning *Give me the cowboy*. And here is an example of the second common order, which states the actor and then the action: "POINT at train GO," meaning *The train goes there*.

Utterances containing three gestures also occur, and in those utterances we find all four meaningful roles in the sentence: the agent responsible for the action, the act, the person or thing acted upon, and the person or thing receiving what has been acted upon. From what source have these Deaf children of hearing parents learned to group gestures into categories like actors and actions and to order them in restricted ways? The surprising answer is, from no source at all. Their mothers produce almost exclusively single gestures while speaking, so they could not have learned this elementary grammar from them. Instead, the ordering of the gestures and their combination into phrases are provided by the children themselves, with very little to go on besides their mother's disconnected gestures. Nevertheless, the result resembles that of children engaged in conventional language acquisition—that is, the phrases seem to reflect semantic/syntactic categories like actor and acted upon. It appears that the child takes the impoverished language input, enriches it, and generates orderly language—incomplete and reduced language to be sure, but language.

Along the same lines, linguists have also studied language acquisition in Deaf children exposed only to systems of manually coded English (MCE). The term MCE system refers to any constructed signing system that represents words in English sentences with signs from ASL, along with invented signed translation equivalents for English grammar words, prefixes and suffixes. Investigators report that children exposed only to MCE systems manage to master parts of ASL, such as pronouns and spatial verb agreement, even though these are not to be found in manually coded English.[12] How can we make sense of this? Where can the ASL be coming from if the children do not see ASL? It must be coming from the minds of the children; they must be predisposed to invent these parts of ASL.

It appears then, that human beings have a biological capacity for language that involves an internal set of norms. Children construct the grammar of the language they are acquiring on the basis of these internal norms. This is called the *nativization hypothesis*, because the children are using their native ability to construct grammars, to *nativize* the incomplete information they receive. Deaf children are no different from any other children in this regard, since all children hear only a fraction of the possible sentences in their language and yet are able to master its complex rules and use them productively. In other words, *all* first-language learners construct grammars from limited input; that is, they all nativize.

The nativization hypothesis goes some way toward giving an account of why Deaf children without grammatical input generate grammatical utterances, but it leaves unexplained why these same children, who have been exposed not to ASL, but to an MCE system, come up with some patterns that actually occur in ASL, such as verb agreement. Linguists have suggested that Deaf children, using their native human endowment for language, invent systematic changes in verb movement that they have never seen, for example to distinguish among YOU-GIVE-ME, I-GIVE-YOU, and HE-GIVES-THEM, because conveying the person giving and the person receiving by the movement of the verb at the same time the verb itself is signed is a time-saving solution that compensates for the slow movements of the limbs and takes advantage of vision's ability to perceive and analyze complex patterns.[13] So it is predictable, they argue, that children exposed to manually coded English systems, which lack verb agreement, will convert that input into a more natural form for signed language, which has information of several different kinds (such as the action and the actors) flowing simultaneously.

The Deaf child's capacity for nativizing appears to wane with age. Psycholinguists have long postulated a critical period for the acquisition of any language, spoken or signed. However, the hypothesis was difficult to test rigorously with spoken languages, since the rare child delayed in the acquisition of spoken language is usually abused in other respects as well. The typical Deaf child of hearing parents allows a test of the hypothesis because that child is usually not exposed to a conventional language until he or she arrives at preschool or even later—wherever there is a group of peers using ASL. There is growing evidence that Deaf children pay a penalty in grammatical mastery and in sentence processing if their opportunity to learn ASL is delayed, and the greater the delay, the greater the penalty.[14] As we shall see in chapter 4, late learners, who have been effectively without language for many years, often have trouble with parts of the grammar of ASL.[15] Moreover, they do not understand the meaning of ASL sentences as well as early learners. These Deaf late learners differ greatly in their mastery of ASL, but on the average they do less well than native and early learners. Indeed, they even do less well on the average than late-deafened children who learn ASL as a second language in adolescence.[16] These late-deafened children, although they come to ASL as a second language relatively late, have acquired a first language on the normal developmental schedule. That timely acquisition of a spoken language may well be the basis of their greater mastery of ASL when compared with Deaf children who are deprived of the opportunity for first language learning.

The moral is clear. Every child, hearing or Deaf, is able to acquire a full natural language, and it is highly desirable to provide the child with accessible language input as early as possible.

When an American Deaf child nativizes reduced language input, he or she is reenacting the process by which, historically, ASL was formed. Deaf pupils who gathered at the first residential schools in America brought to school home signs from their family and sometimes more elaborate signed languages from small Deaf communities. The schools themselves, however, used quite a different language, based on the signed language used in Paris. With so many different languages in contact, the students ended up speaking a contact language to communicate among themselves. Such contact languages are not the mother tongue of anyone but borrow from languages that are in contact, for example, through trading. They have a simplified grammar and a restricted vocabulary. Because the contact languages of America's early residential schools provided only impoverished language input, the Deaf pupils, according to the nativization hypothesis, enriched that input with norms of their own construction. And the enriched contact language, passed down across the generations, became ASL. Here is how it happened.

HISTORY OF ASL

The history of ASL reaches back to the French Enlightenment, if not earlier. In 1779 a Parisian bookbinder named Pierre Desloges, who lost his hearing when he was seven, published what may be the first book concerning the DEAF–WORLD to come from a Deaf author. His book defended signed language against severe criticisms that had recently been published by a hearing teacher who sought to teach Deaf children to speak.

Although Charles Michel de l'Epée, the French priest who founded the first school for Deaf children in the late 1760s, is sometimes said to have played a critical role in establishing French Sign Language *(Langue des Signes Française,* LSF *), Desloges makes clear that Deaf Parisians had a common manual language well before that time. The abbé de l'Epée, Desloges wrote, learned signed language from Deaf people. It is reasonable speculation that the two Deaf sisters in Paris who, according to Epée, launched him on his career of educating Deaf students (see box), were members of a Parisian signed-language community to which Desloges also belonged.[17]

The Legend of the Abbé de l'Epée,
as Told at the Deaf Club of Marseilles

The abbé de l'Epée had been walking for a long time through a dark night. He wanted to stop and rest overnight, but he could not find a place to stay, until at a distance he saw a house with a light. He stopped at the house and knocked at the door, but no one answered. He saw that the door was open, so he entered the house and found two young women seated by the fire sewing. He spoke to them, but they still did not respond. He walked closer and spoke to them again, but they failed again to respond. The abbé was perplexed, but seated himself beside them. They looked up at him and did not speak. At that point, their mother entered the room. Did the abbé not know that her daughters couldn't hear? He did not, but now he understood why they had not responded. As he contemplated the young women, the abbé realized his vocation.

(Translation from Padden & Humphries, 1988)

While Epée apparently learned of the manual language of the Parisian Deaf community from the two Deaf sisters, he was misled by the great differences between its grammar and the grammar of his own language. Because French grammar relies heavily on word endings and word order, unlike signed language, which relies more on systematically modifying the movements of the signs themselves, he thought that LSF lacked rules. Thus, with the aid of his pupils, he undertook to choose or invent signs for all the word endings in French, for all the articles, prepositions, auxiliary verbs, and so on, until virtually every French sentence had its counterpart in manual French, could be transcribed into it, and recovered from it. He then sought to have his Deaf pupils use this manual French rather than LSF.

* It is not clear that there was a single uniform signed language in France in the 18th century. Our practice of referring to signed languages with national names and capital letters should not be understood to mean that there is evidence of a uniform signed language in each case, as there is with ASL, for example.

The two sisters from whom Epée presumably began learning signs, and to whom he probably taught his manual French in daily lessons at his home, were soon joined by other pupils. In the late 1760s, the class had six students; a decade later, there were thirty; by the time of the abbé's death in 1789, there were over sixty. Perhaps the language these pupils used among themselves was the language of the DEAF–WORLD in Paris to which Desloges referred.

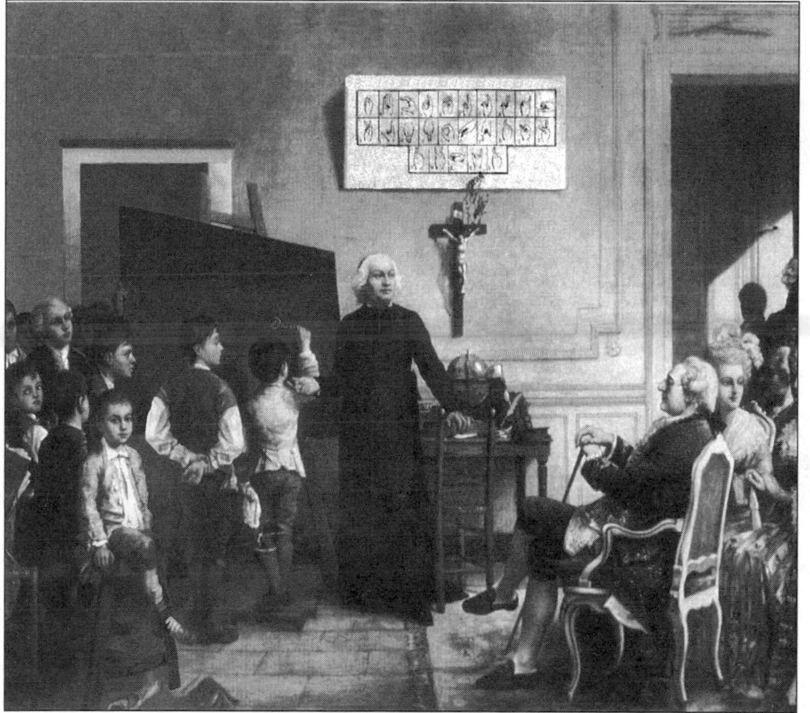

Courtesy, Institut National des Jeunes Sourds de Paris

Fig. 3-1. **The abbé de l'Epée giving a lesson; painting by G. Privat**

During his lifetime, Epée's disciples returned from Paris to their native lands and founded a dozen residential schools for Deaf children throughout Europe, from Rome to Amsterdam, from Madrid to Vienna. It seems likely that most of those disciples learned manual French, which included LSF signs, and possibly LSF itself. Then they took signed language with them when creating schools in their homelands. *Their* disciples and pupils, in turn, used that language in founding yet other schools. This hypothesis would explain the substantial overlap in vocabulary today among signed languages found in just those European capitals where schools were established by disciples of Epée and his successor, abbé Sicard.

On Epée's death, one of his main disciples, abbé Sicard, who had studied with the master for a year and had then returned to Bordeaux to found his own school, took over Epée's school, which had just been nationalized by the new French Republic. In speaking of his prime pupil in Bordeaux, Jean Massieu, Sicard said that they taught each other the words of their respective languages.

Jean Massieu, born Deaf, as were his five brothers and sisters, was appointed head teaching assistant at the Paris school; his autobiography implies that his family used their own home signs. What language Massieu used with his pupils in Paris is not known; presumably he used manual French in class and LSF outside class. By the time of Sicard's death in 1822, the Paris school housed some 150 pupils who used a common signed language, LSF. Like Epée's disciples a generation earlier, Sicard's disciples, hearing teachers who had observed his classes, carried manual French and possibly LSF back to their native cities, where they founded most of the twenty-one schools in France and some sixty throughout Europe that flourished in Sicard's lifetime. The pupils, too, disseminated their signed language: from the Paris school alone came mathematicians, chemists, painters, sculptors, poets, sailors, soldiers, and Deaf teachers of Deaf students, who traveled throughout France and Europe. Several of the Deaf teachers founded schools of their own for Deaf children.

Seven years before Sicard's death, Thomas Gallaudet, a Protestant minister from Hartford, Connecticut, was sent by philanthropists to London to acquire the art of instructing Deaf people. British schools for Deaf children were operated by a single Edinburgh family, the Braidwoods, who held the teachers in their employ under bond to protect the secret of their teaching methods. Refused admission to one Braidwood school after another, Gallaudet finally had recourse to abbé Sicard, who, as it happened, was giving public demonstrations of his methods in London, aided by Jean Massieu and another of his outstanding pupils, Laurent Clerc.

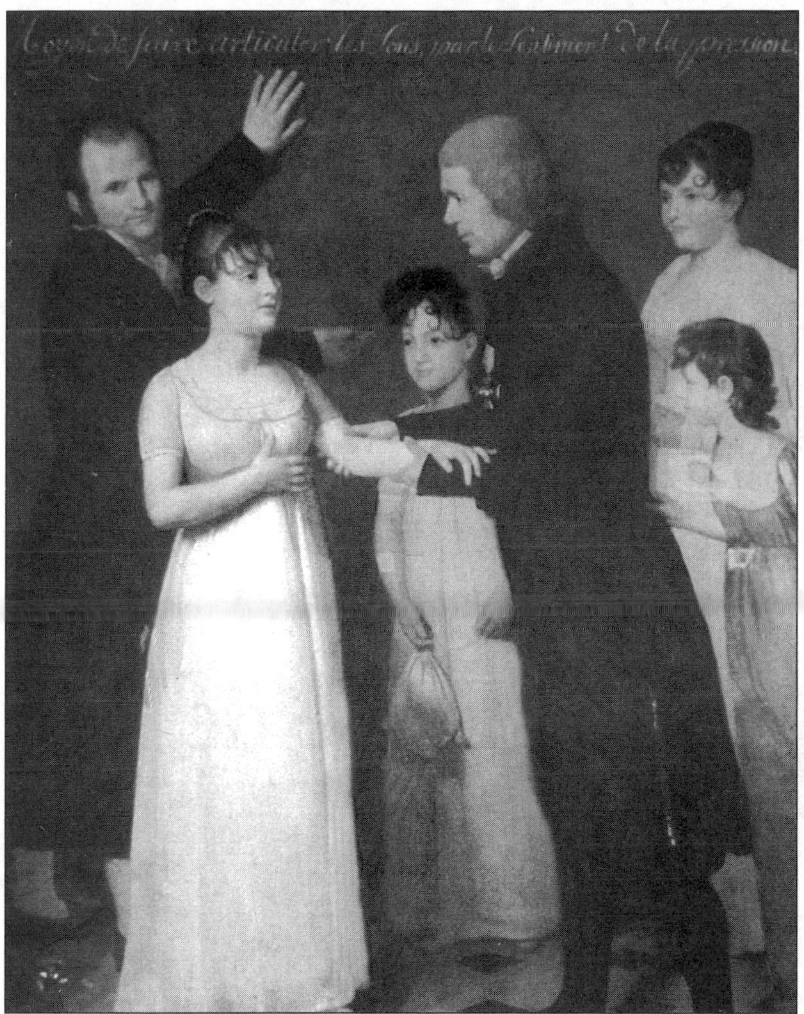

Courtesy, Institut National des Jeunes Sourds de Paris

Fig. 3-2. **Abbé Sicard (on the right) and Jean Massieu; detail from a painting by J. Langlois (1806)**

At Sicard's invitation, Gallaudet soon joined them in Paris and spent a few months studying Sicard's methods, receiving lessons in Epée's manual French from Massieu and Clerc, and attending their classes. In the end, Gallaudet contracted with Clerc to return to Hartford with him to help establish and conduct the first public school for the Deaf in America. (It is interesting to think that, were it not for the Braidwoods' avarice, the language of the DEAF–WORLD in the U.S. would probably be related to British Sign Language rather than to French Sign Language.)

In April 1817, the Connecticut Asylum for the Education and Instruction of Deaf and Dumb Persons opened its doors to seven Deaf pupils from various New England cities, several from families with other Deaf members. The language of the classroom was apparently Clerc's manual French adapted to English, which will be referred to here as manual English. Clerc taught the system to the early hearing teachers employed by the school, who were also in constant contact with the pupils. Soon Clerc was giving private lessons in signed language to nearly a dozen hearing teachers from as many eastern cities. All had journeyed to the school to learn Clerc's language and methods. Those teachers went back to several states to found schools in turn. By the end of the first year at the Hartford school, there were thirty-one pupils from ten different

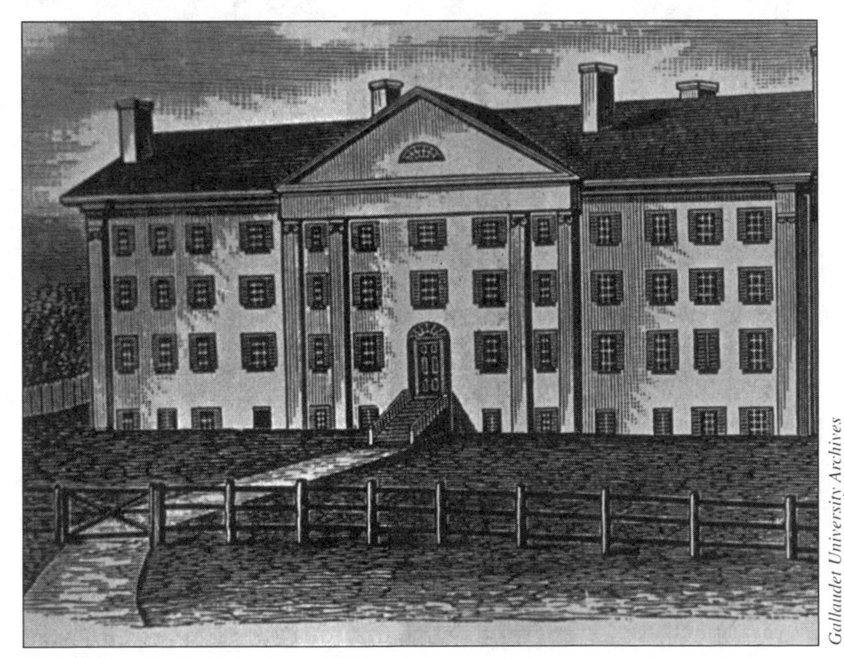

Gallaudet University Archives

Fig. 3-3. **American Asylum, 1821**

states. Among the possible sources for the language they used among themselves, in the dormitories and at play, if not in the classroom, should be listed Clerc's manual English, his LSF, the home signs they brought from their families and from small scattered Deaf communities, pantomime, and new signs generated in the setting of the school.

A comparison of dictionaries of modern LSF and ASL has found fifty-eight percent cognates in a sample of eighty-seven signs; that is, a majority of the signs with similar meanings in the two different languages resemble one another.[18] Such a high degree of overlap in the absence of any significant contact between the two Deaf communities other than through Clerc suggests that, located at the hub of American Deaf education, Clerc exercised great influence indeed. On the other hand, you might well ask why as many as forty-two percent of the words are so different, since ASL came from Clerc's LSF originally. It seems that ASL could not have become so different from its parent in just 180 years without some external force operating on it.

That force must have been the Deaf students in the Hartford school and other American residential schools. Of the first one hundred pupils at Hartford, the vast majority had become Deaf before learning English and a little over a fourth came from families in which there were other Deaf children. Some came from full-fledged Deaf communities, such as there were on the island of Martha's Vineyard in Massachusetts, and at Henniker, New Hampshire. Those children arrived at school with their own manual communication and their own vocabularies of signs. Linguists hypothesize that, under their influence, a contact language arose at the school. This manual contact language would then have been passed on as a native language to the next generation by Deaf teachers and by Deaf pupils if, when adults, they had Deaf children of their own. Since contact languages are no one's native language, they tend to have simple sentences, restricted use, and low status. Contact languages that are passed down across generations, however, undergo structural expansion through nativization, a process called *creolizing*. A creole is a language that is derived from a contact language but has a more complex syntax and a broader range of uses. Thus, as this theory would have it, was ASL "born": a creole of Clerc's imported LSF and indigenous signed languages and home signs.

What transpired in Hartford, in the early 1800s seems to have been representative of what transpired in many other lands: the presence of social institutions, notably schools, bringing Deaf people together creates out of numerous signed dialects and even distinct signed languages a common signed language of broader communication. That development, in turn, contributes to the development of Deaf society and culture. The coalescing institution is commonly a residential school for the Deaf, so the importance of those schools to the DEAF–WORLD is enormous, a topic we will discuss in depth in later chapters.

Besides Laurent Clerc's LSF and the languages of America's Deaf communities, another force shaping ASL as a creole was, and continues to be, successive generations of Deaf people from hearing homes.[19] The home sign that they developed in childhood to communicate with their parents, which had a simple grammar and consistent word order, mingled with the ASL they learned on arriving in school.[20] Yet another historical force at work on ASL is a tendency for signs to lose their iconic characteristics as they become regularized by the grammar of the signed language. Comparing shared entries in dictionaries of LSF and ASL across the ages, beginning in 1856, linguists have concluded that signs passed down across the generations tend to become more symmetrical, more centrally located in the signing space, and more fluid in execution.[21]

In America, as in France, the mother school sent its teachers and Deaf graduates throughout the country to teach in various Deaf schools and to found new ones. As early as 1834, a single signed dialect was recognized in the schools for Deaf students in the U.S. By the time of Clerc's death in 1869, over fifteen hundred pupils had graduated from the Hartford school, and there were some thirty residential schools in the United States with 3,246 pupils and 187 teachers, forty-two percent of them Deaf. Most such pupils and teachers married other Deaf persons and had children. This, too, helped to disseminate ASL.

Through these developments, toward the middle of the nineteenth century, was ushered in a golden era in the education of the Deaf. That is not to say that everything was perfect in the residential schools. However, instructed in the national language and all the traditional branches of knowledge through the vehicle of their primary language, their signed language, Deaf children throughout Europe and America completed elementary education in growing numbers. "High classes" were then launched by the Hartford, New York, and Paris schools, among others. Deaf students gifted in the liberal arts pursued their schooling for another four years, many going on to become themselves teachers of the Deaf. To allow graduates of the high classes to continue their education, Thomas Gallaudet's son, Edward Miner Gallaudet, founded in Washington, DC, in 1864, the first college for the Deaf in the world, known today as Gallaudet University.

The more the signed languages of the Deaf flourished in Europe and America, however, thc more their role was contested by hearing educators convinced of the greater value of the majority spoken language. One approach was to graft the grammar of spoken language onto signed language. As we have explained, Epée and Sicard claimed that the "language of the Deaf" lacked grammar. However, by rearranging the order of signs and by inventing new ones, the signed language would take on the grammar of French. French sentences could be expressed manually, and the students could acquire the world's knowledge through French. But after Sicard's death, manually coded French rapidly fell into disuse. American schools likewise largely stopped using manually coded English in the 1830s. Teachers called it "unwieldy," "cumbrous," and "a dead weight." (As we shall see in part 2, some educators in recent decades, apparently unfamiliar with this history, have reintroduced manually coded English systems in the schools.)

The second approach to ousting signed language was to supplant Deaf peoples' signing with speech. Efforts to teach the Deaf speech have a long history, dating from at least the sixteenth century, when Pedro Ponce de León, a Spanish monk, taught the Deaf scions of noble families to speak, read, and write. This astonished scholars in Spain and, as word spread, throughout the rest of Europe. Ponce de León's method probably served indirectly to guide the three men who are generally considered to have founded oral instruction of the Deaf: Jacob Pereire in the Romance-speaking countries, John Wallis in the British Isles, and Jan Conrad Amman in the German-speaking nations. All three labored under conditions similar to those of Ponce de León, as did their many disciples, well into the nineteenth century. Typically, a wealthy family has a son who becomes Deaf at an early age (Deaf daughters were commonly sequestered at home or in convents). The family hires a tutor, often a man of letters, who works to maintain, perhaps restore, the boy's speech and to expand his knowledge of arts and sciences. The boy makes progress; a philosopher notes it; the tutor publishes letters announcing his achievement, but withholding his method. The tutor goes on to other things; the boy, generally, does not. Desloges' book in 1779, defending signed language, was written to rebut one such tutor, a disciple of Jacob Pereire, who wished to have Deaf pupils speak French and not LSF.

The first serious inroads of the majority oral language in American schools for the Deaf coincided roughly with the abandonment of manually coded English, as if the forces of English dominance, blocked on one route, took an alternate and more ambitious path—outright replacement. In 1843, two leading American educators, Samuel Gridley Howe and Horace Mann, who had no familiarity with Deaf people, returned from Europe with great praise for the schools for the Deaf in Germany, which used spoken German exclusively. So the New York and Hartford schools dispatched their own inspectors, who returned steadfastly in favor of signed language, but advocating some training in spoken English as a supplement for those pupils with partial hearing, especially those who had lost their hearing after acquiring speech.

The next major developments awaited the late 1860s when, at Howe's instigation, an oral school for the Deaf (that is, one requiring that spoken English be used exclusively) was organized in Massachusetts; it is now known as the Clarke School. Shortly thereafter, another oral school was founded in New York, one in London, and one in Paris. In the 1870s, Alexander Graham Bell added his considerable prestige, his tireless labors, and his fortune derived from the invention of the telephone, to the "oralist" movement. Bell's chief adversary, Edward Miner Gallaudet, espoused bilingual education of Deaf students: ASL and written English, with spoken English for those who were capable of it.

During the French Universal Exhibition of 1878 a small meeting of instructors of the Deaf, all hearing and almost all French, was hastily convened.[22] The group dubbed itself the Universal Congress to Improve the Lot of the Blind and the Deaf. The meeting, sponsored by Jacob Pereire's millionaire son and grandson, resolved that only instruction using the national spoken language could fully "restore the Deaf to society," although signing could be a useful auxiliary.[23] The Paris meeting decided to hold a second congress in Milan. In that city were to be found two schools for the Deaf where signed language had formerly been used but where, for the ten years prior, instruction had been given in spoken Italian by hearing teachers. The head of one of the schools was made president of the Milan congress, and the leading instructor of the other was made secretary. Two days before the opening of the convention, and every afternoon of the convention, were devoted to carefully stage-managed public examinations of pupils, conducted in spoken Italian by their teachers. Although the American delegates thought the exercises a sham, their reservations were not shared by most of the 164 delegates, all of them hearing, seven-eighths of whom were from Italy and France. All but the Americans voted for the following resolution exalting the dominant oral language, and "dis-barring" the minority signed language in whatever nation:

1. The Convention, considering the incontestable superiority of speech over signs, for restoring deaf-mutes to social life [and] for giving them greater facility of language, declare that the method of articulation should have preference over that of signs in the instruction and education of the deaf and dumb;

2. Considering that the simultaneous use of signs and speech has the disadvantage of injuring speech and lip-reading and precision of ideas, the convention declares that the pure oral method ought to be preferred.[24]

In the closing moment of the congress, the special French representative cried from the podium *Vive la parole!* (Long live speech!)

In Europe, delegates to the congress returning to their nations' capitals reported the death sentence for signed languages as part of the rise of modernity. Deaf teachers were fired en masse, older Deaf students who had been contaminated by signed language were quarantined in the residential schools, and draconian measures were imposed on newly admitted students in an effort to prevent them ever from using their signed language.

In America, the New England aristocracy had resisted all along the education of their Deaf children, many of whom had once spoken, in the ranks of the poor, congenitally Deaf and by the exclusive means of signed language. Moreover, with the rise in immigration to the U.S. in the late nineteenth century, and the shift in its origins to poorer southern and eastern Europe, the "old" immigrants, particularly those from Britain and Germany, clamored for restrictive immigration laws; for eugenic reduction of the "unfit," including the Deaf; for language uniformity; and for English-speaking day schools for Deaf children. The nation's leading champion of all these causes was Bell, who, in 1890, founded the American Association to Promote the Teaching of Speech to the Deaf (now the Alexander Graham Bell Association), with the underlying goal of promoting Deaf people's assimilation into hearing society and discouraging their intermarriage. (See also chapter 14.) Bell was a tireless advocate for the founding of oral day schools, which attracted many Deaf children of hearing families who otherwise would have entered the residential schools. In the wake of Milan and Bell's efforts, ASL was soon banned in the residential schools, which increasingly came under the control of hearing people with no ties to the DEAF–WORLD. In 1867 there were twenty-six American institutions for the education of Deaf children, and all taught in ASL as far as we know; by 1907 there were 139, and none did. (A few manually taught classes for the "oral failures" survived in some schools.) The fraction of the teachers who were Deaf themselves, and who for the most part would be expected to communicate with the pupils in ASL, fell equally precipitously, from forty-two to seventeen percent by the turn of the century, and most of the latter taught manual trades. (Nowadays an estimated seven percent of teachers of the Deaf are Deaf.)

The National Association of the Deaf defended vigorously but unsuccessfully the role of ASL and Deaf teachers in the schools. National and international congresses of the Deaf in Europe proved equally unable to stem the tide, and the languages of their DEAF–WORLDS, many of them "cousins" to ASL, sharing roots in LSF, were banished from schools for the Deaf everywhere. In a culture that, as we have seen, cherishes its language so dearly, and in which Deaf children come into their linguistic heritage in the schools, no more crushing blow could be struck than to banish signed language from the schools. The Congress of Milan has become emblematic of evil in the culture of the DEAF–WORLD in the U.S., as in that of many European nations.

The ostracism of signed language from the schools continues to the present, although certain developments in linguistics and allied disciplines are leading to change. Word that ASL possesses the properties of natural languages (based initially on William Stokoe's work in the 1960s), along with increasing American tolerance for cultural pluralism, has inspired a resurgence of ASL prestige, instruction, and use. Deaf teachers are once again in demand. Congresses, workshops, books, and journals about ASL are appearing at a high and growing rate. There is an increasing interest in the culture and art forms of the DEAF–WORLD, such as theater, storytelling and poetry in ASL. A few schools for Deaf children have reintroduced signed language in the classroom. Mainstreaming—the practice of putting Deaf children in schools and classrooms for hearing children—has discouraged ASL use in education, but alternatives to mainstreaming seem to be recovering some lost ground. It may be that the United States is now on the threshold of an era in which ASL will again flourish. We will examine this evolving role of ASL in culture and education in later chapters.

LANGUAGE DIVERSITY IN THE DEAF–WORLD

Although signed language has been suppressed in education for over a century in many lands, it could not be banished from the lives of Deaf people; most of them continued to take Deaf spouses and to use their manual language at home, with their children, and at social gatherings. As prominent as signed languages have remained in the lives of Deaf people after Milan, the national spoken languages have also exerted a certain influence on the DEAF–WORLD. After all, ASL speakers, for example, have been engulfed by the English-speaking majority in school, at home, and in the workplace, for many decades. This was and still is bound to have considerable consequences for language use in the DEAF–WORLD. For one thing, some adult members of the DEAF–WORLD acquired English aurally before they became Deaf: six percent of Deaf children in a recent survey became Deaf after age three.[25] Many in the other ninety-four percent studied English intensively at home in their early years, and most have studied English at school. For those who learned ASL relatively late in life, their signing reflects their prior fluency in English as well as their late acquisition of ASL. In short, there is considerable variation in the signed language that one encounters in the American DEAF–WORLD. Linguists have shown that this variation is systematic, and it is related to the circumstances in which the speaker acquired ASL: Deaf people with Deaf parents and early learners of ASL tend to use a grammar different from that used by hearing people, Deaf people with hearing parents, and other late learners whose grammar is more closely related to English grammar.[26]

In addition to family and educational background, geographic region contributes to variation in ASL grammar and vocabulary.[27] When a sample of native signers scattered over the U.S. was asked to give ASL signs for a long list of English words, they produced three or more different signs for four-fifths of the words. *Peanut* for example, elicited nine regional variations.[28] There is also a Black variety of ASL; used by Black Deaf adults in the South, it arose in part in the schools for Black Deaf children that existed before desegregation.[29]

When members of the DEAF–WORLD address hearing English speakers who have limited knowledge of ASL, such as parents or students, they frequently change to a different signed language variety, as they may do on occasion with other Deaf speakers when it facilitates communication. They may utter some English words while using ASL; they may alter the word order of their signed sentences so that they are more like English sentences. This *contact sign,* which has arisen from contact between ASL and English, is an important source of language variation in the DEAF–WORLD. Linguists studying it in the 1970s labeled it *Pidgin Sign English* (PSE).[30]

Contact signing differs from the ASL used by monolingual native speakers—let's call it *heritage* ASL[31]—on the one hand, and from English on the other. For example, English has the articles *a/an* and *the*. To distinguish *a* and *the*, ASL uses pointing, eye-gaze and location. Contact sign fingerspells *a* and *the*. (Fingerspelling represents English words by assigning to each of the letters in the alphabet a distinct handshape. The set of 26 handshapes is called the *manual alphabet.*) Like many spoken languages, ASL does not have a separate word for *be*; contact sign uses the ASL sign glossed as TRUE to mean *be*. For example, to express the progressive, *is running, was going*, etc., ASL modifies the movement of the verb according to rule. English also modifies verbs according to rule, using the suffix *-ing*, for example. Contact sign, on the other hand, frequently uses the word TRUE in addition to the ASL sign for the verb. This is an example of the reduced grammar characteristic of pidgins.[32]

Linguists have recently disputed whether contact sign is best considered a pidgin, on the model of contact between spoken languages.[33] Briefly said, contact sign is unlike English-based pidgins in that it has far too many characteristics of ASL, such as the use of space, eye gaze, and inflected verbs. Thus it is not "reduced English," as spoken English pidgins are. Also, the social situation in which contact sign is used does not conform to the pattern that gives rise to pidgins. For example, when slaves were brought together to Jamaica from various West African nations, they learned enough of the language of the British rulers to be able to communicate among themselves across language barriers and with the rulers themselves; however, they were rarely allowed to socialize with the British and master their language. Thus a pidgin English arose. In contrast, the contact language in the American DEAF–WORLD arises because of the varying degrees of bilingualism of its speakers, some of whom are fully bilingual. Another respect in which contact signing is quite unlike pidgins is in its occasional use of elements from both languages simultaneously. When a signer produces an ASL sign and simultaneously speaks, whispers or mouths its English gloss, he is doing something that no user of a spoken language can do. Different members of the DEAF–WORLD will use the resources of contact signing differently depending on their bilingualism, their conversational partners, and the topic of conversation.

The influence of English on ASL takes several other forms. These are available to ASL speakers depending on the nature of the contact situation, and in particular on the language skills of the conversational partners.[34] The speaker may use fingerspelling, following written English. In addition, some fingerspelled words have been transformed into signs over time. An example is JOB, which began as a fingerspelled word J-O-B, with three separate elements. Although ASL WORK has both a noun and a verb form (as in English), ASL speakers apparently felt the need, perhaps because of their knowledge of English, to have a separate form that was a noun. The sign JOB elides the original *O*, allowing a smooth transition between *J* and *B* and giving it a closer resemblance to other signs.[35] Another influence of English can be seen when speakers utter signs and at the same time mouth their English glosses. In a classroom with Deaf children, some teachers may, moreover, use one of the invented systems of manually coded English, uttering one or more signs for each English word in an English sentence. Or they may actually speak the English words outloud. The consequences of contact between English and ASL can also be seen when members of the DEAF-WORLD have a TTY conversation: the stream of English words across the screen sometimes conforms so closely to ASL that one can recover the intended message best by imagining the ASL sentence that would have given rise to it.

A related source of language variation in the DEAF-WORLD is called *register*. Register refers to variation in language according to the formality or informality called for by the social situation. Linguists distinguish several levels of register, with decreasing use of ellipsis and colloquial language: intimate, casual, consultative, formal, and frozen (formulaic). Early linguistic studies of register in ASL proposed a continuum between two registers: at one extreme, the formal register, or "high variety," of ASL reflected heavy English influence; at the other, the colloquial register, or "low" variety, approached the ASL of Deaf people with Deaf parents.[36] This proposal probably oversimplifies the linguistic situation,[37] but it captures the social situation that long existed in the American DEAF-WORLD, in which English was highly valued and ASL held in low esteem. Although that situation has changed in the wake of linguistic research on ASL and the movement for Deaf rights, some Deaf people still refer to others who use ASL as "low verbal," and to their language as "broken language," or "slang." A Deaf friend of ours referred to her signing in ASL as "low sign"; for her, "high sign" took on more properties of English. Other informants have referred to ASL as "broken English" or "bad English." Nowadays, linguists are investigating ASL registers, and interpreters and ASL speakers are taking classes to master them.

When oral Deaf adults or hard-of-hearing people mingle in the DEAF-WORLD, they may use spoken English (or Spanish, etc.) with selected conversational partners. Written English (and Spanish) are also in use. Recent immigrants will bring their own signed languages to the DEAF-WORLD and, until they have sufficiently mastered ASL, will communicate in a kind of reduced pantomime with borrowings from their signed language and from ASL.

Finally, there are some members of the DEAF–WORLD who have not been able to acquire any language. We recently met a Deaf man, the son of hearing parents, who had been wrongfully institutionalized as a young boy in a state hospital for mentally retarded people. When he was released a few years ago, he had at his command a keen desire to communicate and some skill in pantomime; that repertoire is often called *minimal language skills* (MLS). Deaf people in formal and informal situations have been communicating with him in MLS, teaching him ASL, and endeavoring to acculturate him to the DEAF–WORLD.

To summarize: The DEAF–WORLD in the U.S. embraces wide variation in language use. Speakers range from ASL monolinguals or ASL dominant bilinguals to English-dominant bilinguals. There are people with minimal language skills. National, family and educational background; age; and geographic region all contribute to the variation in ASL encountered. So do the situations in which communication takes place, depending on the conversational partners, the appropriate register, and the topic. Most of these forms of language diversity apply equally to spoken languages. They apply to English in the U.S., for example, which varies with region, ethnicity, social setting and so on. Two noteworthy exceptions: Two spoken languages cannot be intermingled in quite the same way as a spoken and a signed language. Also, it is extraordinarily rare, thank goodness, for accessible language to be withheld from a hearing child, so hearing children rarely are reduced to the near-absence of a language.

THE ROLES OF ASL IN THE CULTURE OF THE DEAF-WORLD

Language has fundamentally three roles in bonding a group of speakers to one another and to their culture. It is a symbol of social identity, a medium of social interaction, and a store of cultural knowledge.[38] ASL fulfills all these roles in the culture of the DEAF–WORLD.

A symbol of identity

ASL is a very powerful symbol of identity in the DEAF–WORLD, no doubt in part because of the struggle of ASL-speakers to find their identity in a hearing world that has traditionally disparaged their language and denied their culture. Deaf sociolinguist Barbara Kannapell, a pioneer in the American Deaf Rights movement, has written of ASL: "It is our language in every sense of the word. We create it, we keep it alive, and it keeps us and our traditions alive."[39] And further, "To reject ASL is to reject the Deaf person."[40]

We recognize such evident pride in one's language. In France, to take just one example, the French Academy (and legislature) have labored for centuries to protect the purity of French from the inroads of other languages. Speakers of several minority languages in France—Breton, Alsatian and Arabic among them—struggle for acceptance of their language and distinct identity. Closer to home, Native Americans have been struggling for the protection of their languages, and identities; in 1990 Congress enacted a law encouraging the use of Native American languages in the instruction of Native American children. When Laurent Clerc was an old man and looked back with satisfaction at his long career, at all the Deaf and hearing teachers he had taught his LSF and all the pupils he had educated, he was pained to realize how much those teachers and pupils had reshaped his language, "corrupted it," as he felt. Just as the French believe their language is central to their culture and heritage and must be protected from alien influences, so Clerc and countless Deaf leaders after him have been concerned with protecting the purity of the signed language, acting on the conviction that manual language was central to their Deaf culture and heritage. In 1913, the National Association of the Deaf, fearing for the very survival of ASL under the scorched-earth policy of oralism, commissioned films of great Deaf American orators; these are a magnificent repository of formal ASL signing and of cultural transmission in the early twentieth century. Recently, the Deaf filmmaker Charles Krauel, who began making films of the DEAF–WORLD in 1925, reminisced about the old days and commented on ASL: "Back then signs were better, you know, natural, but now with all these *is* kind of signs and all that . . . My [old] signs are more abbreviated [and] much clearer."[41]

A medium of social interaction

ASL is also a medium of social interaction in the DEAF–WORLD. This is surely one reason for its power as a symbol of identity. Most Deaf children lack any effective medium of social interaction until they encounter ASL. That encounter not only provides a basis for identifying with the members of a culture, transforming an outcast individual into a participating member of a society, it also enables full and easy communication for the first time. No wonder the discovery of Deaf culture is a central theme in personal history and in DEAF–WORLD legend. Here is an example from personal history. In his autobiography, Deaf American pioneer Edmund Booth—teacher, farmer, Gold Rush miner, journalist—recounted his childhood arrival at the American School for the Deaf in Hartford in the early nineteenth century, accompanied by his older brother Charles, who was hearing. The principal, Thomas Gallaudet, was unable to communicate with Edmund, since the boy knew only home signs. Then, Booth recounts, "Charles and I went into the boys' and next the girls' sitting rooms. It was all new to me and to Charles it was amusing, the innumerable motions of arms and hands. After dinner, he left and I was among strangers but knew I was at home."[42]

Why do Deaf people feel at home when communicating in ASL? Barbara Kannapell asks. And she answers: Deaf people can understand each other all the time in ASL but they only get fragmentary information or one-way communication outside the DEAF–WORLD. ASL comes easily and naturally to most Deaf people. It allows Deaf people to share meanings, that is, common experiences, cultural beliefs, and values.[43] These common experiences arise, in part, directly from being Deaf, where one depends on vision, not hearing, and uses ASL for easy communication.

Common experiences also arise from being Deaf in a hearing society. For example, there is growing up in a hearing family (or, less often, a Deaf one), attending a school for the Deaf, getting a job with the help of Deaf friends. Deaf people share common experiences as well from being Deaf in Deaf society: refurbishing the Deaf club; winning for the club team; finding one's spouse, and countless more. Much of Deaf people's knowledge of life and the world has been communicated to them by other Deaf people speaking their signed language. Because signed language is the medium of social interaction for most people in the DEAF–WORLD, it is also their medium of education and self-instruction: nearly all their knowledge of the world has come to them through signed language.

A repository of cultural knowledge: Values

Finally, the constituents of Deaf culture—its values, mores, history, and artistic expression—are stored in signed language, so to speak, for transmission across the generations. When a Deaf child becomes acculturated to Deaf culture in America, for example, what cultural knowledge does he or she acquire? In the first place, there are values. Deaf identity itself is highly valued; Deaf people seem to agree that a hearing person can never fully acquire that identity. Even with Deaf parents and a native command of ASL, the hearing person will have missed the experience of growing up Deaf, including attending a Deaf school, and that person is likely to have divided allegiances. Speaking and thinking like a hearing person are obviously fine, if one is hearing. And speech skills may be helpful in dealing with hearing people in some circumstances. Within Deaf culture, however, between one Deaf person and another, speaking and thinking like a hearing person are disparaged, as are mouth movements when signing (unless they are called for by the ASL signs).

Deaf people who adopt hearing values, perhaps even looking down on other Deaf people, are regarded as traitors. "We are all in the same family," said one Deaf leader, and, indeed, the metaphor of *family* is fundamental and recurrent in the DEAF–WORLD. (Remember Edmund Booth finding himself "at home" among strangers.) The DEAF–WORLD is, by hearing standards, a heterogeneous family, but the salience of Deaf identity attenuates differences of age, class, sex, and ethnicity that would be more prominent in hearing society. Likewise, there is a penchant for group decision-making, and mutual aid and reciprocity figure importantly in Deaf culture. Consistent with the metaphor of family, there is deference to older Deaf people and their achievements in relation to the DEAF–WORLD. Informality is valued (except on formal occasions). One expert on American Deaf culture, Marie Philip, points out that it normally won't do to appear at the Deaf club in a suit, or to bring shrimp and champagne to a Deaf picnic. Everyone brings food to such Deaf social events in the U.S., but macaroni and cheese are closer to the norm. Physical contact is valued; Deaf people like to get together and see one another and, in the U.S. at least, give one another hugs of *hello* and *goodbye*. All in all, promoting unity is a fundamental value in the

DEAF–WORLD. Informality, hugging, team sports and other joint activities all serve to promote this unity.[44]

Residential school ties are also exceedingly important, and graduates are likely to return frequently for alumni events. Hearing people might mistake this for the fondness for one's alma mater sometimes found in hearing society, but in fact it goes much deeper. The school is home, since home is where your family is from. When asked where they are from, Deaf people will often reply with the name of the residential school they attended; it invariably comes up in introductions (as it did when Ben introduced himself in chapter 1). An interview with a Deaf couple in their eighties eloquently testified to the lifelong importance of school ties. Said the wife: "You see those people sitting over there? Those are my classmates from the Berkeley School. [I went there] when I was nine. They all befriended me, and we have been tight ever since. Of course, once we all started families, we didn't always see each other as regularly as we do now that everyone is retired. It's hard on my husband; he's from out of state and didn't grow up with us, so he feels kind of left out."[45]

There is fierce group loyalty in the DEAF–WORLD, no doubt reinforced by the shared experience of being Deaf in a world dominated by hearing people. This loyalty may extend to protectively withholding from hearing people information about the DEAF–WORLD's language and culture. The members of the DEAF–WORLD believe, as do members of other cultural groups, that one should marry within one's minority: marriage with a hearing person is frowned upon. Deaf marry Deaf approximately nine times out of ten. The DEAF–WORLD collectively values Deaf children highly; Deaf adults in rural areas, for example, will drive great distances to see Deaf children when invited, especially if the children might otherwise lack such contact. To culturally Deaf people, each Deaf child is a precious gift and, as noted in chapter 2, many expectant Deaf parents hope their child will be Deaf like them. This reminds us that we are on a journey into another culture, the culture of the DEAF–WORLD, which places a positive value on being Deaf. The shared identity and sense of family in the DEAF–WORLD crosses national borders: many culturally Deaf people feel they have closer ties to other Deaf people halfway around the world than they do to hearing people in their own country.

Visual perception, and the visual language of the DEAF–WORLD, are valued. As the Deaf Rights movement has spread around the world, one of the first activities of newly empowered Deaf societies has been to publish a dictionary of their signed language. Understandably, attempts to repair, supplement or restructure the signed language are viewed with hostility. Deaf linguist Carol Padden affirms that, in American Deaf culture, "hand gestures must convey some kind of visual meaning"; Deaf people resist nonsense use of hands, for example in cued speech, where hand movements near the mouth aim to clarify speech sounds.[46] ASL literature, including history, stories, tall tales, legends, fables, anecdotes, poetry, plays, jokes, naming rituals, sign play, and much more, are highly valued, and the literature of ASL commonly reaffirms the values of the DEAF–WORLD.

Deaf culture is engulfed by the culture of the surrounding hearing society and frequently takes on many majority values. In the U.S., Deaf values concerning religion, work, money, and family, among others, may derive in significant measure from the hearing society.[47]

A repository of cultural knowledge: *Customs*

Culture is a part of a society's adaptation to its physical and social environment. Some customs are rather transparent adaptations, while others seem, on the face of it, more arbitrary. Most customs are some of both. Clothing, for example, is clearly adaptive: cultures in the tropics prescribe light clothing, those in the polar regions, furs. However, dismissing the Indian's sari as mere adaptation would be a mistake; after all, within each climactic zone, clothing takes on different shapes and colors depending on the culture. So it is with customs in the DEAF–WORLD. Some may seem transparently related to the environment, but it would be a mistake to dismiss them for that reason. Here's an example. Partings in American Deaf culture can take a very long time and proceed in stages. First there are the good-byes in the living room at the end of a successful party. The actual departure may take place more than an hour later. Upcoming events and, especially, plans to see each other again, are discussed. Last remarks continue as departing guests retrieve their things, progress out the door, down the steps, and along the street to their car (of course, the signs are getting larger as they get more distant from their hosts). Even after the guests are in their car, they may wind down the window and sign a few last words.

Indeed, they may continue to sign as they drive off. Likewise, Deaf people almost invariably linger in restaurants and at Deaf public events; they will be seen in the lobby, for example, long after the performance has ended. Some writers see in this custom the natural adaptation of a community that was long unable to use the telephone to stay in touch and had to rely on personal contact. Perhaps that is one of the reasons the custom originally arose. Before we accept this hypothesis, however, we would want to see evidence from other Deaf cultures. If it is so, then why isn't the custom dwindling in the U.S., now that Deaf people have TTYs and access to telephone relay services? And how will that hypothesis account for the fact that American Deaf culture disparages abrupt departures and even temporary unexplained departures (for example, slipping away to go to the bathroom)?

Like partings, introductions in American Deaf culture have particular characteristics. Here is the canonical form, from which particular introductions may deviate in practice. When person C introduces people A and B, C typically positions himself at the vertex of a triangle and says to both, "I'll introduce you." C then turns toward A and fingerspells B's first and last names, followed by B's name sign. (More about name signs below.) C tells what school for the Deaf B attended and may add some salient information relevant to the DEAF–WORLD, such as B's Deaf relatives or someone A might know who also attended B's school or lived in the general area of the school. Then C turns toward A and makes the complementary introduction. B is then free to address A directly. They will not use each other's name signs, however; name signs are used for people who are absent.

Another noteworthy custom in American Deaf culture, one that frequently startles hearing people who have begun mingling in the DEAF–WORLD, is the requirement for frank talk. In hearing society, especially in more formal situations, it is considered rude to come directly to the point and state it explicitly. The hearing student dissatisfied with a grade, for example, is more likely to say to the teacher, "Excuse me, I would like to talk with you about my grade," than "You gave me a C. Why?" Hinting and vague talk in an effort to be polite are inappropriate and even offensive in the DEAF–WORLD. The custom of clear communication is often to be seen in ASL literature. Stories are rich in detail, start at the beginning and end at the end, and they speak directly and candidly on their topic. A principle of etiquette in the DEAF–WORLD seems to be "always act in a way that facilitates communication." Hence, blunt speech is not rude, but sudden departures, private conversations, and breaking visual contact are.[48]

As might be expected, members of this culture have quite distinct rules for attention-getting, turn-taking, polite discourse, name-giving, and other behaviors related to language.

Consider name-giving. Names and naming are significant in many cultures and are subject to many rules; think of all the ways custom constrains the choice of a name in the United States. The giving and receiving of a name sign is also an important event in acculturation in the DEAF–WORLD, and the name sign itself frequently reveals much about Deaf culture. In *The Book of Name Signs*, Deaf scholar Sam Supalla explains that there are basically two classes of name signs: those that are purely descriptive (less common), and those that incorporate a handshape from the manual alphabet.[49] Laurent Clerc had a descriptive name sign: two fingers brushing across his cheek, where a scar remained from an accident in infancy. Embodying American Deaf culture's predilection for plain talk, descriptive name signs frequently speak quite bluntly about a person's appearance or behavior. No offense is intended or taken. For example, a somewhat corpulent (sign FAT) Deaf leader has as his name sign a claw handshape placed over an inflated right cheek.

In his own name sign story, Dr. Supalla relates his mother's consternation when she learned that she had a new baby boy, not a girl as expected, and that his father had chosen the name Samuel, inscribing it on the birth certificate. With that name, Sam's name sign would have to contain the handshape from the manual alphabet that corresponded to *S*, and it would have to be located on the chin because all the members of the family had their name signs there, signifying family unity. (In many cultures where names show family relations, family members' names share common features.) The problem was that the handshape and place were already taken by brother Steve—*S* on the chin. If Sam was to have a name sign beginning with *S*, it would have to be placed outside the family location, leaving him ostracized from birth! Brother Ted soon came home for the holidays from the Washington School for the Deaf and learned about the family's quandary. It was he who gave Sam his name sign: an *S* that moves from one side of the chin to the other.

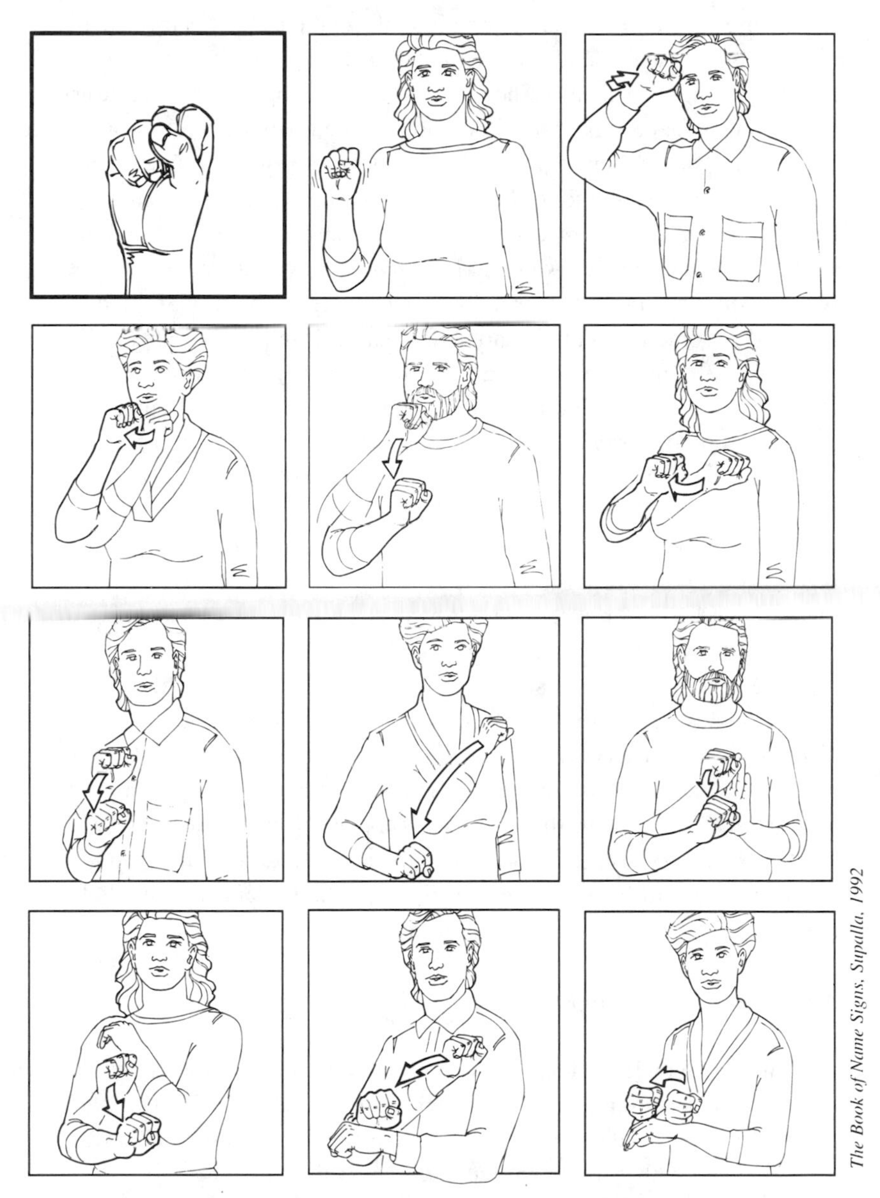

Fig. 3-4. **Some name signs with the closed fist handshape**

Sam Supalla's name sign contains information about Sam and his family, his language and his culture, but it is all encoded. In other words, his name sign is not iconic. The most extreme example of how arbitrary the form of a name sign can be, and how packed with cultural meaning, comes from the Lexington School for the Deaf in New York, where Deaf pupils' name signs used to be their locker numbers. One misguided writer assailed this practice as revealing the depersonalization of Deaf children in the residential schools. Alumni of the school, however, see it differently, and still use their locker-number name signs. A similar practice occurred at some residential schools for the Deaf in France, where children's name signs were their registration numbers. Far from pejorative, such name signs identified them as having attended a residential school, and thus as particularly authentic members of the DEAF–WORLD.[50]

There are many examples in ASL literature of playing with name signs for artful or humorous effect. For example, the ASL sign meaning *to lie* is executed with the *B* handshape (bent thumb, four fingers touching) brushing horizontally across the chin. The name sign for former president Richard Nixon replaced this *B* handshape with an *N* handshape, to represent the first letter of his last name.

The giving of a name sign is a rite of passage. Deaf children from hearing homes frequently arrive at the school for the Deaf without a name sign. As their mastery of ASL and their acculturation proceeds, they receive their name sign. Frequently the honor of conferring a name falls to an authority figure in the DEAF–WORLD, or an older classmate with Deaf parents. Hearing people who learn ASL and mingle in the DEAF–WORLD will be given a name sign as well. Students at schools for the Deaf may secretly assign their teachers derogatory name signs.[51]

A repository of cultural knowledge: Information

Cultural knowledge consists not only of values and customs but also of cultural information. We expect people acculturated in the United States to know who Paul Revere was, where you can buy toothpaste, and how to find a phone number. Different cultures expect their members to possess different information, although the types of information are to some extent cross-cultural. Cultural knowledge specific to the DEAF–WORLD includes such matters as the hours at the Deaf club; the names of important Deaf leaders, including the presidents of the various associations of Deaf people in the state; how to use the telephone relay service; major figures in American Deaf history; and how to manage in various trying situations with hearing people (for example, when your car is stopped by a police officer, do not explain yourself with rapid hand movements).

Sharing information is highly valued in the DEAF–WORLD. Exactly where the universal penchant for gossip ends, and the DEAF–WORLD custom of keeping one another well-informed takes over, may be hard to say, but observers agree that an important social role in the DEAF–WORLD is to pass information along. Secrecy is considered rude and signed conversations are normally quite visible, so necessarily private conversations must be held in private places. When we get together with our Deaf friends, the conversations frequently begin with bringing each other up-to-date on DEAF–WORLD information. A has been hired by the New England Home for the Aged Deaf. B has taken a post at the Austine School. The team from the Boston Deaf Club won the women's softball tournament. They are threatening to close down the Pennsylvania School for the Deaf. And so on. Sharing not only respects the rule of etiquette to facilitate communication, it also promotes unity.

ASL plays so many vital roles in the DEAF–WORLD, as a symbol of identity, medium of interaction, source of values, customs and information, that it is impossible to imagine Deaf culture without it, and it is painful to imagine a Deaf child without it. It is understandable, then, why Deaf people, like the members of other language minorities, are so ferociously attached to their language and have struggled valiantly to preserve it throughout their history. Although the roles that ASL plays in the DEAF–WORLD are much the same as the roles fulfilled by other minority languages in their communities, the form that ASL (and other signed languages) takes is different, since it is a visual and spatial language. That difference in form has wide-reaching consequences for how Deaf people express themselves in conversations and in art forms, and how they perceive, think and remember. These consequences are the subject of the next chapter.

Chapter 4

Form and Function in ASL

THE members of the DEAF–WORLD are more fully visual people than hearing people are, as this chapter and several more will document. Their knowledge of the world—people, places, things, events, language—comes primarily through the visual sense, and theirs is a visual-manual language. Although, as we have seen, signed languages are in many ways like spoken languages—in their acquisition, in their roles as purveyors of identity, values, and information—they are, of course, unlike spoken languages in their form. English and ASL, for example, are quite different: one makes audible words using the small muscles and articulators of the mouth and throat, the other makes visible words moving the larger articulators of the limbs and body around in space. Moreover, they are two different languages, as are, say, French and Navajo, each with its own rules for speaking grammatically.

As many speakers of oral languages are aware, spoken words are made up of a small inventory of vowels and consonants strung out in a row according to rules. If we think of vowels as various movements from one consonant to the next, we find an interesting parallel between the construction of words in spoken and signed languages. Some ASL signs consist only of a movement; others are stationary; but many consist of a series of movements and holds. For example, the sign ME consists of a movement (pointing hand approaches chest) and a hold (hand rests on or near chest). Just as each spoken language has rules for composing syllables from vowels and consonants, signed languages have rules for composing signs from movements (M) and holds (H).[1] In signs, what is moved from one location to another is a handshape with a particular orientation. Fig. 4-1 sketches three ASL signs with the same handshape and movement but different locations: SUMMER, UGLY and DRY.

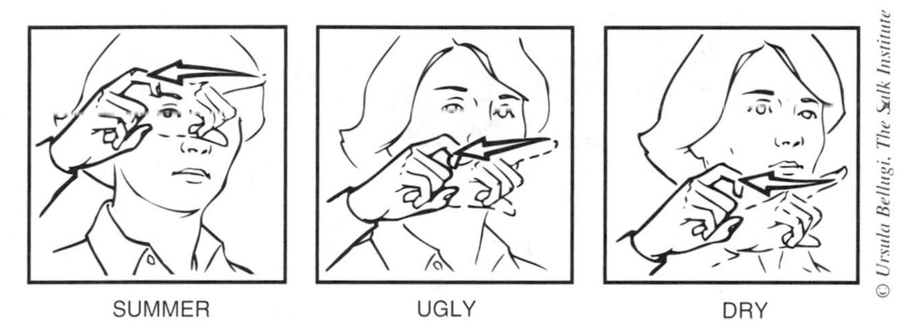

Fig. 4-1. **Three ASL signs contrasting in location**

Using a fully spread hand with the fingers pointing straight ahead, touch your thumb to the side of your forehead twice; that's the ASL sign for FATHER. Repeat the sign but with your thumb touching your breast and you get FINE in ASL. Repeat the sign for FATHER but replace the two taps with an arcing movement away from your forehead; that's GRANDFATHER. Put the spread handshape on both hands facing out in front of your waist, cup your hands a little, and wiggle your wrists; that two-handed sign means TO-CHAT-IN-SIGN. Clap the cupped hands together, and you have signed MARRY.

As with spoken languages, each signed language has its own particular inventory of handshapes, orientations, locations and movements. For example, we can make a clicking sound, sometimes written as *tsk*, but it is not an allowable consonant in English words, although it is one in several other spoken languages, such as Zulu. Similarly, ASL does not have any signs made in the armpit, but Hong Kong Sign Language does—including one meaning WEDNESDAY![2]

Just as there are rules in English that restrict the allowable sequences of vowels and consonants (e.g., if a word begins with three consonant sounds, the first must be *s*), so there are rules that restrict the composition of signs—and apparently for the same reasons: simplicity of execution and of perception. One such rule in ASL requires that if both hands are moving in a sign, then the handshapes, locations, and movements of the two hands must be the same. To illustrate, sign WONDERFUL; open both hands fully and place them, palms facing outward, comfortably close to your shoulders; now advance both hands slightly and return, two times. If the two hands in a sign have different handshapes, then one must be stationary. Furthermore, only six of the score of allowable handshapes in ASL are permitted on that stationary hand. An example is DISCUSS, where an extended index finger strikes an open palm.[3]

There are many more parallels between the production of words in spoken languages and in signed languages. For example, spoken languages frequently adjust the production of a consonant or vowel in a way that makes an easier transition into the following speech sound. Thus, in English, the *k* sound is articulated more back or forward in the mouth depending on whether the following vowel is more back or forward in the mouth (compare *cool* to *keep*). In ASL, one location (or handshape, or movement) in a sign may come to resemble the next one; thus in the contraction of SHOULD NOT, SHOULD is no longer produced in front of the signer at about waist level but anticipates the production of NOT on the chin and is executed high in front of the chin. Compounds in either language are much faster than their separate components, and this speed is achieved by reduction of movement.[4] Consider the compound in ASL comprised of the signs FACE and STRONG, meaning *resemble*. FACE is signed with a circular movement of the index finger in front of the face, ending with a hold (MH where *M* = movement, *H* = hold). STRONG has a held fist, a contraction of the arm, and a second hold (HMH). In the compound, the holds at the end of FACE and at the start of STRONG have been deleted, leaving the circular and contracting movements and the final hold (MMH).

In a classic experiment, psycholinguist Ursula Bellugi and linguist Susan Fischer had hearing children of Deaf parents, who were fluent in both English and ASL, tell the same story in each of the two languages.[5] Since it requires much more time to move the large limbs of the body than the small articulators of the mouth, you might expect that signs would take longer to articulate than words, and that therefore a story would be longer in sign than a corresponding spoken one. You would be only half right; signs do take longer than words, but in Bellugi's and Fischer's experiment, the two versions of the same story generally lasted about the same amount of time. The reasons for this bring us to the heart of the differences between signed languages and spoken ones, and between ASL and English in particular. Here we will describe several reasons for the greater succinctness of ASL, which are all linked to ASL's use of space and vision: its spatial way of expressing verb agreement (assigning roles to people and things in sentences); its use of movement to convey inflections (grammatical information about the timing and distribution of events); its use of classifiers (pronouns) and their incorporation into ASL verbs; and its use of facial expression to convey grammatical information concurrent with signing.

The Succinctness of ASL

Verb agreement

Signed languages exist in space and naturally take advantage of spatial reasoning to convey messages. A great many messages in any language involve someone performing some action that affects or is directed toward someone else. To convey *I show you*, for example, English requires three words. In ASL, *I show you* is one sign moving outward from the signer; *You show me* moves inward toward the signer. Suppose an ASL speaker wants to talk about his quarrelsome cat and dog. He signs DOG and points to the left; then CAT and points to the right. Now he can attribute qualities unambiguously to the dog or the cat by making the signed attributions either to the left or to the right. For example, *The dog bites the cat* can be rendered by a single sign moving from left to right (see Fig. 4-2).

Many ASL verbs, such as those glossed in English as GIVE, NAME, PREACH, SAY-NO-TO, ASK, HATE, and MOCK, are executed with movements that incorporate who is doing the action to whom. Some spoken languages, like English, rely on word order to provide this information about roles in the sentence. Other spoken languages are more like ASL in that they reveal who is doing what to whom by modifying nouns and verbs, frequently with suffixes. Since the role of each sign in the sentence is revealed in the modified sign itself, ASL, like many spoken languages such as Russian, does not have to restrict word order, as English does, in order to indicate roles. The signs CAT, DOG and BITE (or equivalent words in Russian) might be arranged in any order in ASL (or Russian), and there would still be no doubt about which animal was biting which. Word order in such "heavily inflected" languages is available, therefore, to serve other purposes; thus, an ASL speaker might put the topic first and then the comment, as in the sentence with two signs: GIVE-HIM-THE-BOOK, I-DON'T-WANT-TO (*I don't want to give him the book*). However, ASL sentences frequently do have the syntax subject, verb, object.[6]

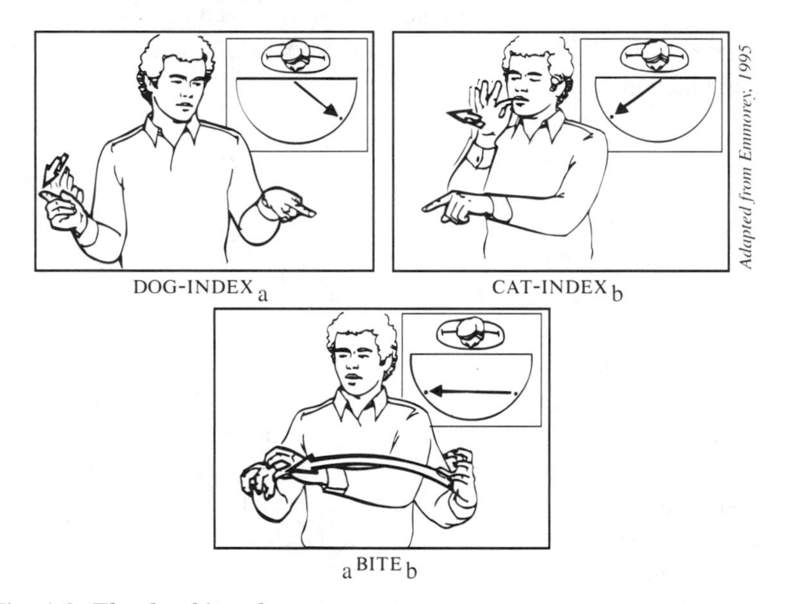

Fig. 4-2. ***The dog bites the cat.***

We have said that when an ASL speaker introduces persons or things into the conversation, the speaker produces the nouns in particular locations in the space in front of him. Then, future pronouns and verbs that relate to the noun may be performed at the noun's location. This kind of spatial verb agreement can be used to convey quite complex relations among people and things, as in this translation from ASL: *John encouraged him to urge her to permit each of them to take the class,* where ENCOURAGE moves from *John* to *him,* URGE from *him* to *her*, and PERMIT from *her* to each of several distinct actors.[7] (A brief caveat before we describe an experiment on the perception of verb agreement in ASL. Not all ASL verbs can have their movements modified to agree with the locations of their subjects and objects. For example, the verb THINK—index finger taps forehead—is illustrative of a class of verbs that are performed on the body and cannot be made to agree. It would be ungrammatical for the speaker to sign THINK at a location in space where the subject of the verb had previously been located. Thus, the subject and object nouns that go with verbs anchored to the body, like THINK, must be repeated each time the verb is uttered or, if they are not, the speaker must abide by a word order in which, as in English, the first noun is usually the subject of the verb.)

An ASL speaker can associate a location with a referent, like *cat*, in several ways: perform the sign CAT at the location; produce the sign CAT elsewhere but point to the location; or gaze in the direction of the location while making the sign CAT. An ASL sentence that involves verb agreement is depicted in Fig. 4-3. Here is the sentence (which we encountered earlier): *I'm a mother, which means a lot of responsibilities; I must take care of the children, feed them, clean them up—there's a whole list!*

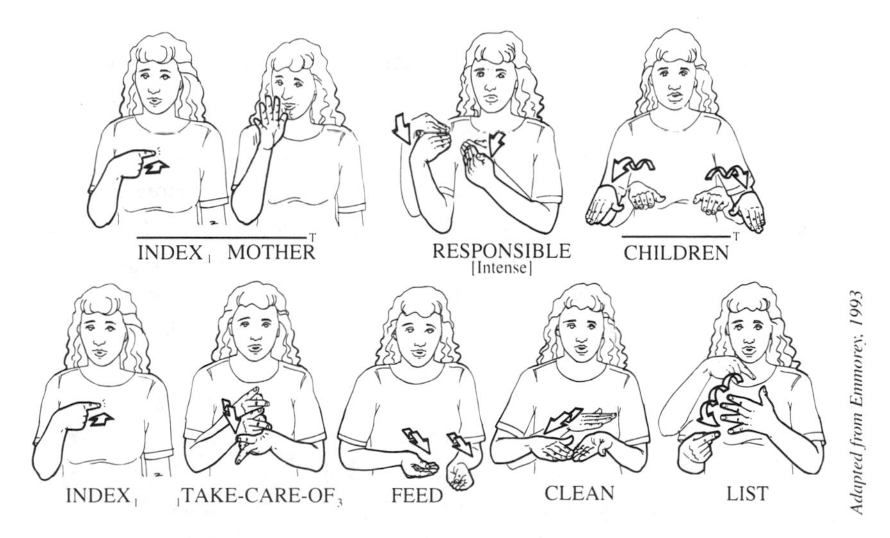

Fig. 4-3. ***I'm a mother, which means a lot of responsibilities; I must take care of children, feed them, clean them up—there's a whole list!***

Note in the diagram that the object of the verb, *children*, has been placed in space out in front of the signer; the subject, the mother, is located at the signer's position, placed there by the first sign in the sentence. The verb TAKE-CARE-OF agrees with the subject and object; that is, it moves (rotates in this case) from the location assigned to the mother (the speaker's location) to the location assigned to the children (out in front of the speaker). If, on the contrary, the children took care of the mother, the speaker would have signed the verb with opposite rotational movement, from the location assigned to the children to the location assigned to the mother, as in Fig. 4-4.

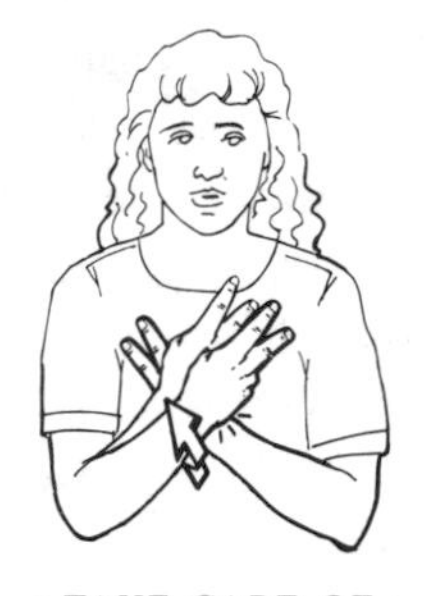

$_3$TAKE-CARE-OF$_1$

Fig. 4-4. **The sign TAKE-CARE-OF moving from the children's location to the mother/signer's location**

The grammar of ASL requires that many verbs move from the subject location to the object location. Psycholinguist Karen Emmorey and colleagues at the Laboratory for Cognitive Neuroscience of the Salk Institute for Biological Studies performed a series of experiments to examine how ASL speakers process the sentences of their language. In one experiment,[8] the verb with incorrect agreement was substituted in the videotaped sentence; so the incorrect sentence read, in part: *I'm a mother, which means a lot of responsibilities; the children take care of me, feed them . . .* ASL speakers were asked to watch the sentence on a TV monitor and push a button as soon as they detected the word FEED. You might reason that the substituted verb agreement, THEY-TAKE-CARE-OF-ME, which is incongruent with the meaning of the preceding clause (the mother has a lot of responsibilities), would surprise the addressees and delay their responding to FEED. Or, on the other hand, you might predict that addressees would not be particularly concerned with verb agreement, especially in sentences like this one, where the meaning of the preceding clause (*I'm a mother . . .*) makes it clear who is the subject and who the object of the sentence (so it is not necessary to rely on the verb agreement to determine that). If the ASL addressees were not paying attention to verb agreement, their reaction times to FEED would be about the same for the version of the ASL sentence with correct verb agreement and for the version with incorrect agreement.

Native ASL speakers (born Deaf to Deaf parents) were tested with one or the other version of twelve sentences like the one in Fig. 4-3. They were told that some sentences might contain mistakes, but they were not tipped off to the purpose of the experiment and no subject saw both versions of the same sentence. On the average, the subjects responded in a little under half a second to the test word (FEED in Fig. 4-3) when the preceding verb had correct agreement (i.e., mother takes care of children); when it had incorrect agreement (children take care of mother), subjects took a reliable ten percent longer. Since the time it took the subjects in this experiment to identify the following word FEED depended on whether the preceding verb had correct agreement, we must conclude that the native speakers of ASL in the experiment were indeed processing verb agreement, even when it was not imperative to do so in order to understand the sentence.

This experiment was replicated with two additional groups (and a larger set of sentences): a group of late ASL learners, who were first exposed to ASL at age fourteen on the average and who had been using ASL for at least ten years, and a group of early but not native ASL users, first exposed at age four, with at least fourteen years' experience. All subjects had become Deaf before learning English, and ASL was their preferred means of communication. The results showed that the presence of an error in verb agreement slowed response times only in the group of native speakers of ASL. Early and late learners of ASL were *not* delayed in recognizing the test word when it was preceded by incorrect verb agreement. It appears that only the native ASL speakers were fully using the grammar of ASL in sentence processing.

Inflections

Where English adds words to a sentence to convey information about the timing and distribution of events, ASL more succinctly changes the movement of the verb in the sentence. Thus, the sign glossed SICK is a single sign, but so is SICK-FOR-A-LONG-TIME-OVER-AND-OVER-AGAIN (long bouts of illness). Classes of verbs in ASL, of which GIVE is an example (Fig. 4-5), can have their movements modified to convey information about timing, such as *repeatedly* and *over a long time*, and to convey information about distribution, such as *to several of them, to each of them, to all of them.*[9]

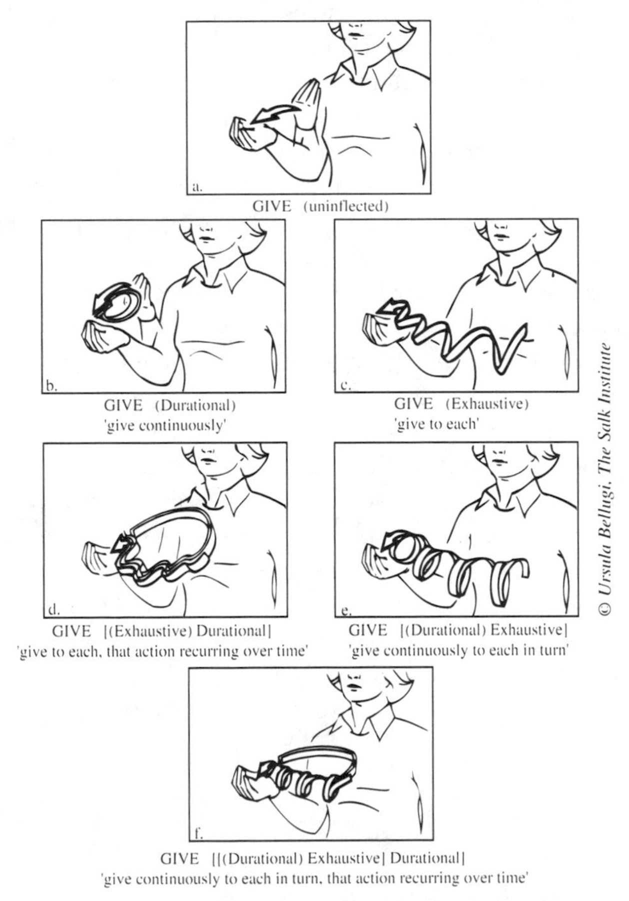

Fig. 4-5. **GIVE shown uninflected and with five inflections**

Movements may be combined to yield, for example, *give to all of them over a long time*—all in a single sign. Movement can also convey grammatical categories; where English would add a suffix to the word indicating that it is a noun or verb, ASL uses tense or relaxed movement and repetition.[10] Thus, SIT is produced by extending the first two fingers on the dominant hand and applying them to the corresponding extended fingers on the other hand. CHAIR, derived from SIT, is produced in the same way but with a double tap.

ASL is not at all unique in having rules to convey roles in the sentence, timing and distribution, and grammatical category; many spoken languages have them. For example, English inflects verbs for tense, modifying their endings. What is unique about ASL is the form of these inflections: they frequently involve changes in the way the verb moves through space, rather than suffixes or prefixes that extend the basic verb. ASL does have some suffixes, however. One type is added to the verb to create a noun meaning *the person who performs that act*. This suffix (two facing hands moving downward in front of the signer) when added to TEACH, for example, yields TEACHER. Suffixes occur in ASL comparatives and superlatives as well.

Linguists have long known that in some languages, a word always appears in the same form whereas, at the opposite extreme, there are languages in which a basic verb may have so many regular inflections attached to it that it conveys as much meaning as an entire sentence. Clearly, ASL has a grammar more like the heavily inflected spoken languages. But it is unlike them in that its inflections are conveyed at the same time as the basic verb, not added on to it. Just as we have evidence, from experiments with verb agreement, that speakers of ASL keep a mental map of the locations of persons, places and things, detect the direction of verb movement toward those locations, and thus arrive at the meaning of the sentence, so, too, we have evidence from experiments with verb inflection that speakers of ASL strip off the timing information in the movement of the verb, identify the meaning of that movement as well as the underlying verb, and integrate that information into an understanding of the sentence.

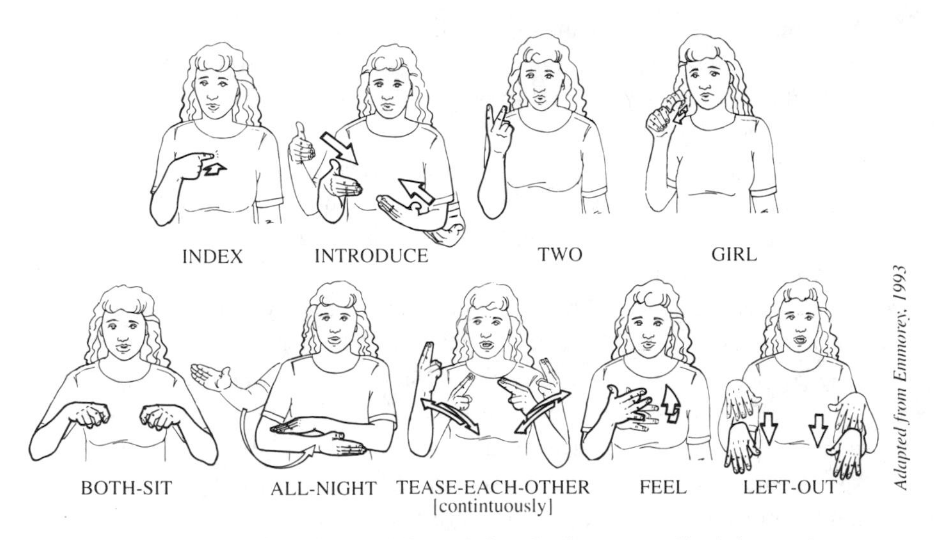

Fig. 4-6. ***I introduced two girls and they both sat up all night teasing each other; I felt left out.***

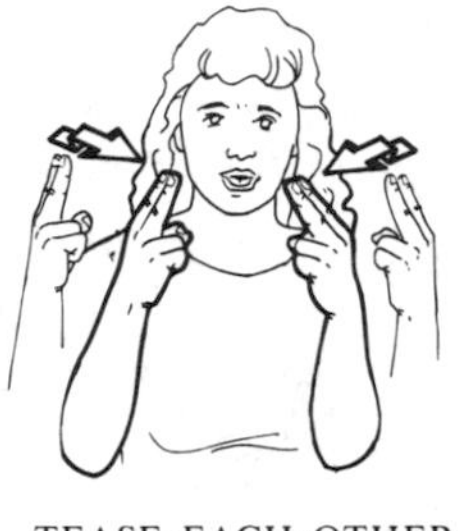

TEASE-EACH-OTHER
(punctual)
ONE-TIME

Fig. 4-7. **The sign TEASE with the inflections [reciprocal] and [punctual] meaning *tease each other once***

Fig. 4-6 depicts an illustrative sentence *(I introduced two girls and they both sat up all night teasing each other; I felt left out)*. Fig. 4-7 shows the verb with incorrect timing information that was produced in the same sentence for testing. Although the first part of the sentence states that the two girls stayed up all night, the erroneous verb movement in Fig. 4-7 states that they teased each other punctually *(teased)*, not continuously *(teasing)*. All three groups of subjects—native, early, and late learners of

ASL—proved sensitive to this kind of error; that is, they took longer on the average to identify the following test word (I-FELT) when it was preceded by the error, than when it was preceded by a verb with the correct timing information. Why are non-native speakers troubled less by errors in the spatial agreement of verbs than by errors in the timing of verbs? Perhaps in the rapid flow of communication they determine the subjects and objects of verbs more from the meanings of the words than from the verb movements between their locations. Focusing on the meanings of individual words, they would tend to overlook the spatial error but notice the error of timing information.

Notice, by the way, how ASL conveys time of occurrence in the sentence diagramed in Fig. 4-6: there is an adverb of time, ALL-NIGHT. Another means of establishing time in ASL is to set up the time at the beginning of the discourse by signing, for example, LAST-YEAR; after this, all events are assumed to have occurred last year until the speaker signals otherwise. Verbs are not inflected for tense as they are in English. Instead, tense is a grammatical category that contains several words of time, like WILL, FINISH (which refers to the completion of an event), and its opposite, NOT-YET. These words specify the tense of the verb, much as they do in English.

To summarize these results: Native speakers of ASL, when processing sentences addressed to them, are sensitive to violations of ASL grammar in both verb agreement and in verb inflections for timing. Non-native speakers are sensitive only to the second of these two types of grammatical error.

Classifiers

ASL has a rich system of pronouns.[11] These are a special kind of pronoun that occur in some spoken languages and that include in their meaning more than English pronouns do; as previously noted, they are called *classifiers.* The correct pronoun to use in English depends on the category or class of the noun to which it refers: if the noun is inanimate, we generally say *it*; if it is animate, our choice of pronoun depends on whether it refers to a female or a male, to one or more than one, and to the subject or the object of the verb. Pronouns in ASL are not concerned with noun classifications such as animacy and gender. Instead, many are concerned with shape and size. So the correct ASL classifier is different if you are referring to, say, a table or a glass (both of which would be referred to by *it* in English). Looking at such ASL classifier handshapes, you know immediately the class of objects, whether large with a flat surface or cylindrical, to which the pronoun refers.

There is a second set of classifiers in ASL that stand in for nouns that have related meanings rather than related shapes. For example, there's one classifier for cars, another one for airplanes, and another for ambulatory persons. Classifiers move from one location to another, and in varying manners. For example, in the ASL translation of *Several boxes of cereal were on the shelf; I took one down,* the ASL verb TAKE-DOWN would be performed with the box classifier handshape. But if one of several balls was taken down from the shelf, the verb would be performed with the small round object classifier (a cupped hand).

Emmorey and colleagues also examined the sensitivity of native, early, and late learners of ASL to errors in verbs that involve classifiers.[12] In videotaped sentences like the one about cereals, they substituted TAKE-DOWN performed with the small-round-object classifier. In other sentences, like *My plane was late; I saw it land,* they substituted the wrong classifier, as in CAR-LAND. Once again, they measured the subjects' delays in recognizing a test word. As it turned out, both native and early learners of ASL were sensitive to both kinds of errors, but again late learners were not. In a further finding, errors in one type of classifier—those that classify based on size and shape—proved harder to detect for all groups of subjects. This is one example where ASL speakers do not appear to process whatever pictorial characteristics signs may have. We will describe more examples in a later section.

Earlier we stated that studies of ASL processing show that late learners are at a noticeable disadvantage. We have now seen that they do not have native mastery of verb agreement and fail to detect errors in the use of ASL classifiers.[13] They also take longer to identify signs;[14] make more errors when repeating ASL sentences or recalling them;[15] and they fail to recognize and perform some required inflections of verb movement.[16] We will explore the implications of these facts for educators and for the hearing parents of Deaf children in part 2.

Facial grammar

We have seen that incorporating right into the sign who is doing what to whom, and in what ways, is a great time-saver. Because signed languages are visual languages, and with vision you can follow many simultaneous streams of information, it is possible for them to have all these different kinds of information displayed simultaneously. Glimpse a novel landscape for half a second, and you could spend a half-hour telling all that you saw, so great is your ability to process all the information that was presented to your eyes almost simultaneously. But listen to an unfamiliar symphony for half a second and you will probably have much less to say, so limited is your capacity to process all the different sounds presented to your ear simultaneously. Signed languages exploit the great capacity of vision for processing concurrent "layers" of information. Thus, there are several more streams of information that occur at the same time as the manual signs in ASL and these come from the face and the body. Facial, eye and head signals in ASL provide information about how the sentence is organized.[17]

As an example of the role of the face in transmitting syntax in ASL, consider sentences with a conditional clause, such as *If it snows today, the trip will be canceled.* The grammatically correct counterpart in ASL requires the speaker to raise his eyebrows and tilt his head and body at the same time as he executes the two signs in the first clause: TODAY SNOW. Then, at the juncture between the conditional clause and the main clause, the speaker pauses, nods his head, lowers his brows, blinks his eyes, and shifts his head and body back to the starting, neutral position. Finally, he signs TRIP CANCEL. If the speaker leaves out those nonmanual signals on the face and body, the ASL sentence not only looks odd, but also the person addressed understands something quite different: *It's snowing today; the trip is canceled.* Eye-blinks not only signal conditional clauses, they commonly occur after most clauses and sentences. Just as a speaker reading a text aloud will postpone taking a breath until arriving at the end of a clause (and with that breath pause, signal the end of a thought), so a signer will likewise postpone normal eye-blinks until the end of a clause.[18]

Nonmanual signals are also important in the various kinds of questions and commands, in negative and declarative sentences, and in signaling the topic of a sentence. Wh-questions (Who, What, Where, etc.) are accompanied by a lowering of the eyebrows and a frown; Yes/No questions are expressed with a raising of the brows. ASL, much more than English, uses rhetorical questions *(Pat works at Gallaudet but lives where? Miles away!)*. They are accompanied by a brow raise and a tilting of the head. Negation is marked by shaking the head and furrowing the brow while executing the manual sign; hence the sign NOT is often not present. As mentioned earlier, ASL (like several spoken languages) characteristically introduces a topic at the beginning of a sentence and then makes a comment about it *(That movie, we went to it but we didn't enjoy it)*. Topics are marked by characteristic facial expressions: Brows are raised during the topic, the head is tilted, and the speaker makes eye-contact with the person spoken to; then, after a pause, the facial expression is changed for the comment.

Facial information occurring at the same time as the signs can also convey adverbs. Consider two facial shapes that accompany signs in ASL: the first was named by linguists *mm*, because the lips are positioned as in humming; it means everything is normal and proper (devices work as they should, people are relaxed and comfortable). The second is called *th*, because the tongue is placed between the teeth as in *thin*; it means carelessly, inattentively. Now consider the two-sign sentence MAN FISH [continuous]. (The brackets indicate that the verb FISH has been inflected for continuous action.) If the verb is accompanied by the facial configuration *mm*, the sentence means: *The man is fishing contentedly*; if accompanied by *th*, it means: *The man is fishing obliviously.*[19] Finally, facial expressions are parts of particular signs, like NOT-YET (which requires a protruding tongue) and RECENT (raised shoulder and protruded lip). And of course, as in spoken languages, the face can add emotional coloring to the message, conveying feelings like surprise, disgust, joy and so on.

Eye-gaze has several roles in the grammar of ASL.[20] Some signs require an eye-gaze that is related to a manual portion of the sign. For example, when signing LOOK-AT (a *V* handshape, palm down), the fingers move and point to the location assigned to the object of the verb, and the speaker gazes in the same direction. Eye-gaze may also modify the meaning of a sign performed at the same time; thus *tree*, signed with eye-gaze skyward, means *tall tree*. Eye blinks (opening and closing the eyes), can also be meaningful. For example, the degree of opening of the eyelids can convey a sense of proximity or remoteness in association with a sign. Eye closure concurrent with signing can also mark emphasis.

At the sentence level, eye-gaze is used something like a pronoun to refer to a previously mentioned person, place or thing. The most common way of referring to a noun that has already been mentioned is by pointing the index finger (or thumb) at the place in space that was associated with that noun, but eye-gaze can stand in for the pointing finger. Eye-gaze may also function to mark the subject of a clause as the most prominent: the speaker shifts body position—including head, shoulders and eye-gaze—toward the position where the subject of the verb was produced.[21]

Eye-gaze is also used to signal a change in the speaker's role. In written English, we use quotation marks to indicate that a character in the narration is now speaking, and not the person narrating the story. In spoken English, voice inflection may be used to signal role shift. In ASL, the speaker may shift position toward the location in space to which the character was previously assigned and gaze away from the addressee to *assume* the role of the character, saying what the character should say, and reenacting what the character does. The speaker now uses the first person, and the audience understands that it is the character who is speaking and not the narrator.[22] Thus the story is not merely related, it is partly enacted in front of the audience. Shifting eye-gaze allows the storyteller to move rapidly between the narrator's perspective and direct depiction of events through the eyes of a character.

One literary effect achievable with eye-gaze creates a kind of rhythm of the sort used in ASL poetry; it also helps to maintain the attention of the audience. It involves rhythmically shifting eye-gaze among the audience, the position of a character in the story, and the narrator's hands.[23]

Eye gaze plays a critical role in taking turns to speak. When Henry is speaking ASL to Laurel, for example, he looks at her from time to time, especially at natural breaks in what he is saying. If Laurel wants to initiate a turn, she will wait until Henry gazes at her and then start signing. If Henry is not ready to relinquish his turn, he will avoid looking at Laurel, depriving her of a chance to interrupt.[24]

MEMORY FOR SIGNED LANGUAGE

Iconicity and short-term memory

We noted earlier that most people overestimate how iconic signed languages are. At the same time, they tend to overlook evidence of correspondence between form and meaning in spoken languages. One example of such iconicity in spoken languages is onomatopoeia, in which the sound of the word resembles the sounds made by the referent, as in *bow-wow* and *tintinnabulation.* But there are several other ways in which the relation of form to meaning is not arbitrary in spoken languages. One concerns the relation between the ordering of clauses in sentences and the ordering of events to which those clauses refer. Thus, in English it is easier to process *He spoke before he left* than *Before he left he spoke.*[25] In the former sentence, the ordering of the clauses corresponds to the ordering of the events described. Nevertheless, spoken languages don't have very many ways, really, of using sound to reflect the visual-spatial world around us, with its arrays of people and things and their movements from one place to another. That is to say, at least they don't have as many ways as languages that are visual-spatial themselves. The greater resources of a visual-spatial language for describing what is a visual-spatial world probably explain why newcomers to signed languages assume that signs must depict what they refer to. After all, why would signed languages pass up such a great opportunity!

How transparent are the meanings of signs? Not very, according to two studies with hearing non-signers. Ninety signs were presented to one group and, for most of the signs, not even one viewer guessed their meanings correctly, although there were a few exceptions (BED, BUTTON, EAR, and EYES, for example).[26] Next, the right and wrong guesses were presented in the form of a multiple-choice test to another group of hearing non-signers who viewed the signs. Constrained to pick the right answer from among one right and four false alternatives, the group performed at chance levels, answering correctly only about twenty percent of the time. However, in a third study, nonsigners were given the same set of signs *and* their English translations and asked what the relation was between sign and meaning. For example, they were shown ASL GIRL (closed fist, extended thumb brushes the cheek twice) and told the meaning. Many viewers independently said the connection between form and meaning in this case was "the soft cheek of a girl." Thus, we should conclude that many ASL signs incorporate elements that are representational to some extent. You might say, the meaning of a sign is not often transparent, but it may be translucent.

There is another kind of iconicity in signed languages that deserves our attention. All languages, both spoken and signed, make extensive use of words about space to talk metaphorically about things that are not inherently spatial. There are countless examples in English, such as *high-level discussions, forward-thinking people, deep depression* and so on. Now, signed languages can express those spatial metaphors directly in their spatial properties. For example, positively valued things and states tend to be signed with upward movements in ASL HAPPY, THRILLED, EXCITED, CHEERFUL, LAUGH), and negatively valued things with downward ones (SAD, CRY, DEPRESSED, CHEAP, LOUSY). Temporal concepts in English commonly rendered in spatial terms (the past is behind us and the future ahead), are implemented using physical space in ASL: events in the distant future often are signed well in front of the signer; the near future, closer to the body; and the past behind (leaning back, or slightly behind the shoulder).[27]

Although in analyzing signs we can see these spatial components that express their literal or metaphorical meanings, it is an important question whether such iconicity actually makes a difference to ASL speakers. Native speakers of ASL asked to remember lists of rather iconic signs like TICKET and TREE were no better and no worse at it than when asked to remember lists of non-iconic signs, like MOTHER and COLOR. What did make a difference was not the iconicity of the signs in the list but rather the similarity of the signs to one another. When a list is made up of signs that have the same handshapes, as in FINE and FATHER, or the same movements or locations, the signs prove easily confused in memory.[28] Something comparable is true of spoken languages: English speakers asked to remember lists of words composed of similar vowels and consonants have more trouble recalling them than heterogeneous lists.[29]

Why should this be true? The obvious inference is that one step in processing a spoken or signed message involves elements that are smaller than a word—that are, in fact, the vowels and consonants, or handshapes, locations, orientations and movements that make up the words. This inference is supported by the errors people make recalling such lists shortly after learning them. They tend to recall words that were not, in fact, on the list they just learned, but were on an earlier list or on no list at all; but the mistaken word often resembles the right word. An English speaker might misrecall *tea* as *key* for example, or an ASL speaker PAPER for MOVIE. It is as if, having seen PAPER, the ASL speaker represented it mentally (but not consciously) as a set of components (flat open-palm hands facing each other, location in front of chest, up-and-down movement, etc.); then, in a later part of the experiment, told to remember MOVIE, the speaker stored that, too, in its components (flat open-palm hands, location in front of chest, to-and-fro movement). Finally, during storage or recall, the movement of PAPER was substituted as the representation of MOVIE.

When lists were presented to ASL speakers for recall that contained either signs similar in meaning or, as in the prior experiment, similarly constructed, the latter proved more difficult, confirming again that storage in short-term memory is in terms of the elements that make up the sign rather than in terms of its meaning.[30]

These findings led psycholinguists to wonder whether, when it comes to more complex signs, the simultaneous layers that convey information like manner, number and time, described earlier, are also separated out in memory. When ASL speakers were presented lists of inflected verbs to memorize, such as BLAME-REPEATEDLY and PREACH-FOR-A-LONG-TIME, they frequently remembered the verbs in the right order but confused the inflections (recalling BLAME-FOR-A-LONG-TIME and then PREACH-REPEATEDLY), or they remembered the inflections in the right order but confused the verbs (recalling PREACH-REPEATEDLY and BLAME-FOR-A-LONG-TIME). Another example: Given a list including TAKE-ADVANTAGE-OF-THEM (which has a movement indicating *several*) and PAY-ME (which has a movement directed toward the signer), recall errors included TAKE-ADVANTAGE-OF-ME and PAY-THEM.[31] When short sentences in ASL rather than lists of signs were to be remembered, many errors in recall shared components with the word originally presented, as in the preceding experiment, but many other errors of recall were related to the original word not by form, but by meaning. In an example of a recall error based on meaning, one subject misremembered *I looked everywhere for my younger brother,* as *I looked everywhere for my older brother.* The earlier in life the subjects learned ASL, the greater the proportion of their errors that were based on meaning.[32] We infer that the late-learners of ASL stored the original sentences according to their form and, when tested shortly thereafter, made errors in recalling that form. On the other hand, the early learners of ASL stored the original sentences according to their form but more rapidly determined the meaning of the sentences, then discarded their forms. When tested for recall, these early learners no longer had the forms of the sentences available in memory but they did have their meanings, and these were the basis of their errors in recall. This result leads us to conclude that the earlier in life you learn a language, the more you are able to move rapidly from the stored form of the message to its meaning. We will return to this topic after considering briefly the performance of Deaf subjects when remembering in their second language, English.

Deaf people and memory for English

To this point we have seen that ASL and English speakers have in common that, when asked to learn and later recall lists of words in their primary language, they store those words initially in memory in terms of the elements from which they are constructed. Consider the implications of this finding first for the native English speaker who is learning ASL. The hearing student of ASL must come to see, not necessarily consciously, the components of signs—handshape, location, orientation and movement—before that student can use the strategy ASL speakers use to retain signs. Until that time, the ASL-learner is presumably stuck with only two possibilities when remembering a series of signs: remembering the signs as unanalyzed wholes, which is rather like remembering a set of pictures (no easy task), or remembering the English translation of each sign, committing the English words to memory in the regular way, and translating back from English to ASL when asked to recall.

Now consider the implications for the Deaf ASL speaker who is learning a list of English words. The Deaf student must come to know the components of words before that student can use the strategy English speakers use to retain words. But here's a problem: Most Deaf students can't hear and don't know what the consonants and vowels are in English words. So it seems that they have to remember the written words visually, or use the translation strategy. In fact, there's evidence that they do all three: remember the words by their printed shapes, by translating them into ASL, and by their sequences of vowels and consonants in English.

Evidence suggesting that some Deaf people are influenced by the written letter-shapes of English words comes from a study that presented two kinds of possible but nonoccurring English words. One kind was constructed using letters common to each successive position in a normal English word; for example, the test word might begin with *r*, since that is a common initial letter in English; in second position, *e* is quite common. Following this pattern yielded the nonoccurring English word *remond*. In the other kind of test word, letters were chosen that were uncommon in each successive slot, yielding, for example, *endrom*. Deaf subjects were presented with a test word, then a letter, and asked if the letter had occurred in the test word. The subjects were better at the task if the test word contained letters that commonly occurred in their respective positions than if it did not.[33] Moreover, on a spelling test, good Deaf readers, like hearing ones, did better with words that contained suffixes than with comparable words that did not (*picnickers* vs. *torpedo*).[34]

Deaf children learning to write and fingerspell words also give evidence of recalling written words influenced by the sequence of written letters. Recall that fingerspelling represents English words by assigning to each of the letters in the alphabet a distinct handshape. (We represent fingerspelled words here with capital letters and hyphens.) Deaf six-year-olds make writing and fingerspelling mistakes that are generally close to the target. The misspellings, while resembling the original, are not random permutations of the letters. Instead, letter sequences predominate in the errors that predominate in English. Thus, *girl* is frequently misspelled G-R-I-L, possibly because *gri* is a more common sequence in English than *gir*.[35]

Evidence that Deaf people remember English words by translating into ASL comes from a study in which they were given two kinds of English word lists to remember: one set had translations in ASL that were similar (like PAPER and MOVIE), the other did not. Of course, nothing was said about that to the ASL speakers. Nonetheless, they found the set of English words with similarly constructed signs in ASL much harder to recall.[36] This suggests that the ASL speakers were using their knowledge of ASL to store the English words.

Finally, evidence that some Deaf people remember English words using their vowels and consonants comes from a study of Deaf college students, ASL speakers who were good readers. When those students were given lists of visually dissimilar printed words to recall, the lists that rhymed proved the most difficult; lists of nonrhyming, visually similar words, and lists of words whose sign translations are visually similar, proved easier to recall. Thus, these relatively skilled readers, who knew ASL, appeared to use knowledge of the vowels and consonants of English and their allowable sequences in reading and remembering the lists of words.[37] Deaf college students asked to think of words that rhyme with a given word can frequently do it; interestingly, words that they claim rhyme look alike in lipreading. They also know how to pronounce invented words like *flaim.*[38] On a spelling test, good Deaf readers, like hearing ones, do best with words that are written the way they sound.[39]

In sum, it is possible for Deaf people to use knowledge of word formation in reading, and such use is characteristic of good readers. What is relevant is not how well the Deaf person can speak but rather how well he or she has mastered the elements and regularities of English words. If, on the contrary, speech were what mattered, good Deaf readers would be good English speakers. In fact, a study conducted with one hundred teenagers with profound hearing loss who had received an oral education found no correlation between their speech intelligibility or speech perception and their reading achievement.[40]

That we have evidence for Deaf people using the visual shapes of English words and their translations into signs in order to remember them is not surprising; what may be surprising is their use of some representation connected with how the words sound. There are many ways in principle in which the profoundly Deaf child could learn about the elements of spoken English words and their regularities: from articulation, to the extent that the child has such skills; from lip-reading; from fingerspelling; from a distillation of experience with the writing system, that is, by learning the regularities in the sequences of letters.[41] When Deaf children and adults are asked to write something down, they frequently fingerspell the word to themselves, producing a hand configuration for the letter before beginning to write it.[42] All in all, it appears that the best Deaf readers use some such strategy to represent English words; readers with intermediate levels of skill call on their knowledge of signs; and the poorest readers are unable to use any of these strategies.

Semantics and long-term memory

Psycholinguists have long known that words are stored in memory in terms of their components only for a limited time; after that time, the forms of the words are no longer available to recall, but their meanings are. Long after someone has told us some information, we forget their exact words but remember the gist. So it is with ASL. In one experiment, ASL sentences were presented to native ASL speakers twice: once for learning, and again to see if they could recognize that they had seen them before. Between the original and the second presentation, some of the sentences were altered either in form only or also in meaning. To change the form but not the meaning, some signs were replaced with synonyms, or the order of the signs was changed in sentences whose meaning did not rely on word order. To change the meaning, an inflection was moved from one sign to another, or sign order was changed in such a way that the meaning of the sentence changed. The subject had to say whether each of the test sentences was exactly the same as one seen previously or whether, on the contrary, it was novel. So that there was no advantage to guessing, half the sentences were reproduced exactly, while the other half, in random order, were changed. When the Deaf subjects were tested for recall immediately after the learning presentation, they spotted as novel equally often sentences that had undergone changes in form and those that had undergone changes in meaning. But when the subjects were tested after a delay of just forty-five seconds, they detected the novel sentences that had undergone a change in meaning more accurately than those that had undergone a change in form.[43]

Findings like these have led psycholinguists to conclude that words or signs are first stored in short-term memory in terms of their components, but then speakers retrieve the meanings of those words from their knowledge of vocabulary and syntax and transfer that semantic information into long-term memory, where it can be structured into their knowledge of the world and the gist can be retained indefinitely. There is evidence that this shift from form to meaning, from short-term memory to long-term memory, occurs at sentence boundaries, at natural breaking points in sentences where, for example, one might pause when speaking slowly.[44]

Signed Language and the Brain

Below are excerpts of interviews with two English-speaking patients. What do you notice about the disturbed language of patients "Brian" and "Warren" and how are they different?

Examiner: Tell me, what did you do before you retired?
Brian: Uh, uh, uh, puh, par partender, no.
E: Carpenter?
B: (Nodding, yes). Carpenter, tuh, tuh, tenty year.
E: Tell me about this picture.
B: Boy . . . cook . . . cookie . . . took . . . cookie.

◆ ◆ ◆

Examiner: Do you like it here in Kansas City?
Warren: Yes, I am.
E: I'd like to have you tell me something about your problem.
W: Yes, I ugh can't hill all of my way. I can't talk all of the things I do, and part of the part I can go all right, but I can't tell from the other people. I usually most of my things. I know what can I talk and I know what they are, but I can't always come back, even though I know they should be in, and I know should something eely I should know what I am doing.

You may have noted that Brian understood the examiner's questions well, but had trouble finding words. Moreover, his speech reads like a telegram: all the words and endings that reflect grammar are omitted. Finally, he makes some errors in the components of words; for example, when he said *partender* for *carpenter*, he substituted the sounds *p* for *k* at the start of the first syllable, *t* for *p* at the start of the second syllable, and *d* for *t* at the start of the third syllable.

Warren is quite different. He doesn't seem to understand the examiner's questions, but he has fluent answers—answers, however, that make no sense.

Using the x-rays of the brain called CAT scans allows neurologists to determine which areas have been damaged. Both Brian and Warren suffered damage to the left hemisphere of the brain, but to slightly different areas. Language difficulties traceable to brain damage are called *aphasias*. Brian, with *expressive aphasia*, has damage to a part of the brain named Broca's area, in honor of the French doctor in the last century whose post-mortem examination of his patients' brains led him to conclude that this area must be responsible for expressing language. Warren, who has problems with language reception, a *receptive aphasia,* has damage to the section of the left hemisphere called Wernicke's area, named after the doctor who recognized that the sort of problem Warren has is fundamentally different from Brian's and is the result of damage to the part of the brain where incoming messages are understood.

How does this relate to signed language? To understand why psycholinguists are particularly interested in learning about the hemispheric specialization of the brain in ASL speakers, you need to know one more important fact: whereas the left hemisphere is specialized for language processing (in right-handed people), the right hemisphere is specialized for visual and spatial processing. Patients with right-hemisphere lesions (tissue damage) have trouble drawing and responding to spatial tasks. Since ASL certainly involves visual-spatial processing, and yet is a language, only the brave were ready to predict beforehand which way the coin would fall. Psycholinguists Howard Poizner and Ursula Bellugi and linguist Edward Klima searched systematically for native ASL speakers who had suffered brain damage, usually as a result of a stroke. Here is an excerpt from an interview with one of their patients, who had damage to her left hemisphere.

Examiner: What else happened?

Gail: CAR . . . DRIVE . . . BROTHER . . . DRIVE . . . I . . . S-T-A-D . . . [Attempts to gesture *stand up.*]

E: You stood up?

G: YES . . . I . . . DRIVE . . . [Attempts to gesture *goodbye*.]

E: Wave goodbye?

G: YES . . . BROTHER . . . DRIVE . . . DUNNO . . .
[Attempts to wave *goodbye*.]

E: Your brother was driving?

G: YES . . . BACK . . . DRIVE . . . BROTHER . . . MAN . . .
MAMA . . . STAY . . . BROTHER . . . DRIVE.

E: Were you in the car?

G: YES.

E: Or outside?

G: NO.

E: In the car.

G: YES.

E: You were standing up with your mother?

G: NO . . . BROTHER . . . DRIVE . . . [Points in back]
DEAF BROTHER . . . I . . .

E: Your brother didn't know you were in the car?

G: YES.

E: Your brother was driving and saw you in the back seat?

G: YES, YES. [Laughs.]

E: Oh, I see.

The resemblances between Gail's language disturbances in ASL and Brian's in English are striking. Gail, like Brian, has ungrammatical language, consisting mostly of single words; her ASL lacks all the inflections and other kinds of grammatical layering in ASL that we have been examining; classifiers are also absent, as pronouns were absent from Brian's speech. It seems very much as if Gail has Broca's aphasia and, indeed, various neurological tests confirmed that she had suffered damage to Broca's area of the left hemisphere. Two other ASL speakers with left hemisphere damage also showed language disturbances that were traceable to the particular locations of their lesions.

Many scientists would be very pleased to stop there, having provided strong evidence that the left hemisphere in our species is specialized not for spoken language but for language in general, and that the same brain areas that serve language production and comprehension in spoken-language users serve those functions in signers. But not Poizner, Bellugi and Klima. They went on to find three ASL speakers who had suffered right hemisphere damage. And indeed, those Deaf patients, like comparable hearing ones, could not manage spatial tasks such as drawing at all, just as expected. But they could do one very special spatial task—signing and understanding ASL! For example, the investigators asked one Deaf patient with right hemisphere damage to describe in ASL her living room and the placement of furniture. She was very bad at it. The items of furniture were stacked one on top of the other in her ASL description and the left-hand side of the space was entirely empty. However, when the same patient was speaking in ASL on ordinary nonspatial matters, she placed her nouns out in space in front of her and made her verb movements agree with their locations as required by ASL grammar. So her right-hemisphere lesion did not affect her use of space for syntax, only for representing nonlinguistic spatial relations.[45]

The evidence that left-hemisphere damage causes aphasia in ASL-speakers, while right-hemisphere damage disturbs only the non-grammatical use of space, is strong evidence indeed that the left-hemisphere is specialized for the processing of language, regardless of the modality of the language.

USING SPACE TO TALK ABOUT SPACE

People in all cultures, including Deaf culture, frequently speak about space, literally and metaphorically. Where English uses prepositions and phrases like *facing toward the house* to express location and, more generally, spatial relations, ASL uses space itself. As we shall show, this unique ability of signed languages to talk about space using space is yet another way in which they achieve succinctness. One method of conveying spatial relations in ASL involves those classifiers mentioned earlier: handshapes that are used to stand in for nouns. For example, extend your hand, palm down, fingers touching and thumb fully bent under the palm; this classifier (let's call it the *flat surface classifier*) stands for rectangular flat-topped objects, like tables or sheets of paper, whose tops are prominent. Describing the locations of furniture in a room, an ASL speaker who had previously described the room might say: TABLE-IT-THERE, signing TABLE in front of the chest, then extending an arm with the flat surface classifier pointing toward the location of the table. Whereas in verb agreement, ASL grammar places people and objects in space in arbitrary locations, when talking about space itself, ASL places people and objects in locations that map real spatial relations. So ASL uses space in two different ways, both to refer and to map, and these two uses of space often overlap in ASL discourse.

Because English speakers use many separate words to convey spatial relations in complex and approximate ways (words like *near,* phrases like *on your left,* etc.), sometimes it is quite difficult to recover the intended spatial relations from an English sentence. Suppose you are giving a lecture and you look into the audience at two adjacent people, Will and his wife. You might say, *Will is to the left of his wife*. But in that case, you can also say, *Will is to the right of his wife*, meaning he is on his wife's right. Which is it? Is Will to the left or the right of his wife? Anna, who is seated behind them, disagrees with you; Will was never to the left of his wife. If you followed that and think that English is clear, although complicated, about left and right, try this: Arrange Will, his wife, and Anna so that Will is to the left of his wife, his wife is to the left of Anna, and Will is to the right of Anna.

English speakers give different accounts of the same spatial array depending on the speaker's point of view. If you say that Will is to the left of his wife but Anna says he is to the right of his wife, you are not puzzled long by her claim if you know her location. There are cases where it is not necessary to know the speaker's point of view in order to understand the spatial arrangements; that is when the scene has a built-in orientation. However, many things, such as trees, tables, and heaps, do not have fronts and backs. Sometimes the speaker's point of view and the built-in orientation give different accounts of the same spatial arrangement. Imagine you and a friend are seated at the start line of a dog race. As the dogs leave the gate, the only dog you can see is the dog closest to you, which is, of course, in front of the other dogs; but it may be behind them as well. The rabbit that runs around the inside rail of the track is behind all the dogs up to the turn, even though it is always in front of them.

One of us (Harlan) decided to explore the differences between spatial descriptions in English and those in ASL, and an informal experiment was conducted.[46] Because space talk is so common, any of countless tasks could have been used for this experiment: explaining how to find an address, tie shoelaces, make a soufflé; describing the solar system, a V-8 engine, or the rules of baseball. A doll house was selected that came with a few pieces of plastic furniture and a picture on the box showing how to arrange the furniture in this two-story home. There was a sofa, a TV, a stereo, a picnic table and two chairs, and a barbecue. With the house assembled and the furniture piled in front of it, the speaker in each pair of subjects was to look at the picture and tell the other subject where to place each item of furniture so as to reproduce the arrangement shown. The furniture mover was asked not to talk, and the speaker was videotaped. A representative transcript for a native speaker of English doing this activity appears in the left-hand column of the box below.

When pairs of signers were asked to do the experiment, they were not only quicker at it than English speakers, they followed a different strategy: they created a verbal map of the doll house by naming fixed parts of the house and locating those parts in space. Then they named the movable items that had to be placed by their partner and positioned them in the verbal space they had just created. This result reveals yet another interesting difference between English and ASL when it comes to portraying space.[47] In English, the object to be located, called the *figure*, comes first, and the setting in which the object is located, the *ground*, comes second: *The cereal is on the shelf*, but not *The shelf is under the cereal* (unless, of course, the shelf is the intended figure, as in *Where's the shelf? Under the cereal)*. In ASL, however, the ground comes first and then the figure, so the structure of the sentence would be: *On entering the store, there's an aisle whose shelves are full of cereal boxes*. It may have occurred to you that placing the ground first and then the figure is particularly logical in a visual-spatial language. It remains to be shown, however, that numerous other signed languages are like ASL in this regard.

Talking About Space in English and ASL

Transcript of English	Translation of ASL
"Okay, we'll start with the table and chairs on the bottom floor. In front of the house, um, there's a patch of green, like a patio, and the round table goes in the—in the—uh—top corner of the pa—of the green square. Okay. And in front of the—at—in front of the table—um—between the ladder	"Okay, take the round white table and put it outside, in front of the house, in the green area. The two chairs go next to the table. So the table's here and the chairs are one here and one here in front. Now, the cooking grill, you know, with the black hood that opens—the table's

and the table—goes one of the red chairs. Okay. And across from that red chair, on the other side of the table, goes the second red chair. Okay. Now, the barbe—the barbecue goes on the strip of patio between the green square and the house. Um, um, over to the left, almost in the left corner. Not quite. Okay, now let's go upstairs. Oh, excuse me, we have to go back downstairs; I forgot the record player. Now we're in the house, and as you face the house, it's a—the—the right—your right corner; okay, that's where the record player will go. Against the wall, well, against the wall in the corner. Okay? Now let's go upstairs. Okay. Now, on the second floor—the floor's divided into a terrace and a bedroom, and just where the terrace and the bedroom are divided there's—no—there's a frame but no wall there, and the couch or the little red seat goes in that frame, at an angle, so it's mostly in the room but it seems to stick out onto the terrace just a little bit. Okay. And the television goes—okay the floor in that room is separated by—there's a little ridge that sticks out of the floor, so the couch is on one side of the ridge—the television goes in the area that's separated with the other side of the ridge—and it's facing so that the person who is sitting on the couch can't see the tv screen—in other words, the tv screen is facing into the—is facing out of the house. Okay. Sort of facing the ladder. Okay. So we're done."	here, the grill goes here. The round table goes here, the chairs go here, the grill goes here. Now, the stereo—careful, it's heavy; **find the living room wall with the bookshelves and the mirror and put it there in the corner**, like this. Now, the TV—go upstairs, up the steps, enter where the roof begins, see where there's a dresser, pictures, and a lamp—put the TV there. Now, the chair, which folds open like a bed, it's red and white, take that upstairs. You see where the TV, the dressers, and the lamp are? Put it there. That's it."

In describing the arrangement of furniture in the doll house, ASL speakers first established the ground, the parts of the house, then identified each object of furniture and, after each, positioned it with respect to the ground using a classifier verb: for example, TABLE-IT-THERE. How can we convey the ASL description using an English transcription when our point is precisely that ASL uses space to describe space and English does not? We cannot. Whenever an ASL speaker used a classifier and located it in space, we have transcribed the verb as *go there*. The right-hand column of the box gives a transcript in its entirety for an ASL speaker, who was typical of the group we recorded. To give you a clearer idea of what was actually said in ASL, we have depicted in Fig. 4-8 below the ASL signs comprising one sample clause.

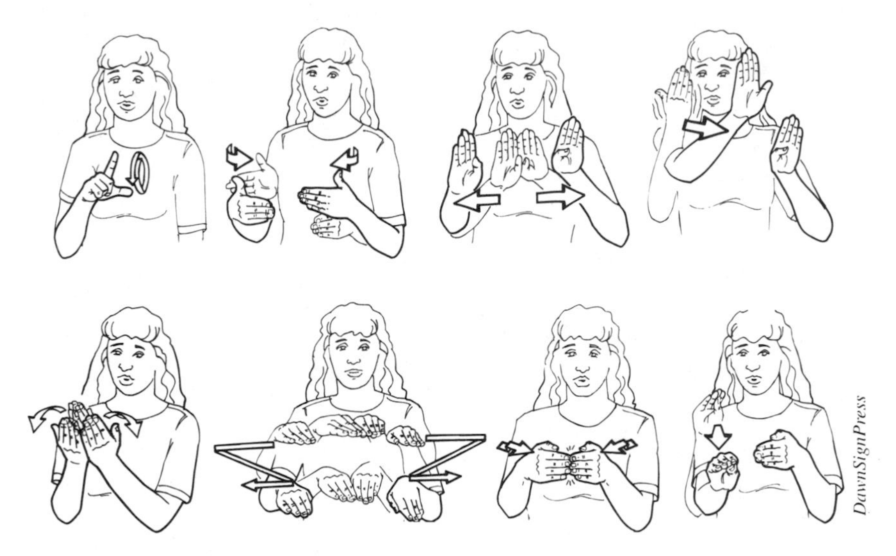

Fig. 4-8. **The ASL for *Find the living room wall with the bookshelves and the mirror and put it there in the corner***

You will note that the ASL instructions transcribed in the box have many fewer words than the English instructions. In a carefully crafted experiment using doll house descriptions, Emmorey and colleagues found that English speakers take thirty-five percent longer than ASL speakers on this task.[48] You may recall that, in the classic experiment by Bellugi and Fischer, signed and spoken stories took about the same time. Presumably ASL speakers had the clear advantage on the doll house task because it is so spatial in nature. ASL does not need to be as "linearized" as English: both hands can be used simultaneously with two different classifiers, and the positions of the hands against the ground represent the location and orientation of the objects referred to.

The present discussion has found it necessary to distinguish space in the grammar of ASL, used for reference, from space that is mapped out in ASL when describing physical space.[49] In the experiment with ASL speakers who had suffered damage to their right hemispheres, the patients had difficulty with spatial mapping but not with using space for the grammar of ASL. A follow-up study with a fourth such patient, an ASL interpreter, strongly suggests that the use of space for referring is mediated primarily by the left hemisphere of the brain, while the use of space for spatial description is mediated by the right hemisphere.[50] Emmorey and colleagues asked this patient, identified as DN, to draw complex figures from memory and to construct patterns from colored cubes. She had difficulty with these tasks. Despite these visual-spatial impairments associated with her right hemisphere damage, she had no language problems in ASL (or English). In ASL, she could name signs, repeat phrases, understand complex commands, and so on. She even did well on a test of understanding ASL verb agreement, where, as we have seen, the addressee must keep track of which nouns are placed where in space, and interpret the verb agreement with those locations as indicating subject and object (as in *The dog bites the cat*).

Although she was not impaired, then, in the use of space in ASL to refer, DN was severely impaired in its use to map the real world. She had great difficulty retelling descriptive narratives, like one about how the furniture was arranged in a dentist's office. She remembered the actual items well, but she failed to place them properly: she correctly located only about a third. In the story of the dentist's office, she tended to pile all the furniture in the center of the room. She also had problems with the correct use of classifiers, which you will recall frequently correspond in size and shape to the nouns they stand in for. Thus she used a bucket-type classifier in her description of a magazine rack. The investigators tried something quite clever: They asked DN to repeat stories that they had signed intentionally without using space. How could they do that? They relied on word order to indicate who was the subject and who the object, and they selected verbs for their signed stories that normally require agreement in front of the chest. When repeating such no-space stories, DN introduced space to mark linguistic relations: she placed objects and people out in space and correctly moved verbs among those locations. In short, DN, like several other patients, provides eloquent testimony to the fundamental difference in mental processing between the two basic uses of space in ASL.

A little earlier, we described experiments showing that what one remembers of sentences over the long haul, whether in English or ASL, is not their exact form but the gist of their meaning. This suggested another approach to studying the difference between referring and mapping in ASL. When the locations assigned by the ASL speaker have meaning as part of a description of some space, the addressee must remember them to remember the gist of the message. When the locations just function for common referencing (serving as "hooks"), they are commonly arbitrary and there is no value in integrating them into the long-term understanding of the message. On the contrary, one ought to "erase" them as soon as the discourse has switched or ended. To see if this reasoning was correct, Emmorey and colleagues presented blocks of ASL sentences to subjects who had to say after each sentence if it had been seen previously. Some of the sentences had indeed been seen previously but had been edited in one of two ways. In the first type of change, meaning was preserved: the subject and object were simply assigned different locations. In the second type of change, a new noun was substituted for one in the original sentence, changing the meaning. If subjects remembered the meaningful gist of sentences better than the surface forms, noun substitutions would be more obvious than changes in the locations chosen for them. However, the substitution in location should really be striking if the sentence uses space to map some real-world arrangement such as the furniture in the dentist's office, because that would be to change the meaning by locating things in different places. As predicted, the ASL speakers detected noun substitutions very well. And they were less good at noticing the spatial changes, except when the locations of the nouns in the sentence corresponded to real-world locations.

Several lines of evidence thus converge to suggest that the unique capacities of signed languages like ASL to use space for grammatical functions, and at the same time to talk about space *in* space, are associated with distinct processing systems, with their own mental representations, and with localizations in the two different hemispheres.

Nonlinguistic Spatial Processing

Think for a moment about the mental processes required of the person being addressed in an ASL conversation. For example, suppose Jake and Henry are chatting. Henry must recognize the basic signs and their inflectional movements. When Jake assigns nouns to locations in space, Henry must remember the several locations and the people or things assigned to them; otherwise, he would not know the subject or the object of the verbs that move among those locations in verb agreement. When Jake positions a classifier in some location (and then immediately removes it), Henry must remember that assignment and the noun indirectly assigned there by the classifier. If Jake refers to someone or something that moved to a new location, Henry must keep in mind the new place in signing space to which it has been relocated. If the topic of the conversation is spatial itself, Henry must build a mental map of the layout of the space described. Yet another degree of complexity arises if Jake reports what someone else has said or, more generally, changes the point of view in his narrative.

When speakers talk about space, whatever their language, they tend to prefer their own viewpoint. Within a story, however, the viewpoint may shift to that of one of the characters. English speakers convey shifts in point of view by changing pronouns (e.g., *I* to *he*), or voice (e.g., active to passive), by using indirect discourse (Jesus said, "I am the light and the way"), and with changes in speaking style. ASL can also use space for this purpose. In ASL, the speaker may shift body position toward the locus where an actor in the story has previously been located and the speaker will then produce sentences from that shifted position (with appropriately changed facial expression) that are to be attributed to the actor previously placed in that location. Other more subtle ASL ways of indicating a change in viewpoint are changes in eye-gaze and head position. As long as the viewpoint has shifted, the path that verb movements take will also be shifted.

An ASL comedian whom we recently saw tells the story of an overweight customer, a flirtatious waitress, and an uncooperative hamburger at a McDonald's. First the narrator takes the role and hence the position and demeanor of the customer placing an order, then those of the waitress noting down the order, those of the cook preparing it, those of the waitress delivering it, and then those of the customer again, now getting ready to devour an oversize hamburger. Then he shifts his torso toward the hamburger's position (rotating, leaning down, and looking up at the customer) and pleads for mercy. A rapid return puts him in the role of the startled but implacably hungry customer. In the ensuing dialog between the burger and the customer, the narrator needs only to shift eye-gaze up or down and turn his head slightly to indicate who is talking, the hamburger or the customer. Notice that the audience has to recognize the signs that have been placed in space, keeping a mental image of them and where they were located in order to interpret verb agreement and classifiers. The audience also has to transform spatial relations with each successive shift in narrative roles, all the while processing the grammar and meanings of the sentences. Notice, too, that transformations must include mirror reversals; that is, when the audience sees the speaker place a person or thing on the audience's left, for example, they must understand that it is on the character's right.

Role shifting not only occurs in storytelling but also is quite common in everyday discourse in ASL. Accordingly, you might expect that ASL speakers are particularly adept at generating and transforming mental images, and you would be right.[51] In one image generation task, subjects saw and memorized block letters on a grid (Fig. 4-9). Next they saw a series of grids, each containing an *x* mark and each preceded by a lowercase letter prompt. They were then to decide as quickly as possible if the corresponding upper-case letter would cover the *x* if it were superimposed on the grid. Some of the letters presented were simple and some were complex, with four or more segments. As the graph of results shows, native speakers of ASL were the fastest at this image generation task, hearing speakers of ASL were only a little slower, and hearing control subjects who knew no ASL took the longest of all to generate the images, especially when they were complex.

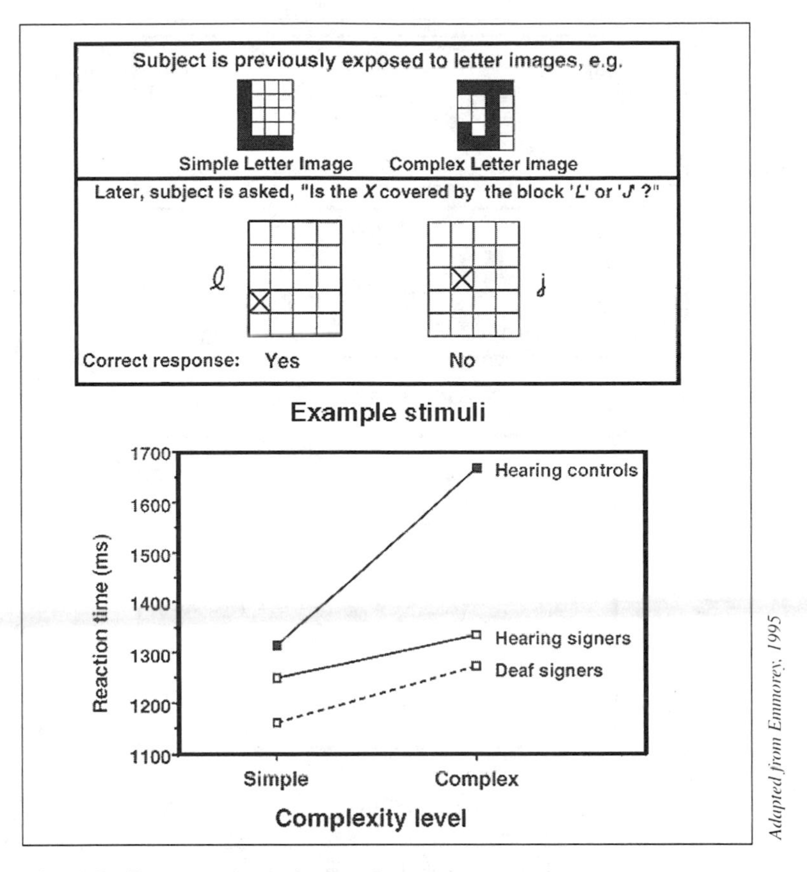

Fig. 4-9. **Image generation task**

In a similar test of image-rotation ability, subjects were shown angular shapes made of cubes (Fig. 4-10, p. 114) and had to decide as quickly as possible whether a target and a comparison stimulus were the same or mirror images, regardless of rotation.

Fluent speakers of ASL proved to be much faster than hearing subjects who knew no ASL when it came to identifying mirror images, no matter how many degrees the comparison had been rotated away from the target. Furthermore, native speakers of ASL proved to be more accurate than non-native speakers.

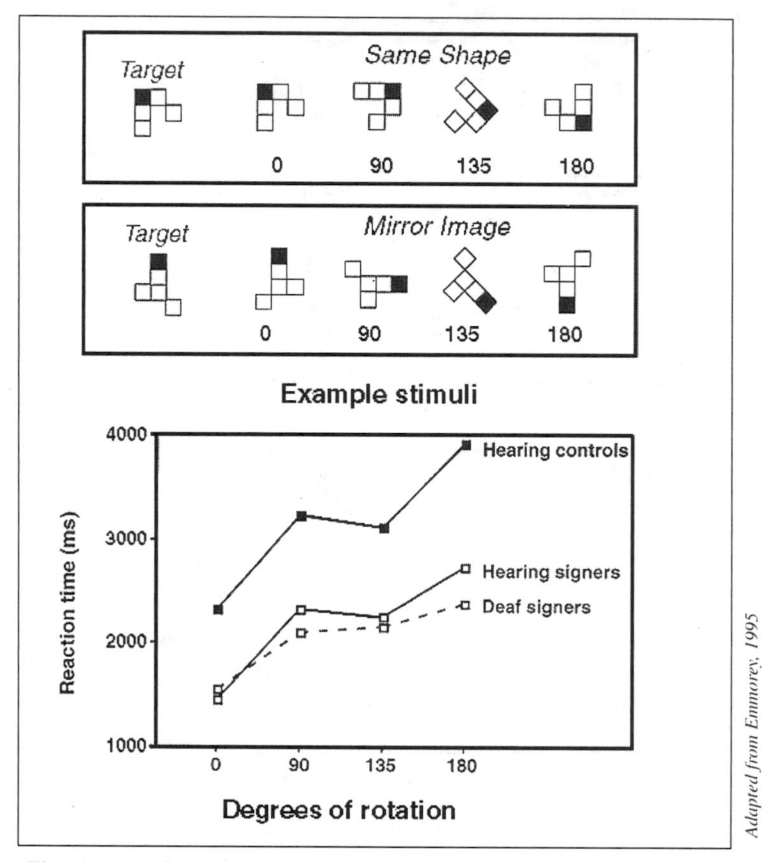

Fig. 4-10. **Mental rotation task**

Nonverbal IQ tests consist in part of spatial cognition tasks such as these. For example, the Block Design subtest of the Wechsler Intelligence Scale for Children consists of colored, three-dimensional blocks that the child must arrange so that the top surface of the block arrangement matches a colored picture. Several studies have found that Deaf children score higher than hearing children on this and other nonverbal IQ tests.[52]

Image generation of letters, transformations of cube forms and block design are only three of several non-linguistic spatial tasks on which ASL speakers have been shown to have a decided advantage. Recall that the face carries extensive grammatical information in ASL, including signals for relative clauses, conditionals (if . . . then), and topic marking. Moreover, the face conveys expressive information and helps to signal roles in ASL. There have been several studies of face recognition with Deaf children and adults, hearing speakers natively fluent in ASL, and with hearing control subjects who know no ASL.[53] When subjects have to choose a target face from an array of six faces with different orientations and shadowing, ASL speakers out-perform those who know no ASL.

Another example of enhanced non-linguistic visual-spatial abilities among ASL speakers may be related to the practice in ASL conversations of fixing one's line of sight on the face of the speaker much of the time.[54] As everyone knows, our vision is most acute in the center of the visual field, so this practice aligns the smallest movements coming from the speaker (changes in facial expression and hand movements on the face) with the greatest resolving power of the addressee's vision. It also means that the addressee must perceive many other signs in the periphery of the visual field where visual acuity is reduced. However, signs produced in the periphery favor two-handed signs, larger movements and more open handshapes, so they are more readily perceived than a representative sample of signs would be.

In order to study how the brains of Deaf people process peripheral visual stimuli, neurolinguist Helen Neville and colleagues looked at electroencephalogram tracings of brain waves associated with attention.[55] The waves were evoked by presenting a flashing square that appeared to move on the edge of the visual field. The investigators found that their Deaf subjects showed enhanced brain waves coming from a region of the brain that, in hearing people, processes sound. Neither codas nor hearing subjects in the study gave this result, so it was attributed to growing up without hearing, rather than to learning ASL. It is as if the brain reallocated to vision areas that were not serving hearing, and thereby enhanced attention to visual stimuli. This reallocated gray matter may be the basis for some of the Deaf advantage in visual perception. In this study, Deaf people were better on average at detecting peripheral movement than codas and hearing subjects.

Other studies have found that fluent Deaf speakers of signed language are better than hearing controls who know none when it comes to integrating rapidly presented visual information. In one study, invented

Chinese characters were written in the air with a light-emitting diode attached to the hand.[56] The fleeting trails of light created in that way were recorded on videotape and presented to hearing and Deaf Chinese children in the first grade, with a request that they draw the pseudo-character that had been traced in the air. To do this accurately, the children had to maintain in memory the path traced rapidly by the trail of light, then analyze it into its component strokes, and finally reproduce those strokes on paper. In some ways the task resembles identifying an inflected verb from the path of its movement (and handshape). The Deaf signed-language speakers had a large advantage.

The body of research we have just reviewed employed a wide variety of tasks that tapped space perception and spatial thinking in Deaf and hearing people: subjects had to generate and rotate images, assemble blocks, recognize faces, detect peripheral movement, and integrate rapidly presented visual information. None of these tasks required the subject to know or use signed language, and yet the native speakers of ASL had a distinct advantage in performing them. This research gives depth and detail to Deaf people's oft-repeated self-description as "visual people." And it suggests that language and thought sometimes draw on overlapping intellectual resources.

ARTISTIC EXPLORATION OF FORM IN ASL

Because speakers know the grammatical rules of their language, those rules can be violated to artistic effect. Some forms of artistic expression play off rules concerning the surface form of languages, such as the carefully arranged patterns and timing of elements in poetry and their substitutions in puns and spoonerisms. We have seen that the rules of ASL concern shape, space and movement, so you may well ask, Are there poetry and humor in ASL and do they play with the form of the language? It is a most interesting discovery concerning human creativity that the answer is *yes* to both questions. The capacity for language play, then, must have roots deeper than the surface form expressing the play.[57]

It appears that ASL speakers particularly like to play with the simultaneous layering of meanings that we have been describing. For example, there are substitutions of handshape. A Deaf person, when asked if he understood a technical explanation in linguistics, replied *I understand*, but instead of making thc sign with his index finger as usual, he substituted his little finger. The little finger occurs in several signs associated with thinness or smallness, like THREAD; so his meaning was, of course, *I only understand a little*. Sign locations and movements are also interchanged for artistic or humorous effect. Since the signer has two hands, there are rich possibilities for playing with simultaneity. For example, a signer who wanted to convey that he was both happy and sad to be moving to a new city, signed EXCITED with one hand while signing DEPRESSED with the other. Signs may also be blended in the heightened use of ASL. One signer explained ruefully that whenever she is tempted by cookies, she eats them: she signed TEMPT (made by tapping the curved forefinger on the elbow), then slid the curved finger along her arm and up toward her mouth while transforming it into a round shape, index touching the thumb tip (COOKIE); then she gazed at her hand and suddenly "ate" the imaginary cookie. This plays on numerous rules, but perhaps the most basic one is the fundamental difference between a word and its referent. In this case she ate her words!

The distinguished Deaf actor Bernard Bragg illustrated some features of art sign in a translation of an English poem by e.e. cummings, *since feeling is first*. In the literal rendition (see Fig. 4-11), the title line consisted of a two-handed sign (two index fingers touching, SINCE), two one-handed signs (bent middle finger grazes chest, FEELING; index leaves lips, TRUE), and a two-handed sign (index taps thumb, FIRST).

In the art sign rendition, the right hand announces a handshape theme (index finger folds into closed fist at forehead, BECAUSE) which is held throughout the line; in the second sign, the left hand enters (FEELING) and keeps that shape to the end of the line. In the third sign, the closed hand drops to sign ITSELF on the sign for FEELING and then returns to the forehead position (FOREMOST); only one hand has been active in each sign: right, left, right, right. The continuity of the signs is assured not only by the overlapping handshapes, but by making the final position of one sign the starting position of the following one. These techniques can be exaggerated, with the poet selecting locations in space or tempos that superimpose a particular shape or rhythm on the entire poem.

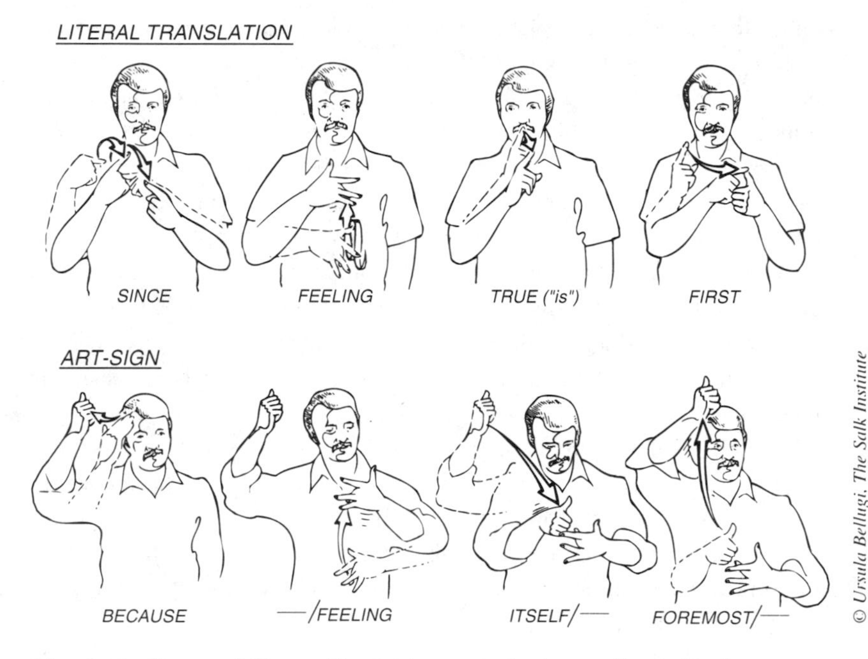

Fig. 4-11. **Bernard Bragg illustrates some features of art sign in a translation of e.e. cummings' *since feeling is first***

There are other stories based on word play, such as ABC stories and classifier stories. An ABC story is a twenty-six sign narrative in which each sign includes a handshape that is similar or identical to each one of the twenty-six handshapes in the manual alphabet, in order. A classic one, *The Haunted House*, begins, in translation, "With pounding heart [A handshape] and careful footstep [B], I opened the door [C] . . ." In classifier stories, the tale is restricted to using only the dozen classifiers of ASL. We take an example from perhaps the most loved Deaf comedian in the U.S., a former member of the National Theatre of the Deaf and a founder of the New York Deaf Theatre, Mary Beth Miller. Miller's talent for mimicking Deaf and hearing people and for side-splitting comedy sketches is renowned.[58] In *The Pinball Machine*, she provides the pinball's point of view; as the rod, released by the force of a compressed spring, hits her in the face, it sends her twirling up a corridor. Next, she slowly begins to spin down the board, veering from one side to the next as she hits the posts.

Finally she rolls free and clear, until hit back up by the flippers. Once more she goes through the head-knocking routine before rolling back past the flippers, where she is able to recuperate in line with her fellow metal balls. Her interactions with all these devices are described exclusively with classifiers.[59]

There is also poetry conceived and performed in ASL. In Ella Mae Lentz's ASL poem *Eye Music,* the narrator, facing the audience, is imaginatively seated inside a moving vehicle, perhaps a train, while telephone lines swoop toward her, past her, and out of view. Lentz uses her spread fingers alternately to represent telephone wires with an undulating movement, and the staff of sheet music with a tense horizontal movement, such that the undulating wires merge into music. The flow of the wires is punctuated by telephone poles (closed fist, index extended) which merge into drum sticks. Vision into sound, *Eye Music*. Here is an excerpt from the English translation of the poem:

> The eye music of the telephone wires
> With the music sheets
> With the lines that rise and quiver
> Sway and lower
> Along with the passing of space and time . . .
> Eyes are the ears
> And the piano and flute are the wires
> And the occasional pole is the drum! . . .

This excerpt may suffice for discussion of the poet's point, and to make one observation about formal devices in ASL poetry.[60] A central claim of this poem is that there is a kind of music in vision, that form-in-movement serves some of the same aesthetic roles in the visual DEAF–WORLD that harmony, beat, and so on serve in the culture and lives of hearing people. As ear music commonly connotes rather than denotes, so, too, eye music creates the mood and nuances of meaning. The form of poetry in English is dictated by the sound of the poetic line—its stress pattern, rhyme, etc.; the form of ASL poetry is dictated by the assonance and dissonance of handshapes, the flow of the movements of each hand individually, and the relations between the two hands. Other formal devices from ASL, such as body shift and facial expression, also play a role.

Linguist Clayton Valli, a leading poet of ASL, has presented an inventory of poetic devices in a recently released videotape of some of his work.[61] The focus is on what is unique about ASL poetry, that is, its remarkable range of formal devices. When we speak of rhyme in spoken languages, we have in mind a patterning of sound. When the components of ASL signs—handshapes, movements, orientations, and locations—are patterned in a poem, the effect is also esthetically pleasing to the native speaker. Figure 4-12 illustrates three signs from the poem *Circle of Life*, along with an analysis of their patterning.[62]

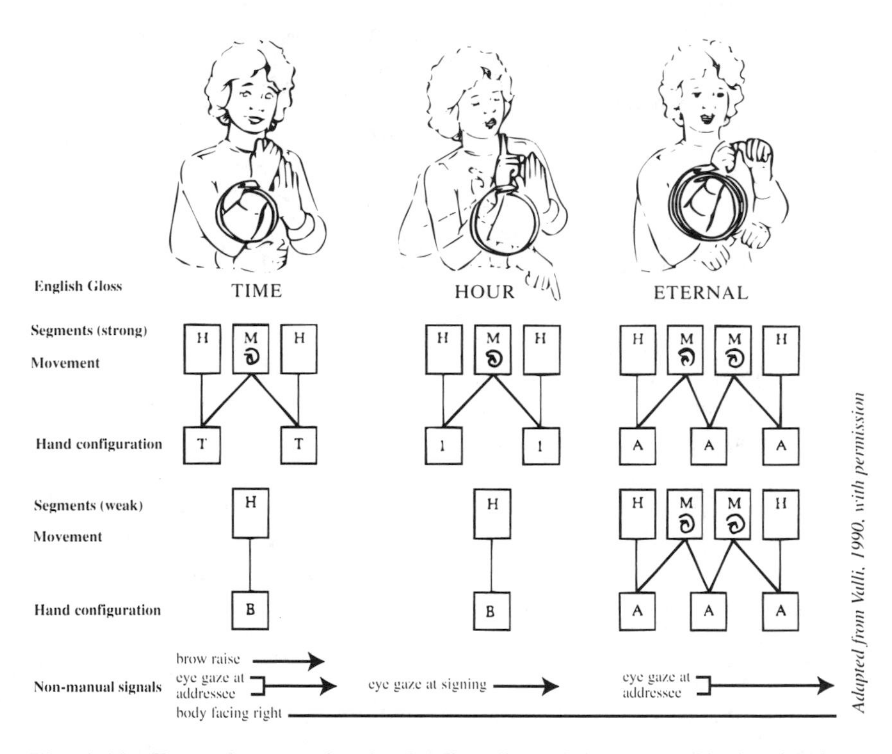

Fig. 4-12. **Formal patterning in the first line of the poem *Circle of Life***

The theme, unending cycles of time, is clearly captured in the movement rhyme, and in the repetition of cycles in the successive signs of the first line, TIME, HOUR, and ETERNAL, which are shown in the drawing. The third row of the figure shows that there is in the first line also patterning of the "holds" (momentary arrests of the hands, H) followed by movement (M). TIME and HOUR differ only in the hand configuration on the active hand, as indicated in the fourth row; then both hands take on the same handshape in the last sign. Notice, too, how the eye gaze (last row) starts on the addressee, moves to the immensity of time, and returns to the addressee. These handshape and movement rhymes recur in the next and subsequent lines, both with variations. Table 4-1 presents, somewhat abridged, Valli's inventory of poetic devices in ASL.

HANDSHAPE RHYME	**METER**	**NON-MANUAL SIGNAL RHYME**
Numeral HS	1. Hold Emphasis	Eye-gaze direction
Selected HS	long pause	Eye-gaze shift
Alphabet HS	subtle pause	Eyebrow movement
Closed HS	strong stop	Mouth movement
Open HS	2. Movement Emphasis	Head shift
Double HS	alternating MVT	Body shift
Worded	repeated MVT	**HANDEDNESS RHYME**
MOVEMENT RHYME	long MVT	One hand
MVT contour	short MVT	Two hand
MVT duration	3. MVT Size	Alternate hands
MVT size	regular	**RHYTHM**
Hold emphasis	enlarged	Rhymes
LOCATION RHYME	reduced	Handedness
Body LOC	4. MVT Duration	Assimilation of HS
Spatial LOC	regular	Choice of sign
Spatial level	slow	Change of sign
PALM ORIENTATION RHYME	fast	Creation of sign
Palm up	jerky	
Palm down	5. Stress	
Palm side up	iambic	
	spondee	
	trochaic	

Adapted from Valli, 1995

Table 4-1. **Poetic Devices in ASL**

Like poetry, humor is frequently creative with the form of its language, and this is part of the pleasure we take in it. A language that is visual in its form opens up remarkable and unique possibilities. It is always daunting to translate humor across the boundaries of language form and of culture, but especially so when translating Deaf humor from ASL into English. For these cultures are quite different, as we shall see, and their languages are in different modalities exploiting utterly different possibilities of form. Unless you know ASL, these examples of humor will probably not strike you as very funny—not nearly as funny as they are to Deaf people; but we hope you will find them revealing about language form and culture, and that they will enable you to see ways in which the visual/manual language of the DEAF–WORLD opens up particular possibilities for humor that have no close counterpart in spoken language.

French Deaf leader and humorist Guy Bouchauveau distinguishes three categories of humor in signed language. The first is a funny story whose punch line inspires laughter—we will come to an example in a moment. Another form is caricaturizing animals or people. The third is the creation of absurd images, something like cartooning. Here is one of Bouchauveau's examples using absurd images. A biplane is flying through the sky, when the upper wing prods the lower to suggest going north. The lower wing demurs. The upper wing then goes north but the lower insists on going south, with disastrous consequences.

Here, translated from ASL, is an example of humor based on a good punchline. It is a funny story, one that is particularly rich in elements of Deaf culture and whose humor lies (in part) in its play with the form of language.

> A huge giant is stalking through a small village of tiny people, who are scattering throughout the streets, trying to escape the ugly creature. The giant notices one particularly beautiful blond-haired girl scampering down the cobblestone street. He stretches out his clumsy arm and sweeps up the girl, then stares with wonder at the sight of the shivering figure in his palm. 'You are so beautiful,' he exclaims. The young woman looks up in fear. 'I would never hurt you,' he signs. 'I love you. I think we should get MARRIED.'

With the production of the sign MARRY the beautiful young woman is crushed. (Recall that to produce MARRY the speaker claps the cupped hands together.) The giant then laments, "See, ORALISM is better."[63]

Note that this tale is, in the first place, highly visual. The horror on the faces of the townspeople, who scatter, the beautiful frightened girl, the difference in scale between the giant and the town, all invite a dramatic performance, with not a word said until the middle of the story. Next, the story calls on the viewers' knowledge of ASL: the sign MARRY ends with the two hands clasped, palm over palm. But the giant's beloved is *in* his palm. Here now is the heart of the humor. It is a truism that words can't kill, meaning that words merely signify actions, and it is the actions that kill. In this story, however, the boundary between signifying and signified is crossed; words do kill, simply by being uttered. That infraction of the rules is funny. Finally, the story is funny on another, sociological level, since oralism symbolizes oppression in the DEAF–WORLD. Tongue-in-cheek, the story supports oralism. "There is something after all to be said for oralism," it seems to say, "provided you are a dim-witted giant with a lady in your hand."

The visual character of the story, the trespass on the axioms of ASL, and the reference to the hated oralism, together serve a larger function: they mark the story as coming from the DEAF–WORLD; they invite the listeners to identify with the culture from which it arises and so enjoy the solidarity of attending, expecting, laughing and applauding. Thus the funny story is validating. Language is perhaps the most important force that bonds the members of the DEAF–WORLD together. However, there is much more to Deaf culture, to which we now turn.

❦

Chapter 5

Deaf Culture

LAUREL, Roberto and Henry are representative of hundreds of thousands of Deaf Americans from hearing families who gradually developed strong bonds with other members of the DEAF–WORLD in the course of growing up. What are the bonds that hold Deaf people together? Collectively, they are called *Deaf culture*. We have seen in the preceding chapters that the members of the DEAF–WORLD are bonded by a common language, as well as common mores and values. Like most people with a common language, there is territory that they share. We continue our exploration of Deaf culture in this chapter by examining that territory, and then two other bonding forces in Deaf culture, namely, its athletic, social, and political organizations, and its artistic expression. Finally, we examine two powerful DEAF–WORLD forces: the unifying force of shared oppression, and a potentially fragmenting force—diversity in the DEAF–WORLD.

THE LAND OF THE DEAF

Language minorities commonly have a keen sense of shared place and the DEAF–WORLD is no exception. However, as we noted in chapter 1, the land of the DEAF–WORLD is not to be found in any single locale. That is probably because most Deaf people come from hearing families and mostly have hearing children. If they came mostly from Deaf families and had Deaf children, we expect they would all gather together in some single shared place, like the large Deaf clans found around the world (see chapter 6). Instead, many small places are surrogates in American Deaf culture for the single land of the Deaf that the culture yearns for but can never possess. It was this fragmentation, we think, that Olof Hanson, president of the National Association of the Deaf from 1910 to 1913, partly had in mind when he wrote that the Deaf are "foreigners among a people whose language they never learn."[1] Where is the land of the Deaf "foreigners"? It is, first of all, in the network of residential schools for the Deaf, which are the foundation of the DEAF–WORLD in the U.S., as in many other lands. For it is in the residential schools that the vast majority of DEAF–WORLD members acquire their shared language and culture. Nine out of ten Deaf people in the U.S. come from hearing homes where Deaf language and culture are rarely to be found. That Deaf Americans should feel they have a place of their own, that such a conception is useful in organizing the prominent facts of American Deaf history, speaks powerfully to the key role of the Deaf schools in American Deaf culture.[2]

The importance of place for Deaf people, and the primary role of the residential school as this place, are reflected in several facts about Deaf culture. Deaf introductions, as we have said, require stating one's school. The DEAF–WORLD favors voluntary separation for Deaf children in residential schools and is bitterly opposed to mainstreaming most Deaf children in local hearing schools. Deaf people have mounted aggressive campaigns to block the closing of residential schools where this has been proposed, for example, by advocates for children with disabilities. Deaf ties formed at school are commonly lifelong, as noted earlier. Deaf people's itineraries on trips around the U.S. frequently include visits to a string of residential schools. Moreover, the first recorded organization of Deaf people in the United States was the alumni association of what is now the American School for the Deaf in Hartford. As each successive school in the residential network developed, another alumni association was formed.

The central role of place in the minds and lives of America's Deaf people could not be satisfied by the residential-school network alone. For one thing, many of the residential schools were founded and directed by hearing people, and late in the last century those people took drastic steps

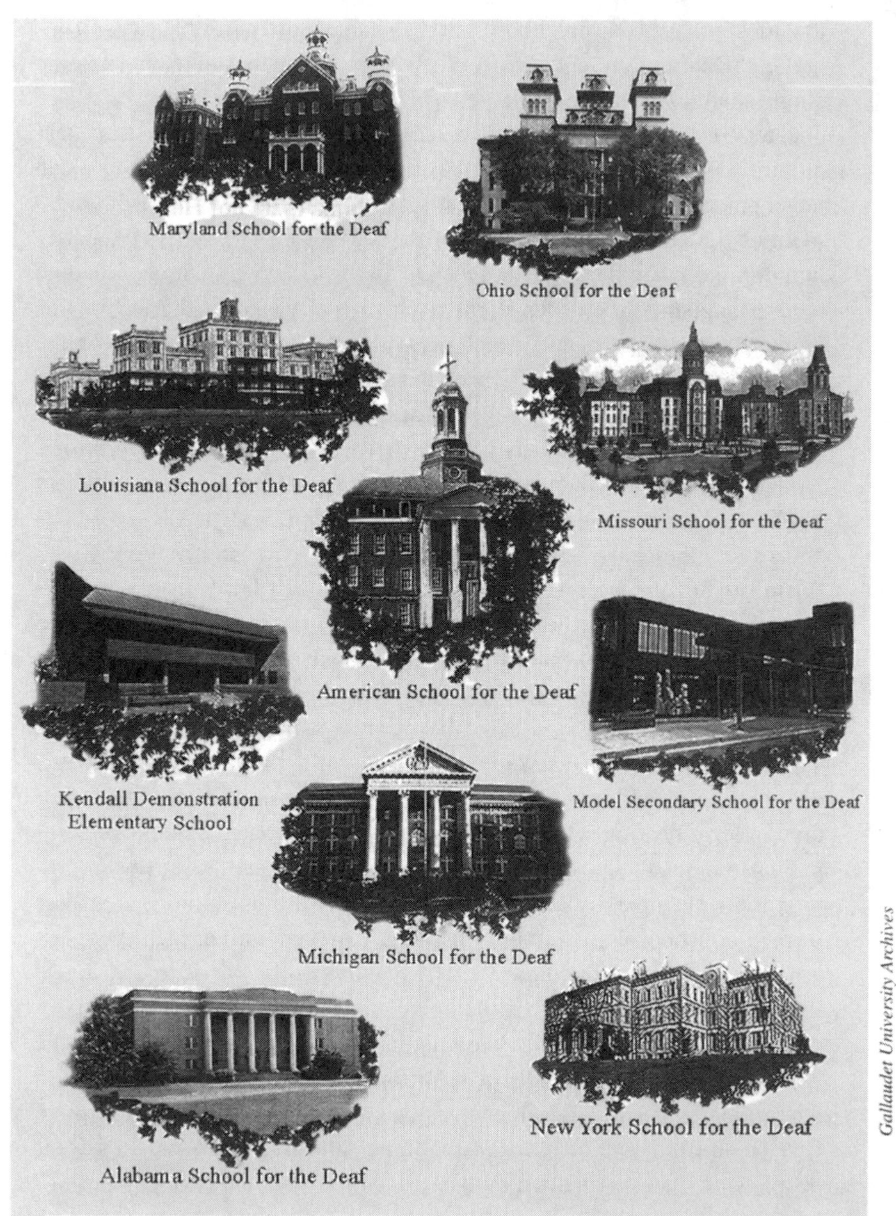

Fig. 5-1. **Main entrances to some residental schools for the Deaf in the United States**

to replace ASL with English and to impose hearing culture. Moreover, the Deaf young man or woman, having developed a deep sense of place at the residential school, then graduated and frequently lived apart from the school and its community (though many stayed on at the school or in the town). The search for a place apart from the residential school led to the establishment of Deaf clubs, tiny reservations of Deaf culture, as it were, across America, where Deaf people govern, socialize and communicate fluently in ASL after the workday ends. The residential schools also have important links with the Deaf clubs and with Deaf sports.

The concept of place is so central to the lives of America's Deaf people that a utopian vision of a "Deaf country," one created by and for the Deaf, has long played a role in American Deaf culture. The idea was put forth in the 1830s by recent graduates of the American Asylum (the school founded by Clerc and Gallaudet, which had changed its name from the Connecticut Asylum after a congressional land grant). These graduates formed an association to purchase land from the federal government; however, employment scattered the group and the project died. A little later, Clerc advocated establishing a Deaf "headquarters" on land granted the American Asylum by Congress. In the 1850s, the desire of American Deaf people for a place of their own surfaced once again; there was an extended debate in the *American Annals of the Deaf* and at meetings of Deaf organizations.[3] Similar utopian plans arose in the British and French Deaf communities in the last century.[4]

The vision of a Deaf utopia has been the inspiration for numerous folk tales in American Deaf culture, the most recent of which is known as *Eyeth* (the name is a pun on the first three letters of *Earth*), as well as a few novels by Deaf authors.[5] A recent editorial in a Deaf newspaper describes a utopia where ASL is the official language, spoken by everyone from store clerks to policemen, bank tellers to dog groomers. In this utopia, everyone assumes you are Deaf, movies are all open-captioned, plays are all in ASL, school classes are in ASL, and kids are not sure who is Deaf and who hearing, nor do they care.[6] What bliss it would be for Deaf people to live in a place like that!

In the absence of a single gathering place for all the members of the DEAF–WORLD in America, the scattered residential schools and clubs have served to bring groups of Deaf people together, ending Deaf isolation. In the middle of the last century, when numerous schools for the Deaf had already been founded by Deaf and hearing educators, a movement arose to found the National Deaf-Mute College in Washington, DC. Since its founding, the college has played a symbolic role as a place belonging to Deaf people, and it has long been called the Mecca of the DEAF–WORLD.[7] Indeed, Deaf people from around the world make "pilgrimages" to this place, now Gallaudet University, toward which they feel some sense of ownership.

However, prior to 1988, most Deaf people, especially university-educated Deaf Americans, did not consider that Gallaudet truly belonged to the DEAF–WORLD. First, it was controlled by hearing people, and second, it promoted a hearing agenda, even if that agenda in some ways overlapped the Deaf agenda. Then, in 1988, the DEAF–WORLD in the U.S. seized control of Gallaudet University from its hearing directors. This act won Deaf students and leaders acclaim around the world and raised the consciousness of Americans concerning the DEAF–WORLD as had no prior event in this century.[8]

The week in March, 1988, that shook the DEAF–WORLD, has come to be known as the *Gallaudet Revolution*. It began with an announcement on Sunday that the governing board of the university, consisting of seventeen hearing and four Deaf persons, had made their selection of the university's new president. For the first time in Gallaudet's history, two of the three final candidates were Deaf; both were accomplished administrators and scholars. I. King Jordan, whose doctorate was in psychology, was dean of the university's College of Arts and Sciences. The other Deaf candidate was the director of a residential school for Deaf children, a child of Deaf parents, and a leader in the U.S. DEAF–WORLD; his doctorate was in education. The one hearing candidate, an administrator at another university, knew nothing of the DEAF–WORLD or of ASL. A small crowd of students and some employees had gathered on campus to hear the announcement. The board had chosen the hearing candidate.

The crowd reacted with shock, anger, disbelief, and tears. Posters and news releases were burned and speeches were made in ASL. The crowd swelled with the arrival of many faculty, staff members, and alumni, and it took to the streets and marched to the hotel where the board was staying to demand an explanation. There, the chairman of the board was understood by student representatives to say that the board had not picked a Deaf candidate because "Deaf people are incapable of functioning in a hearing world." Although she claimed later that her remarks had been misinterpreted, the quote was picked up by newspaper reporters covering the demonstration. It added fuel to a volatile situation.

Hundreds of Gallaudet employees, returning to campus on Monday, found all the entrances to the campus blocked. The university was forced to close down. The students issued four demands that the board would have to satisfy before they would reopen the campus: the board must annul its decision and appoint a Deaf president; the chairman of the board must resign; the Deaf membership of the board must increase to more than half; there must be no reprisals against protesters. The board met with a delegation of students and refused all the demands. The students organized a movement called *Deaf President Now* (we spoke of it earlier when discussing the Deaf pride of the Deaf children of Deaf parents). It began with a rally that filled the stands of the football field. The protesters burned effigies of the chairman of the board and the hearing candidate. *Deaf President Now! Deaf President Now!* became the protest chant. The Deaf President Now Council was formed to coordinate developments, make plans, and oversee the protest. The third day ended with the lines of battle drawn up.

Deaf students, national Deaf leaders, and university staff met with several congressmen, who took their side. The faculty of Gallaudet and the staff voted overwhelmingly to support the students' four demands. The national media swarmed over the campus. The Deaf President Now Council set up a communications center and a team of interpreters for the reporters. That evening one of the four Deaf student leaders, Greg Hlibok, appeared on the ABC News program *Nightline*, along with the hearing candidate and Deaf film star Marlee Matlin. The heavy media coverage attracted much support to the students' cause, including $20,000 in contributions. Letters, telegrams and phone calls poured in. Rallies were held at Deaf schools all over the United States. Later that Thursday evening, the hearing candidate withdrew, acknowledging the justice of the Deaf cause.

Friday's march to the capitol attracted three thousand participants from all over the nation, including busloads of Deaf students and their parents. The march began with a huge banner, lent by an African-American museum, which proclaimed, *We still have a dream!* People along the parade route cheered and waved. Cars and trucks honked their horns in support. Government workers stopped their labors and leaned out office windows to cheer the students on. On the steps of the capitol, congressmen stood in line to address the rally. The students' determination and behavior in the struggle won their praise. Said one senator, "You have succeeded in educating the world about Deafness, the concerns of Deaf people, and the simple truth that we all need and are entitled to dignity and respect." All three candidates for the presidency of the United States sent the students letters of support. Said U.S. Black leader and presidential candidate Jesse Jackson: "The problem is not that the students do not hear; the problem is that the hearing world does not listen."

On Saturday, hundreds of students and their supporters gathered on campus for a "Board Buster Day." There were lectures, a picnic, free food, strategy meetings. Meanwhile, members of the Board of Governors were returning to Washington from their homes around the U.S. to pick another president and to discuss the remaining student demands. On Sunday, the board announced that the seventh president of Gallaudet, and its first Deaf president, would be Dr. I. King Jordan. The chairman of the board had resigned. The board would be reconstituted with a Deaf majority, and there would be no reprisals against the protesters. The board had agreed to all the students' demands. Deaf people had reclaimed their land.

The fruits of that Deaf activism have been copious. Gallaudet University itself has adopted a more Deaf agenda. For example, there are more Deaf personnel at all levels, a new Deaf Studies major, and greater tolerance for ASL. Millions of Americans are aware of the DEAF-WORLD and ASL as never before. Deaf pride is at an all-time high. The Revolution was above all a reaffirmation of Deaf culture, and it brought about the first great worldwide celebration of that culture, a congress called *The Deaf Way*, held in Washington, DC, the following year. Five thousand spokespersons from Deaf communities around the world, including scholars, artists, and political leaders, participated in lectures, exhibits, media events, and performances. On the Gallaudet campus, there was a spectacular display of Deaf arts: mime, dance, storytelling and poetry in manual languages, crafts, sculpture, video, and fine arts. It is clear that Deaf leaders and artists in many nations have, to a degree, a sense of ownership of the Gallaudet Revolution, just as they have a sense of special fellowship with the members of the DEAF-WORLD in the U.S. and around the globe.

Deaf Organizations

Athletic organizations

Sports are one of the powerful bonding forces in the Deaf-World. The love of individual and team sports is nurtured in the residential schools and whetted by rivalry among schools. Sports rapidly become a vehicle of acculturation for the Deaf child, a shared experience, a source of Deaf pride, and an avenue for understanding customs and values in the Deaf–World. Something similar could be said about the role of sports in the acculturation of hearing children in the larger society. However, sports frequently play a particularly important role in the lives of minorities, for they open a path to achievement and distinction where many others are closed by prejudice. In the Deaf–World, moreover, athletics provide a level playing field when it comes to language. The ASL speaker's limited command of English (like that of members of other language minorities) may be a handicap in the classroom, but it is not one on the baseball diamond.

Some Deaf people attend athletic tournaments to play, of course, but they and many more are there for another reason: to be with other members of the Deaf–World (frequently impossible during the work day) and to see old friends who have become separated after graduation or marriage or a move to a new job. Athletics in Deaf culture also serve linguistic and political functions. ASL is a truly national language, in part because of the co-mingling of Deaf people in the residential schools, in the clubs and in regional and national athletics. And athletic programs provide an opportunity for Deaf managers, so often disempowered in the larger society, to further their leadership abilities, to show what they can do, and to broker a certain amount of power in the Deaf–World. At the local level, Deaf clubs are involved in numerous sports, including volleyball, softball, and basketball.

At the level above the individual clubs, there are regional leagues grouped into a national organization, the American Athletic Association of the Deaf (AAAD). On April 13, 1945, representatives of several Deaf clubs met at the Akron Club of the Deaf and founded the AAAD. Why Akron? During the world wars, Deaf men and women were not permitted to serve in the military, so they joined the war industries work force instead. The great rubber companies based in Akron hired large numbers of Deaf workers and, with a critical mass of Deaf people, local Deaf culture flourished.[9] The AAAD publishes *Deaf Sports Review* and supports the Deaf sports Hall of Fame on the Gallaudet University campus. Its affiliates include a score of national Deaf sports organizations from aquatics to wrestling.

In 1924, six national federations of the Deaf sent contingents to the first World Games for the Deaf. During the games, the International Committee for Silent Sports (later, Deaf Sports; Comité International des Sports des Sourds, CISS) was founded to forge a union among all Deaf sports federations. The International Olympics Committee gave formal recognition to CISS as an international federation with Olympic standing in 1955. A few years ago, CISS acceded to the request of the Olympics Committee and joined the International Paralympics Committee. However, it was never the intention to combine World Games for the Deaf with those for people with disabilities. The DEAF–WORLD sees itself as a language minority, not a disability group (see chapter 15) that requires adaptations of sports such as those used by athletes with disabilities in the Paralympics.[10] At the 1995 biennial congress of CISS, members voted to withdraw from IPC and return to the former direct relation with the International Olympics Committee. In the same year, the Committee awarded the Olympic Order, its highest honor, to CISS president Jerald Jordan.

With athletics organized formally in Deaf schools and clubs and at local, regional, national and international levels, and given the role of athletics in social life, leadership training, and cultural bonding, Deaf sports are clearly a major institution in the DEAF–WORLD. There is considerable pressure on Deaf athletes to participate in Deaf sports, for the community is relatively small, and its athletes are thus the guardians of an important cultural institution. That institution is in danger of serious deterioration as increasing numbers of young Deaf people attend mainstream schools where Deaf sports are not offered. The U.S. contingent of outstanding athletes competing at the World Games of the Deaf has reportedly declined in recent decades. Canceled Deaf sporting events are another visible consequence of depriving Deaf children of an opportunity for Deaf pride and acculturation through Deaf sports.

Deaf teams compete with hearing teams as well and often trounce them, challenging the hearing view of Deaf people as limited or isolated.

Some Deaf athletes have achieved national and international recognition, like Eugene Hairston in boxing, and "Dummy" Hoy in baseball. Hoy, outfielder for the Cincinnati Reds, is credited with inventing the hand signals used by major league umpires. Incidentally, the football huddle is said to have originated at Gallaudet University (presumably so the opposing team could not observe the signed description of the next play). Some Deaf athletes have competed in the Olympic Games and some have won medals.

The Legacy of Eugene Hairston, Deaf Boxer

Eugene Hairston boxed against the world's best welterweights and middleweights in the 1940s and 50s, when boxing was the king of sports. Hairston wasn't the first Deaf boxer, but he was the most popular. Before turning pro, he was defeated only once in 61 Golden Gloves and AAU bouts. As a pro beginning in 1947, he won 45 fights, including 24 knockouts in 63 bouts. Hairston defeated two world champions in non-title bouts, outpointing welterweight champion Kid Gavilan in 10 rounds in 1950 and knocking out middleweight champion Paul Pender in 1951. Then suddenly it was all over. A severe gash above his eyebrow forced him to hang up his gloves at the age of 22 in 1952. It was a screeching halt to a short but glittering boxing career. He took too many punches to the head, and one more punch could have left him sightless.

While Hairston retired with his ambition to become a world champion unfulfilled, he left boxing with an enduring legacy—the flashing corner lights that, along with the bell, indicate the end of the round and for boxers to return to their corners for repairs, rest and instruction. Deaf boxers are not the only ones who have problems knowing the round has ended. Boxers who can hear, especially those engaged in furious combat, have often missed the bell and have continued slugging each other. Inability to hear the bell in the heat of action was a problem that lingered for many years, until Hairston came along demanding lights.

(Adapted from Strassler, 1995, with permission)

In a less competitive vein, Deaf people who, like other Americans, are living longer, are more interested than ever before in engaging in leisure time activities. Traditional leisure activities in the DEAF–WORLD include parties, card games, and bingo—small, all-Deaf and usually sedentary events. Increasingly, Deaf groups are participating in recreational activities set up on a larger scale for the general public, including domestic and overseas tourism. In 1986, the World Recreation Association of the Deaf was born to promote such activities as camping, excursions to amusement parks, ski-days, white-water rafting, and the like.[11]

Social organizations

Despite the importance of schools and athletics, undoubtedly the strongest organizational bonding in the DEAF–WORLD has come from the Deaf club. A hearing ethnographer studying a Philadelphia Deaf club recounts how, as she was leaving the club one evening, one of its older members rose to show her to the door. The member said: "Look at me, I act as if this were my home . . . but this is like my home. You know, for Deaf people, the Deaf club is like a second home. Hearing people don't have anything like that."[12] A Deaf man opposed to marriage with a hearing woman significantly uses the Deaf club to convey his cultural antipathy to mixed marriages: "If I married a hearing wife, what would happen to her? . . . Would she visit the Deaf club? Hearing people go to the hearing club—they go to the clubs and dance. Am I going to be able to interact with the hearing? No way. They don't know me . . . So, I'd be just sitting back doing nothing; I'd say, 'I don't want to go to a hearing club,' and my wife would say, 'I don't want to go to the Deaf club.' We'd become opposites. Opposite cultures and opposite lives."[13]

Most major cities have Deaf clubs, and some have several. For Deaf children of Deaf parents like Jake (and hearing children of Deaf parents, too), socializing at the Deaf club starts very early. For a time, the club complements the acculturation taking place at the school for the Deaf. One theory has it that the snack bar at the residential school is a training ground for club managers. (See Figure 5-2.) In managing the snack bar, the Deaf high school student learns how to assure cooperation among the student staff, keep inventory, plan ahead for supplies, keep accounts and so forth—skills that serve the student well in later years as a leader of a Deaf club.

When school days are over, the club is traditionally the key place for further acculturation and socializing. Older members teach younger ones, explicitly or indirectly, about Deaf values, customs and knowledge, ASL, Deaf stories and jokes, and Deaf history. For example, an account of "How We Founded the Club" can be a lesson not only in Deaf history but in ASL, in narrative, and in the values worth striving for, as well. In the Deaf clubs, members seek information about the world, the community, employment, friends. They seek relaxation and easy conversation, participation in sports and leisure activities, and entertainment. There are dances, raffles, banquets, costume parties, beauty contests, lectures, gambling nights (when hearing people are particularly welcome), and anniversary celebrations. There used to be captioned films as well before the advent of captioned television programs. And of course Deaf people find at their club all the activities that keep any club vital: elections, celebrations, business meetings, and distributions of awards recognizing service to the club and community.

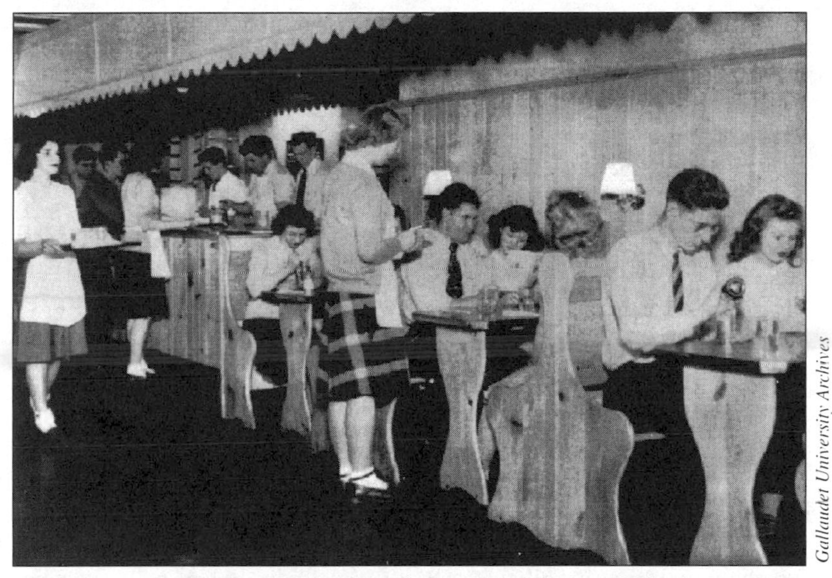

Gallaudet University Archives

Fig. 5-2. **A snack bar at a residential school for the Deaf.** circa 1950.

Reportedly, membership in Deaf clubs has been dwindling, especially among young people, who are the next generation of Deaf leaders. There seems to be no hard data, but if the reports are accurate, the DEAF–WORLD has reason for concern, and its members are searching for causes and remedies. One frequently cited cause is that mainstreaming of Deaf children in local schools delays Deaf children's acquisition of ASL and Deaf culture (see chapter 8). Another reason given is the growing practice of captioning television programs, which makes some entertainment available to Deaf people right in their own home. Others contend that membership may be off in the older urban Deaf clubs, but has grown over the years in suburban clubs.

There are many national organizations of culturally Deaf people in the United States, including alumni associations and organizations of various minority groups within the DEAF–WORLD (of which more later). The National Fraternal Society of the Deaf was conceived by some students at the Michigan School for the Deaf around the turn of the century. At that time Deaf people paid a high premium for life insurance and disability insurance when they could obtain them at all. The society became a fraternal insurance organization which also provided automobile insurance in later years, another form of insurance that Deaf people had difficulty obtaining at standard rates. The society's thirteen thousand members are organized in over one hundred local divisions similar to lodges that sponsor social gatherings, athletic events, and community projects.[14]

Religious organizations have had an important role in the bonding of the American DEAF–WORLD. Thomas Hopkins Gallaudet was a clergyman, as were so many other founders of Deaf education, beginning with the abbé de l'Epée in mid-eighteenth century France. Like Epée, Gallaudet gave the "saving of souls" as a central purpose of Deaf education. He and Clerc raised money for the first charitable institution in the United States, the American Asylum for the Deaf and Dumb, by appealing to the religious beliefs of New England Protestants. The school that they established, like virtually all others to come after it, included rigorous religious instruction. Thomas's eponymous eldest son founded, in the mid-nineteenth century in New York City, the first congregation of Deaf worshippers. It was followed shortly in Philadelphia by a second Episcopal congregation, led by America's first ordained Deaf priest, Rev. Henry Syle. Since that time some fifty more Deaf priests have served Episcopal congregations. The period of greatest growth in their ranks was in the first half of this century, when the ministry was one of the few professions open to members of the DEAF–WORLD. Lutheran, Methodist and other denominational congregations soon followed Syle's; several of them sustained schools for Deaf children. There are national Deaf religious organizations such as the National Congress of Jewish Deaf, and international organizations such as the International Catholic Deaf Association.

Churches with Deaf congregations play a much larger role in the DEAF–WORLD than communal worship alone. These churches sponsor homes for elderly Deaf people, recreation programs, vocational and family counseling, youth camps and more. Despite their Deaf membership, these are not strictly speaking Deaf organizations, however. Historically, Christian churches with Deaf ministries have been led by hearing people, frequently people with limited knowledge of the DEAF–WORLD who view Deaf people as handicapped. Thus, Deaf church-goers have had little opportunity to develop forms of worship that reflect Deaf culture and experience. Moreover, they have been frustrated by poor interpreting, lack of access to the Bible in ASL, lack of support services, and sheer lack of fellow Deaf people. Perhaps these barriers go some way toward explaining why, in contrast with the Black Civil Rights movement in America, Deaf religious leaders have not been in the vanguard of the Deaf struggle for equal rights. In 1984, Deaf and hearing leaders deeply concerned by these barriers issued a manifesto, calling for a view of Deaf culture as a gift from God and for reforms to create a Deaf-friendly church with Deaf leadership.[15] In recent years, the National Council of the Churches of Christ has sought to put those principles into action. Thus, the empowerment of Deaf people is progressing in the church as it is elsewhere.

Political organizations

At about the same time that hearing educators of the Deaf were decreeing an end to signed languages at the Milan Congress of 1880, Deaf people in America representing twenty-one states were gathered in Cincinnati at a meeting of about the same size. They, too, sought to improve the welfare of Deaf people, but they had an entirely different conception of what that was. “The meeting was called the National Convention of Deaf-Mutes,” said Deaf leader George Veditz, who would become president of the National Association of the Deaf, “and that’s that. If oral magicians, who yank educational rabbits out of silk hats and pearls of speech out of the mouths of those who have never heard, choke over it, why bless ‘em!”[16] This group of educators, engineers, businessmen and so on, decided to form a permanent association of the Deaf and set about drafting a constitution. Robert P. McGregor, the Deaf principal of the Ohio School and then the Colorado School, was elected president. Today, the National Association of the Deaf (NAD), which is a federation of state associations of the Deaf but has 22,000 direct members, is a vigorous advocate for signed language and the rights of Deaf people. NAD helped conduct the first census of the Deaf population of the United States. It publishes numerous books, a quarterly monograph, *The Deaf American*, and a newspaper, *The Broadcaster*; it supports a legal defense fund, sponsors an annual youth leadership camp, and backs a Junior NAD for its school-age members. Its biennial conventions include the Miss Deaf America contest, exhibits and theatrical performances, banquets, and business meetings in which resolutions on all facets of Deaf life are voted, shaping NAD's agenda for action. As is the case with athletic events, NAD conventions also have an important social function: they reunite schoolmates and friends who have been scattered around the country.

Many Americans know that there is a national Miss America contest and that a contestant with a hearing impairment won that award in 1995. Fewer people realize that the Deaf–World has its own Miss Deaf America pageant. Evaluations of young Deaf women for the title combine the consensual selection of the storyteller with more formal competitions. The successful candidate often begins as a self-identified performer at a Deaf school, as did the last Miss Deaf America, Maureen Yates. Known as a bright young woman with Deaf pride (she is part of the seventh generation of Deaf people in her family), Ms. Yates was first recruited for the Miss Deaf Maryland pageant. There she presented a narrative skit on a theme in Deaf culture (a child who cannot call for help because her teachers have muted her unseemly voice) and impressed the judges with her knowledge of Deaf culture and of current events, her reflection on important issues confronting the Deaf community, and her beauty. Having won the state pageant, she competed successfully against winners from all the other states in the national pageant,[17] and has become a model to Deaf youth as she travels among the residential schools and is presented at other programs. She is sought after to lecture at Deaf meetings, she participates in ceremonial events, and she often describes her celebrity role in the pages of *The NAD Broadcaster*.

The Arts

The institutions of the Deaf–World, some of which we have just surveyed, are a central part of its culture. The arts also play a critical role in bonding the members of any culture, and the members of the DEAF–WORLD are no exception. In fact, in at least two respects, the arts have a privileged relation to Deaf culture. Deaf people are, as we have seen repeatedly, best thought of as visual people, so it should be no surprise that there has always been a substantial number of Deaf artists, many with worldwide renown. Then, too, ASL is an unwritten language, so literature such as storytelling and humor carry much cultural information that, in cultures with written languages, would be passed down through the generations in books. At Deaf clubs there has traditionally been a variety of cultural activities, including performances, storytelling, skits, and comedies. The flourishing study of signed languages in the last few decades and the associated enhanced empowerment of Deaf people, have fostered a particularly prolific period in the Deaf arts, one might even say a renaissance.

The visual arts

At the outset of modern Deaf history in the mid-eighteenth century, Deaf artists played an important role in creating awareness of the abbé de l'Epée's pioneering efforts and those of his successor, the abbé Sicard. Thus, for example, one of Epée's Deaf pupils was a painter, another a sculptor; each presented a Deaf person's vision of "the father of the Deaf." And ever since then, Deaf artists have continued to present Deaf culture to Deaf and hearing people.[18] Whatever their subject matter, Deaf artists breathe pride into the DEAF–WORLD and serve as role models for young Deaf children. However, it is when the DEAF–WORLD sees itself and its culture reflected in the works of its artists that Deaf art is most effectively a bonding force in Deaf society, so we will focus on Deaf art defined in this way, as a form of cultural expression.

As part of the renascent foment of Deaf culture in the U.S. in the 1970s, an organization called *Spectrum: Focus on Deaf Artists* was started by some hearing artists in Austin, Texas, in 1975. Deaf painter Betty G. Miller left Gallaudet's art department to join them. Two years later, Spectrum was officially launched and twenty-two Deaf artists—dancers, painters and actors from around the country—assembled to collaborate. A Spectrum Visual Arts Institute was established under Miller's direction, which published a newsletter and convened summer conferences on Deaf arts. The American Deaf Dance Company was formed, as was the Spectrum Deaf Theater, directed by performing artist Charlie McKinney, then president of Spectrum. Miller and Deaf painter Chuck Baird organized a major collection of slides of the works of various Deaf painters and sculptors in the U.S.[19]

Miller presented a major exhibit of her work at Gallaudet University in 1972; it may have been the first exhibition in the U.S. devoted to art expressing themes from the DEAF–WORLD. Since much of the work was highly critical of hearing oppression, the exhibit was controversial among both hearing and Deaf audiences. It also introduced many future Deaf leaders to Deaf art for the first time.

A contemporary of Miller's is the acclaimed Deaf painter Morris Broderson, whose work is represented in several major museums across America. Many of his paintings are on religious themes and others reflect his travels in Japan. He is cited here, in relation to art on Deaf themes, because of the series of works The Sound of Flowers, and the inclusion of the manual alphabet in several of his works, reminding us that images reflect both sight and sound.[20]

Growing interest in Deaf art led in 1985 to creation of the professional organization, Deaf Artists of America, in Rochester, New York. Prior to closing its gallery in 1992, DAA organized more than twenty exhibits featuring works by scores of Deaf artists. The organization sponsors conferences, publishes an artists directory and a newsletter and serves as a clearinghouse concerning Deaf art.[21] In 1989, a group of nine American Deaf artists met prior to the Deaf Way International Conference on Deaf Culture, and developed a manifesto in which they dubbed an art form De'VIA (Deaf View/Image Art), meaning one which "uses formal art elements with the intention of expressing innate cultural or physical Deaf experience."[22] The manifesto explains that De'VIA often includes a focus on the hands and face.

In 1993, a major exhibit of Deaf art was presented in Haverhill, Massachusetts, and comparable exhibits accompanied the third and fourth Deaf Studies conferences. Viewers had an unusual opportunity to examine the works of a range of Deaf artists, who varied in their ages, their preferred media, their themes and their visions. There were lithographs, oils, watercolors, acrylics, pen-and-ink drawings, neon sculptures, and animated films. Aspects of the lives of people in the DEAF–WORLD were captured in many stages of the life cycle: the struggle of growing up Deaf with hearing parents; the suppression of signed language; the imposition of oralism; cochlear implant surgery.* These themes were explored at both individual and cultural levels. For example, Susan Dupor's *Family Dog* attracted particular attention: a somewhat imbecilic-looking child, the family pet, lounges on the living room carpet and stares out of the canvas at the viewer; behind her, a barrier (the edge of a coffee table) separates her from the legs of several adults, seated side by side on a couch. Their heads are spinning, their hands "silently" wedged into their armpits. At the cultural level, Deaf Canadian artist Mary Thornley's *Milan Italy, 1880* (after Goya's *Third of May, 1803)* portrays ASL being shot by a firing squad, a reference to the infamous Congress of Milan.

Betty G. Miller's *Untitled, 1994* portrays with mixed media the battle between the medical and cultural understandings of Deaf people. Several contemporary Deaf artists have acknowledged their debt to Miller's work, which can rage against cultural oppression in one canvas, and in the next celebrate the beauty of ASL. Two of those for whom her work paved the way are Harry Williams and Ann Silver. Williams' paintings frequently express his joy in Deaf culture, often using symbols from hearing culture. Thus in his Musical Notes Series, colored flowering dots stand in for musical notes. "Art is our music!" several of his works proclaim. In other words, culture and thought, like language, are not rooted in any one modality. In one canvas, a large decayed ear rests alongside a keyhole. Through the keyhole we see colors, showing that light has entered the mind through the prism of the eyes; a full–fledged mind is at work behind locked ears.

In the painting on the cover of this book, Williams celebrates the discovery of language, a peculiarly Deaf experience, since for most children language comes first and conscious discovery comes later. Williams' discovery of language came when he grasped that the fingerspelled word B-A-L-L matched the picture of a ball; then the door of enlightenment

* A cochlear implant is an electronic device, part of which is surgically implanted in the inner ear. The device converts sounds to electrical signals that stimulate the auditory nerve. See chapter 14.

opened for him. Before, his mind was a desert. After, his vision was transformed by the primary colors (red, blue, and yellow), which were to change his life. The flower in full bloom is Williams' rendering of the moment of discovery: I-UNDERSTAND.[23]

Ann Silver's witty and arresting poster art capitalizes on the evocative powers of road signs and other familiar objects to send messages about Deaf culture and Deaf studies. Poster art is also the vehicle chosen by Elizabeth Morris for her moving protests against childhood cochlear implants. She uses Deaf publicity to counter that of the implant manufacturer. (See Fig. 14-2.)

Chuck Baird's work is sampled and discussed in a recent book commissioned and published by DawnSignPress.[24] Baird attended the Kansas School for the Deaf, Gallaudet College, and the Rochester Institute of Technology, where he earned a degree in studio painting. In many of his paintings, Baird plays with the relation between signifying and signified, between language and reality. Hearing artists before him have written on their canvases; Braque glued lettering in his collages; Magritte presented a pipe side–by–side with the statement that it was not a pipe. However, the form that language takes in Baird's paintings is more evocative, because the ASL signs that he often incorporates into the very objects to which they refer, come from a visual language. Not all of Baird's paintings are on Deaf themes, yet they all seem to contain a Deaf vision, in their vivid hues and engagement with form and light. In recent years, Baird has completed major murals on Deaf themes at Gallaudet University and the Learning Center in Framingham, Massachusetts.

One contemporary sculptor whose work reflects DEAF–WORLD culture is Lee Ivey, a Gallaudet University graduate whose 1992 *Deaf Power* is a celebration of the Gallaudet Revolution. Her *School Memories* of the same year presents a pupil locked in a small room: Did he sign when it was prohibited, or did he fail to use his voice?

Possibly the first architect in the U.S. whose work reflects Deaf culture was Olof Hanson (1862–1933), the NAD president whom we quoted earlier on the alienation of Deaf people in hearing society. In the course of a very successful career, Hanson designed scores of residences, store buildings and hotels, schools and churches, many of them adorned by numerous turrets, towers and chimneys, arched doorways and windows. Hanson was born in Sweden but moved to Minnesota when he was thirteen, attended the state residential school for the Deaf, then Gallaudet College, which awarded him his degree in 1886. He earned a master's degree there three years later, then spent a year studying the architectural sights of Europe and taking classes at the famed Ecole des Beaux Arts in Paris.

On return, he married Agatha Tiegel, the first Deaf woman to earn a B.A. degree from Gallaudet. Hanson took a position as an architect in Philadelphia and designed most of the buildings on the campus of the Pennsylvania School for the Deaf, the first of many buildings he conceived expressly for Deaf people, including the North Dakota and Mississippi Schools for the Deaf, and buildings on the grounds of the Washington School, the Minnesota School, and Gallaudet College. In his designs, Hanson incorporated large double-hung windows on all floors to allow adequate natural light for signed communication. Windows were not placed behind the speaker's platform, however, as that would have obscured the ASL speaker's face and made it difficult to see the facial grammar. Interior windows allowed Deaf people to communicate between adjoining rooms. Lighting controls were placed near the podium, so the speaker could attract audience attention by making the lights flicker, and seating was arranged for maximum visibility. In 1915, Hanson designed the first civic and social clubhouse for Deaf people in the U.S., the Charles Thompson Memorial Hall in St. Paul, Minnesota. Over the years, the club has hosted numerous weddings, banquets, and conventions, as well as presenting silent films and then captioned films. Today this Deaf club includes game rooms, a dining room, a two-hundred seat assembly hall, a bar, and a Deaf-culture salon.[25]

Art historians have yet to focus their trained eyes on Deaf art in the U.S. and abroad, to deliver an analysis of its themes and methods, to inventory the many artists, and to present their works in book form. Deaf artists have yet to be recognized in the larger art world, despite their growing and enthusiastic following in the DEAF–WORLD, and despite the wide attention to the art of other groups such as African-Americans and Native Americans. Perhaps with the growing recognition of the distinct culture of the DEAF–WORLD, this minority's art will finally receive the attention it deserves.[26]

Performing arts

Deaf theater is an expression of Deaf culture and finds a natural audience in the members of the DEAF–WORLD. However, Deaf theater may be the best opportunity that hearing people have of glimpsing the richness of visual life that is the gift of the Deaf experience. Chapter 4 presented some research evidence that speakers of signed languages are particularly adroit at processing visual arrays, recognizing faces, and integrating rapidly presented visual information. We hypothesize that Deaf theater engages those capacities at the same time as it engages the viewer's understanding of the signed message. Thus a dramatic story line proceeds simultaneously with choreography and mime, the artistic use of language, and the recognizable conventions of Deaf culture and of the theater. For the viewer who is able to process so many levels of meaning concurrently, Deaf theater is a dazzling display indeed.

Recent decades have seen Deaf performing artists win Tonys, Emmys, and Oscars in the United States, and comparable awards for outstanding television, theater, and movie performances in numerous nations. The first Tony awarded to Deaf performers was garnered in 1977 by the National Theatre of the Deaf. That institution, which we describe below, helped to lay the groundwork for the most recent Tony Award in the DEAF–WORLD, won by *Children of a Lesser God*, a play that has probably done more to raise hearing consciousness of the DEAF–WORLD in the U.S. (and some European countries) than any other single event in this century (with the possible exception of the Gallaudet Revolution). Deaf actress Phyllis Frelich starred in this winner of three Tony awards, about love between a speech therapist and a Deaf woman proud of her Deaf culture. Deaf actresses Elizabeth Quinn and Emmanuelle Laborit won best actress of the year awards in Britain and France, respectively, for their performances in this play. When the U.S. touring company of *Children of a Lesser God* was formed, Deaf actress Linda Bove, best known from her appearances on *Sesame Street* and an extensive television career, played the leading role throughout the U.S. and Canada. Finally, the play was brought to the screen by Deaf actress Marlee Matlin in an Oscar-winning performance, and millions more Americans learned about Deaf culture and Deaf pride. The award-winning film for television, *Love Is Never*

Silent, co-produced by Deaf actress and director Juliana Fjeld, and starring Frelich and Deaf actor Ed Waterstreet, taught Americans more about Deaf oppression in a tale concerning Deaf parents' struggles to raise their hearing children, an adaptation of Joanne Greenberg's book, *In this Sign*.

The earliest plays by Deaf actors on DEAF–WORLD themes in the U.S. probably originated in the mid-nineteenth century in the residential schools, where plays develop around Deaf school life, Deaf history, and Deaf family situations. In such plays, students are not limited by their abilities in English and can give free rein to their talents in acting and in the expressive use of ASL. In this century, serious drama has flourished at such schools as the California School for the Deaf in Berkeley, the New York School for the Deaf in White Plains, and the American School in Hartford. In the 1890s, St. Ann's Church for the Deaf, founded by Thomas Hopkins Gallaudet's oldest son, also named Thomas, presented plays for Deaf audiences in New York City. The first formal theater production was staged at Gallaudet University in 1884; a male theater group was organized seven years later, and four years after that the female students organized their own drama club.[27] Deaf theater was also to be found in the Deaf clubs (especially informal skits and mime shows), at Deaf literary societies, and at Deaf theater groups. New York City, for example, counted three such groups in the 1950s: the Metropolitan Theatre Guild, the New York Hebrew Association of the Deaf, and the New York Theatre Guild of the Deaf.

Gallaudet University started formal drama classes in 1940. In recent years, its drama department has presented powerful plays about the Deaf experience, some written by its first chairman, Gilbert Eastman. His *Sign Me Alice* (an ASL satire on the use of invented sign systems, based on Shaw's *Pygmalion*) and *Laurent Clerc: A Profile,* have received wide acclaim. Starting in 1985, Eastman co-hosted the Deaf television magazine *Deaf Mosaic*. Produced at Gallaudet University but seen nationwide on cable television, the program won the Emmy Award ten times by addressing such themes in the DEAF–WORLD as Deaf history, cochlear implants for Deaf children, World Games for the Deaf, and ASL poetry; it was discontinued for lack of funds in 1995. The National Technical Institute for the Deaf, in Rochester, New York, also sponsors student productions on Deaf cultural themes and has counted distinguished Deaf actors on its faculty. These include Robert Panara, who founded the experimental theater department in 1973, and National Theatre of the Deaf veteran Patrick Graybill, now an educational filmmaker. As at Gallaudet, most of the productions at NTID are signed language adaptations of plays written for hearing audiences.

Eastman, Frelich, and Bove were among the seventeen founding members of the National Theatre of the Deaf, organized in 1967. NTD has sought primarily to bring hearing theater to hearing and Deaf audiences using Deaf actors, and thus to show to the world their extraordinary talents. Through its plays, workshops, and frequent appearances on television (many Americans have seen the NTD presentation of *A Child's Christmas in Wales*, for example), NTD has not only contributed immeasurably to the development of Deaf theater, Deaf performers and Deaf playwrights, it also has made a growing hearing audience aware of the DEAF–WORLD and the power and beauty of signed language.

The public acceptance of the DEAF–WORLD and ASL is so much greater today that it may be difficult to comprehend what a remarkable departure NTD represented when it was founded. In an era when oral education of the Deaf was dominant and ASL denigrated, NTD performances presented to a large public a language of startling beauty and evident effectiveness, in addition to a cast of witty, smart and attractive Deaf people. The promotion of Deaf culture to the American public has long had ardent opponents, however, as we shall see in detail when we examine the hearing and Deaf agendas for Deaf people, toward the end of our journey into the DEAF–WORLD. An example of that opposition, which might have torpedoed the launching of NTD, should be noted here. The year it was founded, NTD presented the first nationally broadcast television program featuring Deaf performers, NBC's one-hour *Experiment in Television*. When the newspapers announced an upcoming special using signed language, the Alexander Graham Bell Association protested vigorously in a telegram sent to NBC and the members of Congress:

> We are opposed to any programming which indicates that the language of signs is inevitable for deaf children or is anything more than an artificial language, and a foreign one at that, for the deaf of this country.[28]

Today NTD can look back on thirty years of accomplishment with pride. It has to its credit more than fifty touring seasons and twenty-eight foreign tours, more than 6,000 performances of some fifty productions and numerous awards for its work. All these have contributed to the momentum for the recognition and acceptance of signed language here and abroad.[29]

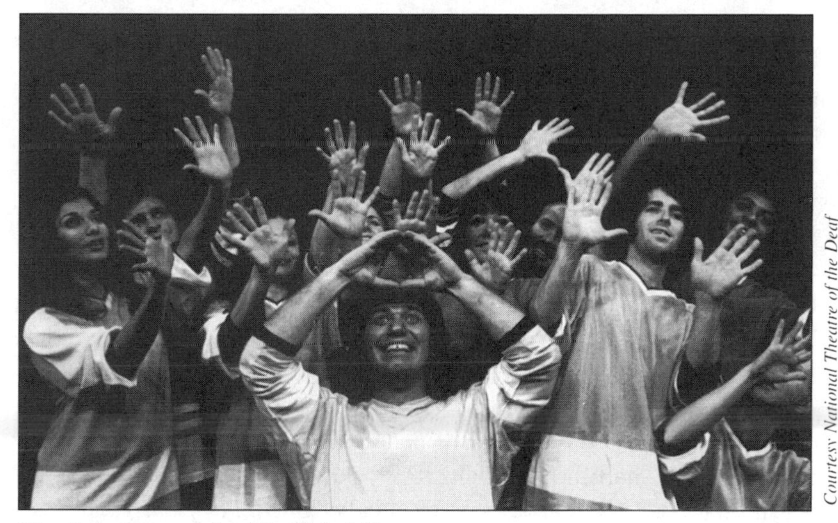

Courtesy National Theatre of the Deaf

Fig. 5-3. **A scene in *My Third Eye***

The NTD troupe has presented the Deaf experience in several of their works, for example in its original company piece, *My Third Eye*, a play in five parts about ASL and Deaf people. One of those segments, co-directed by the late beloved British Deaf actress and poet Dorothy Miles, features a ringmaster who displays two caged hearing people and explains their bizarre ways to the audience ("They see with their ears and sign with their mouths!"). Turning the tables on hearing people in this way is very gratifying to Deaf audiences, who commonly receive *My Third Eye* with a standing ovation. In founding NTD, director David Hays collaborated closely with the great Deaf mime, actor and director, Bernard Bragg, who recruited most of the initial troupe, none of them professional actors at the start. Bragg has had a long and distinguished career that includes many performances for NTD. He has also performed as an artist-in-residence at the Moscow Theater of Sign Language and Mime, and as artist-in-residence at Gallaudet University. Over the years, NTD has launched ten different ancillary programs, such as the Little Theatre of the Deaf and the Deaf Playwrights' Conference. More than eighty plays have been written by members of NTD or participants in the Playwrights' Conference.

NTD has played an influential role in establishing Deaf theater in numerous other countries. Three troupe members, for example, went to Paris to establish the International Visual Theatre (IVT), which proved influential in the renaissance of French Deaf culture, as we will see in the next chapter. NTD tours abroad created the right climate in several countries for the formation of national Deaf theater. Additionally, members of foreign troupes attend NTD professional theater school during the summer. Professional Deaf theater has flourished in recent decades in numerous countries around the world, including Australia, Britain, Canada, Denmark, France, Japan, Poland, Russia, and Sweden. The International Pantomime Festival of the Deaf was organized in 1970 and the first World Deaf Theatre Festival in 1981.

Regional Deaf theater in the U.S. has also had wide influence. A California group, D.E.A.F. Media (including Deaf actors Howie Seago, Freda Norman and Ella Mae Lentz, better known for her ASL poetry[30]), began a televised ASL talk show in 1974 called *Silent Perspectives*. It was the first television program produced in ASL "of, by and for the Deaf." It ran for five years and won an Emmy. That led, in turn, to a program called *Rainbow's End*, the first and, to date, the only nationally broadcast program in ASL for Deaf children.

In 1980 D.E.A.F. Media began a biennial program to promote Deaf culture called Celebration: Deaf Artists and Performers. It features leading Deaf performers, poets and artists. The event combines academic seminars on Deaf culture during the day and cultural presentations in the evening. There are opportunities for artists to discuss their work in progress with their colleagues; for example, one of us (Ben) first presented his ASL story *Bird of a Different Feather* there. Celebration has had an enduring impact on the work of many Deaf artists, poets and performers. "This was an attempt to keep the spirit of the Spectrum experience alive," writes D.E.A.F. Media director, anthropologist Susan Rutherford, referring to the Deaf arts movement in Texas that we described earlier. "But it also had a political purpose—to provide a prestigious venue for the production and recognition of Deaf arts."[31] Indeed, it awakened many hearing people to Deaf culture and nourished Deaf pride in the DEAF–WORLD.

The Northwest Theatre of the Deaf was established by members of the Deaf community in Portland and nearby Vancouver, Washington, in 1974, with the goal of providing better access to theater and cultural events for speakers of ASL. The theater also seeks to educate the general public about signed language and Deaf culture, to provide theater workshops for children and adults, and to give an outlet for the talents of Deaf playwrights and actors.

The Fairmount Theatre of the Deaf, founded in Cleveland, Ohio in 1975, was the first resident professional signed language theater. Recently renamed the Cleveland Signstage Theatre, it has made a mission of informing hearing people about the DEAF–WORLD. Half the works they present are original, most concerning Deaf themes. The theater, directed by Deaf actor and playwright Shanny Mow (whose plays were extensively performed by NTD in the 1980s), also presents bilingual versions (ASL and English) of a wide variety of hearing playwrights, from Molière to Tennessee Williams.

The New York Deaf Theatre was established in 1979 by a group of Deaf actors and theater artists who wanted to create opportunities for signed language theater. Some of their plays are hearing classics adapted for ASL performance, such as *The Gin Game,* directed by Frelich. Others are indigenous Deaf art forms, such as *Lovelost* by the late Deaf playwright Bruce Hlibok. The New York Deaf Theatre sponsors an annual Deaf playwright competition to encourage Deaf writers to tell about the DEAF–WORLD.

The Onyx Theater was founded in 1989 to give greater visibility to minority Deaf performers and themes of minority cultures, especially Black culture, within the DEAF–WORLD. A related undertaking for the film medium, Deafvision Filmworks, was founded in 1991.[32] The same year, Deaf West Theatre Company was established in Los Angeles; NTD alumnus and former director Ed Waterstreet became its artistic director, where he was joined by NTD actors Bove, Norman, Frelich and Graybill, among others. Each season Deaf West presents several original productions in ASL, as well as adaptations of plays written in English, with on-stage actors providing interpretation into English. Thus audiences, like the staff, performers, and the plays themselves, come from both the DEAF WORLD and the hearing community. Deaf West innovated in some performances with hearing actors speaking off-stage, their voices broadcast to those in the audience who wished to hear them wearing receiver-headsets.

There are also several small theater groups and one-man shows focused exclusively on the DEAF–WORLD. An example: CHALB Productions, launched in 1980 by Deaf actors/producers Alan Barwiolek and Charles McKinney. It performs primarily at Deaf clubs, conventions, schools and colleges. SignRise Cultural Arts (Oakland, California) was founded in 1991 and has developed several new plays on the Deaf experience; this is also the purpose of the Rochester, New York, group LIGHTS ON!

Deaf production groups have been established from time to time to make television and film documentaries concerning the DEAF–WORLD. Two that flourished, and made an important contribution, were the Silent Network and Beyond Sound. Both were established in the early 1980s. The Silent Network became the leading producer of Deaf programs for television and won eight Emmys. It evolved into Kaleidoscope Television.[33] Beyond Sound produced a weekly news program and important documentaries, such as a history of the Los Angeles Club of the Deaf.

The various theatrical performances in the DEAF–WORLD can be helpfully gathered under four headings.[34] There are adaptations of hearing theater presented in ASL (such as the NTD's performance of the Babylonian myth *Gilgamesh*, or its adaptation of Dylan Thomas' *Under Milkwood*); these have been called "sign-language theater." There is DEAF–WORLD theater, which presents in signed language stories situated in Deaf culture. Examples include Bernard Bragg and Eugene Bergman's *Tales from a Clubroom*, set in a fictitious Deaf club, CHALB's *Deaf Pa What*, and Willy Conley's *The Hearing Test*. According to leading Deaf theater critic, playwright and director Donald Bangs, the most common themes in original plays in DEAF–WORLD theater are the problem of communication between Deaf and hearing people; the central role of schools in Deaf acculturation and the oppressive attitudes of the hearing authorities in those schools; Deaf dignity; and the beauty and artistry of ASL.[35]

A third genre of theatrical performances, one that is cross-cultural, is exemplified by *Children of a Lesser God*, which combines elements of sign-language theater on the one hand and of DEAF–WORLD theater on the other. Finally, there are hearing plays adapted into Deaf culture, like Eastman's *Sign Me Alice*, adapted from *Pygmalian* and *My Fair Lady*.

Deaf theater, like all minority theater, must grapple with a common financial and moral dilemma. Its sense of mission and natural proclivity is to address a Deaf audience with Deaf themes. Its financial needs, however, and its desire to inform the larger society, make it aspire to be understood and enjoyed by a wider audience. One solution, adopted by the Paris-based Deaf troupe International Visual Theatre, is either to rely on avant-garde visual imagery, or to produce plays in LSF without voice interpretation (as, for example, operas are usually produced in the original language without simultaneous interpretation), thus obliging their audience to enter into the visual world of the Deaf. Other groups incorporate voicing actors or narrators into the signed language performance, sometimes in highly creative ways. One production of an absurdist Ionesco play had voicing actors in the roles of pieces of furniture on the set! For the National Theatre of the Deaf, the eminent American interpreter Lou Fant was one of the hearing actors over the years who provided English translations addressed to the ninety percent of the audience that was hearing and knew no ASL. And then there is the hearing-oriented solution of, notably, *Children of a Lesser God*, which seemed to forget its Deaf audience by creating whole scenes in which hearing characters spoke and there was no ASL interpretation! This Deaf morality play ("our story," as Phyllis Frelich called it) was inaccessible to Deaf audiences on both stage and screen, except when Deaf characters were speaking ASL.[36]

The choice of target audience is not the only financial peril that confronts Deaf theater. Because of the visual nature of its productions, Deaf theater cannot use a large theater house; yet it cannot use a small house and charge high admission, because the target audience often has a limited budget for entertainment. To aggravate the problem, Deaf theater productions can be especially costly because of their need to make the play accessible to both English and ASL speakers.

In the era of silent films, Deaf audiences could also see Deaf culture performances on film as well as on the stage. Moreover, Deaf actors could perform in films alongside hearing ones, and Deaf audiences could attend the theater on a par with hearing audiences.[37] There were several outstanding Deaf filmmakers in that era who chronicled the lives of the members of the DEAF–WORLD. Possibly the earliest films about the DEAF–WORLD in the U.S. were made by the National Association of the Deaf between 1910 and 1920, at a time when it feared for the extinction of ASL in the era following the Milan Congress. More than a dozen films were produced that recorded poems, lectures, and reminiscences by Deaf leaders. One of those films has NAD President George Veditz (1904-1910) speaking grandiloquently in ASL about the importance of preserving the language.

We mentioned earlier the DEAF–WORLD filmmaker Charles Krauel, who filmed Deaf life, especially in the Midwest, during the period 1925 to 1940. Krauel sought to preserve for posterity the social life of Deaf people and made careful film records of the conventions of the National Fraternal Society of the Deaf.[38] The ensuing decades saw the work of several Deaf filmmakers, among them Deaf actor Ernest Marshall, who produced nine feature films between 1937 and 1963 with an all-Deaf company. Some were based on original scripts by Deaf writers. Various Deaf clubs made films in the same era, a priceless record of Deaf people's lives and culture. In more recent decades, however, Deaf-culture films have been blocked in the U.S. by the lack of training of Deaf producers and directors, who have been effectively barred from the motion picture industry. Finally, Peter Wolf, Deaf producer, director, cinematographer and NTD alumnus, received training at Cinemalabs, a professional program in San Francisco. He directed the first two feature-length films on Deaf topics, *Deafula* and *Think Me Nothing*.

Because film is an expression of the cultural values of a society, films for the general public have usually portrayed Deaf people as self-absorbed, sad, and solitary; *The Heart Is a Lonely Hunter* is an example. As is commonly the case in their written literatures, the films of hearing societies, when they introduce Deaf characters at all, do so to advance the plot, and not because the DEAF–WORLD is thought to be of interest to large audiences. In the Hollywood stereotype, Deaf people are individuals who can read lips and speak intelligibly; they live precarious lives and they long for a cure. Such films contain not a hint that there is a Deaf culture, with its own language, art forms, and traditions. Ironically, that culture is particularly strong and manifest in film haven Southern California, where Deaf clubs and other organizations are among the oldest and the most progressive in the nation.

Literature

American Sign Language has a rich literary tradition. The storyteller and the story have an important role to play in the bonding of the DEAF–WORLD and the transmission of its heritage and accumulated wisdom. Storytelling develops early in residential schools for Deaf children, where youngsters recount in ASL the idiosyncratic mannerisms of hearing teachers and the plots of cartoons, westerns, and war movies. (Because these films and television programs were frequently uncaptioned, they used to challenge the young storyteller's craft and imagination more than they do today.) Some children soon emerge as the ones with the most loyal and sizable audiences. Those children self-identify as storytellers, a fact which is confirmed by their audiences. Their craft is perfected as they watch Deaf adults tell stories at home, at school, at the Deaf club, or at various cultural events. In later life, at the Deaf club for example, the self-identified storyteller volunteers to tell a story at some event. This later storytelling is sometimes more formal—for example, bearing witness to the acts and character of important Deaf figures or to significant events (how we founded the club) or relating part of Deaf culture (the abbé de l'Epée meets the two Deaf sisters). In order to become a storyteller, it seems one must be able to control language and nonverbal communication, react to audience response, and make suitable selections from a repertory of stories. Naturally, being a successful storyteller also requires one to be observant and feel the pulse of the DEAF–WORLD, and what one learns is then reflected in the way one selects and relates the stories.

As in many if not all cultures, there are archetypal stories in the DEAF–WORLD. One genre is the "success story," with the following skeletal structure: The protagonist grows up in an exclusively hearing environment, never having met any Deaf people. Later he meets a Deaf person who teaches him signed language and instructs him in the way of Deaf people's lives. He becomes more and more involved in the DEAF–WORLD and leaves his past behind. Carol Padden points out that in much the same way as Americans support and propagate the "American Dream," these Deaf success stories reinforce the belief that it is good and right to be Deaf.[39]

Another widespread genre is the legend of origins. One such story in hearing cultures is that of the founding of Rome, in which a wolf suckles

Romulus and Remus, twins fathered by the god Mars. The Deaf story of the abbé de l'Epée, and how he founded Deaf education, has been told and retold countless times in America as well as in many other lands (the legend as told at the Deaf club in Marseilles, France, appears in this book in abridged form in chapter 3). It tells of Epée's encounter with two Deaf sisters that led him to establish the first schools for the Deaf, which would become small Deaf communities in cities and towns all over the world, where a signed language of broader communication frequently was formed, and where young Deaf children could receive their Deaf heritage. Indeed, the long tradition in France of calling Epée "the father of the Deaf" may have its roots in calling "father" the man who presides at the moment of origin and gives rise to that origin.

There is a legend of origins unique to the DEAF–WORLD in the U.S. It is the story of how Thomas Gallaudet met the little Deaf girl, Alice Cogswell, and was led to found the first school for the Deaf in the U.S. It is striking to notice the parallels. Both Epée and Gallaudet are humble hearing people, both are seeking a calling in life, and both are quite ignorant of the DEAF–WORLD and its unfair exclusion from education. Both have an epiphany, thanks to young Deaf women. They must acquire the signed language, symbolically enter the DEAF–WORLD that far, and then they are in a position to help Deaf people get access to education and, most important, to one another. Both genres, the success story and the legend of origins, move from the individual to the social, from silence to communication.

The same affirmation of community and redemption through identification with the DEAF–WORLD can be seen in the classic American Deaf folk tale, "Sign Language Saves a Life," recounted in Jack Gannon's *Deaf Heritage*. Here is the basic story line: A teenage Southern boy, Joshua Davis, was squirrel hunting on his hearing parents' plantation during the Civil War when he found himself surrounded by Union soldiers. Davis pointed to his ears and gestured that he was Deaf. The soldiers shoved him to a nearby house where his parents said that he was indeed Deaf. But the soldiers believed he was a spy "playing Deaf" and prepared to hang him. Then an officer arrived and, when told about the prisoner, fingerspelled to him "Are you Deaf?" The boy assured him he was and they conversed in signed language; it later came out that the officer had a Deaf brother. Davis was freed and after a while moved to Texas, where he raised seven children, five of them Deaf, and lived to eighty-four, never forgetting how close he had come to death when he was eighteen. As Padden points out, the story tells what will save you if you're Deaf—signed language; what will not—relying on primitive gestures or on speech; and who will save you—someone with a Deaf connection. All in all, DEAF–WORLD knowledge can save your life.[40]

The list of literary forms in the DEAF–WORLD is long. In chapter 4, we touched on ASL stories based on word play, and on ASL poetry and humor. In addition to theater, narratives, and legends, there are *anecdotes*, tales about the material culture of the Deaf community, such as mechanical clocks rigged with weights that fall at the appointed hour and awaken the Deaf owners with their vibrations. There are even tall tales, such as when the weights waken all the Deaf people in the town![41] There are allegories, like Ben's *Bird of a Different Feather*, the ASL fable of a Deaf child born into a hearing family. The story is rich in caricatures of hearing people: the bogus doctor who confirms the baby eaglet's defective straight beak and later recommends surgery; the priest and the faith healer; the principal of a school in straight beak education. Straight Beak's predicament, hovering between two different cultural "worlds," is reified in two different settings: the eagle world on the mountain with his biological parents, and the straight-beaked bird world of the valley, where his adoptive family lives.[42]

In common with the literature of many other minority cultures, DEAF–WORLD literature is recorded in part in the majority language, as well as in its own language. In the last century, at the same time as stories, legends, poetry and humor were passed down face-to-face in the DEAF–WORLD, there began to appear a DEAF–WORLD literature written in English. For example, John Carlin, born Deaf, attended the Pennsylvania School for the Deaf and became an accomplished draftsman and painter, a prominent spokesman in the DEAF–WORLD, and a poet. The first stanza of an 1847 poem by Carlin:

I move—a silent exile on this earth;
As in his dreary cell one doomed for life,
My tongue is mute, and closed ear heedeth not;
No gleam of hope this darken'd mind assures
That the blest power of speech shall e'er be known.[43]

A poem published by Raymond Luczak in 1992, *Learning to Speak Part I*, is also part of Deaf literature in English but, written a century and a half after Carlin's, it speaks in a quite different voice about a quite different cultural understanding of Deaf. The Deaf narrator of the poem recounts boyhood scenes in a small town where there was only one other Deaf person, Gramps, a peddler. Resignedly, the boy's parents hire a signed language teacher for him. The last stanza:

Mary Hoffman, didn't you know what
you had begun when
you agreed to teach me my first, and then, the
next sign until I couldn't stop, not until
I became Gramps, not mute but raging instead,
hands howling volumes?[44]

A 1987 meeting devoted to ASL poetry in Rochester, New York, gave rise to the more encompassing ASL literature conferences, held at the National Technical Institute for the Deaf in 1991 and 1996. These gatherings of poets, storytellers, playwrights, literary critics, and others, promote the creation, study and teaching of the literature of DEAF–WORLD culture. They are contemporary counterparts of the Deaf literary societies that, in the U.S., date from the last century, and offer to their members storytelling, poetry, drama, debates and monologues, some serious, others humorous.

We have spoken about humor in ASL in chapter 4, where we focused on ways in which the visual/manual modality of ASL creates special opportunities for humorists to play with the rules of grammar and to entertain and enlighten us. Such humor, as we pointed out, also contains cultural messages and plays an important role in cementing the society. There is likely to be humor when Deaf people gather for banquets, conventions, dances and the like. Because humor is deeply embedded in culture, if it is presented in translation, readers or listeners who do not share the author's culture are likely to find it not funny. This is no doubt what Sarah had in mind, in *Children of a Lesser God*, when she snapped at her speech therapist boyfriend, James, who had been boasting of how funny he was: "You're funny in hearing," she signed, "not Deaf."[45] French Deaf comedian Guy Bouchauveau makes the same point about the embedding of Deaf humor in Deaf culture. He noted that when Deaf adults laugh, a Deaf child can laugh, but if the adult is a hearing person, the child is commonly excluded from the understanding and the laughter.[46]

Deaf humor is frequently about oppression, as in this Deaf tale, translated from ASL:

> Three people are on a train: one Russian, one Cuban, and one Deaf person. The Russian is drinking from a bottle of vodka. She drinks about half the bottle, then throws it out the window. The Deaf person looks at her, surprised. "Why did you throw out a bottle that was half full?" The Russian replies, "Oh, in my country we have plenty of vodka." Meanwhile, the Cuban, who is smoking a rich aromatic cigar, abruptly tosses it out the window. The Deaf person is surprised again and asks, "Why did you throw out a half-smoked cigar?" The Cuban replies, "Oh, in my country we have plenty of cigars." The Deaf person nods with interest. A little while later a hearing person walks down the aisle. The Deaf person grabs the hearing person and throws him out the window. The Russian and the Cuban look up in amazement. The Deaf person shrugs, "In my country we have plenty of hearing people!"[47]

Deaf humor can be found not only in funny stories, caricatures, and absurd images, but also in cartooning. It is often said that Deaf people love comic strips. After all, their language is visual and comic strips, although they may contain some print, are a largely visual means of communication. Professor Lynn Jacobowitz of Gallaudet's School of Communication has sifted through a great many Deaf cartoons and finds that their themes fall into seven categories: visual; can't hear; linguistics; hearing dogs (a dog specially trained to respond to noises and alert owners); interpreters; politics; and response to oppression.[48] As with the humor of other minorities, some of it is an outlet for anger over oppression. Some is self-deprecatory and some self-congratulatory. All of it evokes the cultural recognition response and the associated glow of solidarity.

For more than a century, publications have been an important force bonding the members of the DEAF–WORLD in the United States. Publications kept scattered Deaf people informed about the lives of their peers, school friends, and leaders. They informed Deaf people about social and political gatherings, about athletics and opportunities for employment.

Since the Deaf have had limited access to the telephone, publications and gatherings were the two main ways of staying in touch. Because printing was a leading trade taught in the residential schools, numerous schools had their own newspapers that chronicled current events, reprinted stories from other newspapers and magazines, published poetry, and included items about prominent Deaf people such as "Dummy" Hoy, the baseball star. There were editorials, too, and discussions of Deaf education and signed language. In 1893, an organization of all the school newspapers was founded, the *Little Paper Family Editorial Association*. Other newspapers were established by Deaf publishers to serve the interests of the DEAF–WORLD. *The Silent Worker* began early in the twentieth century as a newspaper, but was transformed into a magazine, taken over by the NAD, and renamed the *Deaf American* in 1964. In addition, many state associations of the Deaf and various agencies publish newspapers and newsletters. One that we particularly enjoy is the *DCARA News* from the Deaf Counseling, Advocacy and Referral Agency in San Leandro, California. Nowadays, leading DEAF–WORLD newspapers nationally include *Silent News* and *The NAD Broadcaster*; leading magazines, *Deaf Life* and *Gallaudet Today*.

An important development in DEAF–WORLD publishing in the U.S., no doubt a consequence of the growing acceptance of ASL and Deaf culture here in recent times, has been the advent of publishing houses that publish books, videotapes and other materials exclusively concerning the DEAF–WORLD. Some of the longest-standing publishers include Gallaudet University Press, TJ Publishers, and the National Association of the Deaf. However, a new breed of more focused publishers has been growing since the mid 1980s, for example, DawnSignPress in San Diego, California (emphasis on ASL study, art, poetry, and literature, including Ben's *Bird of a Different Feather*), and Sign Media in Burtonsville, Maryland (ASL and Deaf culture, including an ASL version on videotape of Harlan's *When the Mind Hears: A History of the Deaf*). To facilitate the dissemination of publications relating to Deaf culture, distributors have proliferated, among them Harris Communications and the GLAD (Greater Los Angeles Council on Deafness), DCARA, NAD, and Gallaudet University bookstores.

Shared Oppression

Four common characteristics of minorities that underpin affiliation are (1) the group shares a common physical or cultural characteristic, such as skin color or language, (2) individuals identify themselves as members of the minority and others identify them in that way, (3) there is a tendency to marry within the minority, and (4) minority members suffer oppression. The DEAF–WORLD finds unifying force on all four counts. First, its members share a common physical characteristic: their primary source of information is vision. This is of the greatest importance as a solidifying force, for as long as human variation engenders visual people, there will be a constitutional basis for affiliation and there will be a manual-visual language. Put in other words: The DEAF–WORLD is the one minority that can never be totally assimilated or eradicated.

To a large extent, members of the Deaf minority also share a common language (ASL in the U.S.) and, because of their common physical characteristic, that language will never die out. On the second count, Deaf people do indeed identify themselves as culturally Deaf and, third, they marry Deaf nine times out of ten. Finally, Deaf people do indeed suffer oppression. Both Carlin's and Luczak's poems, for example, reflect the oppression that members of the DEAF–WORLD experience. On the face of it, Carlin came to see himself, living in a hearing world with hearing parents, as many hearing people saw him: isolated, limited, yearning for his "tongue to be unbound" in heaven. If so, then Carlin had internalized the oppression of the DEAF–WORLD. Luczak, on the other hand, rages against it, "howling volumes."

Oppression is a unifying force when sufficient numbers of the oppressed minority are, like Luczak, raging, for their appeal goes forth to minimize differences within the minority in the effort to vanquish a common enemy. In some ways like the members of other language minorities that have been colonized, members of the DEAF–WORLD frequently find themselves subjected to the wishes of outsiders pursuing an alien agenda that enhances the outsiders' economic and social standing. The Deaf person is cast in the subservient role of pupil, patient, client and employee, while the outsider, from the majority culture, takes the dominant role.[49] The list of professions serving the Deaf is imposing and includes administrators of schools for Deaf children and of training programs for Deaf adults, teachers of Deaf children and adults, interpreters, some audiologists, speech therapists, otologists, experts in schools, mental health and rehabilitation counselors, psychologists, psychiatrists, librarians, researchers, social workers, and hearing-aid specialists. These interventions and services on demand are well-intentioned, and some are valued highly in the DEAF–WORLD, but the fact remains that they are predicated on an imbalance of power that can be, and all too often is, oppressive. The point is not missed by many of the professionals involved, who individually and through their organizations have been trying to redress the balance. We will return to this theme later in our journey into the DEAF–WORLD.

Discrimination against Deaf people in employment has been a constant part of life in the DEAF–WORLD and has contributed to longstanding cultural customs, such as seeking jobs with the help of employed Deaf friends. This also ensures continued contact in job situations which, with the Deaf club and Deaf spouse at home, are the sequel to the Deaf school as settings for Deaf socializing and socialization.

The struggle in childhood and adolescence for language and identity is particularly keen in the DEAF–WORLD, as we have seen, because most Deaf children, born Deaf, cannot receive from their hearing parents their Deaf language and Deaf cultural heritage. Hearing parents might well protest that their child's heritage, whether the child be Deaf or hearing, is *their* culture and *their* language, and they are quite able to pass it on. But logic and experience teach otherwise. Where there are cultures whose members have a characteristic physical constitution, all the children with that constitution are seen as the rightful recipients of that culture to some degree. As we see it, Black children, for example, however raised, have Black heritage from the day they are born. Accordingly, the National Association of Black Social Workers is opposed to trans-racial adoption on the grounds that it will deprive such children of their heritage. We need not decide at this juncture whether it is more important for these Black children to be adopted as quickly as possible or to take possession of their heritage; the relevant point is that they *do* have such a heritage at birth. Similarly, the Deaf child, however raised, has a Deaf heritage from birth. The child's life trajectory will normally take him or her into the DEAF–WORLD. The Deaf child can be deprived of the opportunity to acculturate to that world, as can the Black child, but the child's potential travels with the child. Reasonable people might, and do, reason differently on this adoption issue, but experience with regard to Deaf children is more univocal. Most children who cannot communicate well in spoken language will, when allowed to, learn signed language, become acculturated to Deaf culture, marry Deaf, and identify themselves as members of the DEAF–WORLD.

A distinguished otologist has contended that Deaf children start out in mainstream hearing society and enter the DEAF–WORLD in adolescence.[50] Yet, how could Deaf children start out in hearing society when they do not speak the language of that society and have not become, through the language, acculturated to it? No, they are Deaf, even though they are frequently not allowed to take possession of their Deaf heritage until either they attend school with Deaf peers or are old enough to make their own decisions. In ethnic minorities, where culture and constitution are usually congruent, one's first loyalty may be to the family, which is the setting for acculturation as well as nurture; loyalty to the ethnic minority comes second. But most children in the DEAF–WORLD cannot communicate with their parents who know no signed language, and while their home may be nurturing, it cannot be substantially acculturating. We speculate that those conditions engender a special measure of loyalty and commitment to the DEAF–WORLD, where acculturation can finally take place.

The anomaly of having culturally different parents is then both a centrifugal and centripetal force in the DEAF–WORLD. It tends to splinter and separate Deaf people in several ways. It discourages their pride in their minority identity. It delays their language acquisition. It may well lead to their education, isolated from other Deaf pupils and role models, in the local hearing school. It frequently commits them, through articulation drills and cochlear implant surgery, to values and behaviors repellent to members of the DEAF–WORLD. At the same time, the anomaly propels Deaf people toward the DEAF–WORLD, since identification with the DEAF–WORLD offers pride, language, instruction, role models, a culturally compatible spouse, and more that cannot be had elsewhere.

DIVERSITY IN THE DEAF–WORLD

Since visual people are found in all ethnic groups and walks of life in the U.S., our DEAF–WORLD is extraordinarily diverse. In a nation committed to the principle that we are all created equal, it is heartening to see one community that embraces its diversity so extensively (though not utterly without bigotry). At a recent meeting of the Boston Deaf Club, for example, gathered to celebrate its fiftieth anniversary, we noted Black, Hispanic and Asian members of the DEAF–WORLD. There were many women members (including the president), and numerous older members (some of the founders were given plaques on this occasion). There were Gay and Lesbian members. There was a table of Deaf–Blind members, each accompanied by a Deaf interpreter, and there were members with other disabilities. To some degree, then, shared language, culture, and experience attenuate the differences in the DEAF–WORLD that are so divisive outside it.

Although there are many forces that bind Deaf people together in the DEAF–WORLD, there is also discrimination when it comes to gender and sexual orientation, ethnicity and disability. Thus, women did not gain equal standing with men in the DEAF–WORLD for a long time. It was one hundred years after the founding of the NAD when it elected its first woman president, Gertrude Galloway. Today there are distinguished Deaf women political leaders, scholars, actresses, artists, athletes, business people, teachers, and so on.[51] There is also a social, political, and charitable organization to promote the interests of Deaf women, called Deaf Women United, Inc. (DWU). Nevertheless, stereotypes about women endure in the DEAF–WORLD, as they do in our larger society. A Massachusetts survey concerning gender roles in 1993 found, for example, views on ironing clothes particularly marked. Deaf women definitely thought it was their job. Deaf and hearing men agreed that it was women's work, but to a lesser degree than the Deaf women. Hearing women were much less convinced that ironing was women's work, though they, too, rated it slightly more a female task than a gender–neutral task.[52]

Black Deaf Americans have a triple heritage. Their lives are shaped historically by Black culture in America. The U.S. Black community is highly diverse, embracing people with French, Spanish and African heritages. Then there is the Deaf heritage that Blacks share with other members of the DEAF–WORLD, to which this chapter is addressed. In addition, there is a long Black Deaf tradition in America's Deaf community, which reaches back to the special residential schools for "colored" children that were founded in the mid-nineteenth century and abolished about a century later. A distinct Black dialect of ASL arose in that setting, as we mentioned in chapter 3, and continues in use. It is only partly intelligible to most white Deaf speakers of ASL.[53] In the early 1950s, thirteen states were operating separate and segregated schools for Black Deaf children, where the emphasis was on vocational training. As late as 1963, eight states still had separate schools for these children. Many of these schools had close and valuable ties to historically Black colleges, from which vocational and academic teachers were often recruited; those ties were broken when desegregation closed the schools and sent the pupils into formerly all-white schools for the Deaf. Numerous Black clubs have been founded over the years, most recently by and for Black women, an outgrowth of the women's rights movement of the 1970s.[54] Studies of Black people in the Chicago and Washington, DC Deaf communities in the 1980s reported that clubs and congregations were segregated, and the races rarely intermingled.[55] The history of Black Deaf culture cries out for scholarly investigation, but it has received very little indeed.

Today, the National Black Deaf Advocates (NBDA), along with several regional programs, pursues the agenda of their double minority.[56] NBDA, founded in 1982, now has nineteen chapters serving over 700 members. There is much to do. There are low expectations of Black Deaf children. There are too few Black Deaf teachers and other professionals. There is a lack of Black interpreters (the National Alliance of Black Interpreters counts sixty-eight members). There is little awareness of Black Deaf history and culture and of the achievements of Black Deaf leaders, such as rehabilitation expert Glenn Anderson, chair of the Gallaudet University Board of Trustees.[57]

Earlier we emphasized the common bonds in the DEAF–WORLD that unite minorities within the minority. However, the continuing segregation of some Deaf clubs, and the decision of Black Deaf people to form their own national organization, remind us of some of the tensions on those bonds.[58] A sampling of the Black Deaf community in Washington, DC, found that eighty-seven percent identify themselves as Black before they identify themselves as Deaf.[59] (Of those who identified themselves as Deaf first, the majority had Deaf parents and had attended a residential school for the Deaf.) Black Deaf leaders point to facts such as these: Gallaudet University admitted its first Black Deaf student, Andrew Foster (of whom more later, when we examine the world Deaf scene) only in 1951, nearly a century after Gallaudet opened its doors. In 1964, there was only a handful of Black students on campus.[60] Twenty-five years later, one hundred fifty of Gallaudet's two thousand students were Black.[61] There were no Black members of the National Association of the Deaf until 1965. In short, practices in the DEAF-WORLD, as in other minorities, have reflected the massive discrimination against Black people in the larger hearing society.

Black and Hispanic children comprise a disproportionate one–third of Deaf children in the United States. In the South over half the Deaf students surveyed in a 1989 study were Black. In the West, nearly half were Hispanic. In California, sixty-one percent were from minorities. Thus, minority Deaf children are actually in the majority in some regions, and their numbers are growing rapidly.

Double minority children may face double prejudice in education. Deaf children from non-English speaking families are three to four times more likely to be labeled learning disabled, mentally retarded or emotionally disturbed. It is impossible to say to what extent this labeling reflects faulty means of evaluation or downright prejudice, and to what extent it reflects real differences in prevalence of disabilities. However, as we shall show in chapter 11, Deaf students are seriously disadvantaged in psychological and achievement testing because of the English-language and cultural bias of the tests; Hispanic Deaf students are doubly disadvantaged. Likewise, Black and Hispanic Deaf children score well below white peers on achievement tests. They are more likely to drop out of high school or to be tracked into vocational rather than academic programs. Those who finish high school are less likely to go on to college. Minorities comprise thirty-seven percent of all Deaf schoolchildren but only seven percent of their teachers. Hence there is a near absence of role models for many of the children, who find little in their curriculum that relates clearly to their identity and their lives. These educational handicaps of minorities within the DEAF-WORLD take their toll on life fulfillment, economic success, and minority leadership in the subsequent years.

Black and Hispanic Deaf children are less likely than white Deaf children to have a signed language used at home. Therefore, as a group, they have less than average opportunities for communication, and this may contribute to their academic disadvantage. Perhaps they are less likely to have Deaf family members, or perhaps their parents are less able to find signed language classes that suit their schedules and neighborhood. Language plays a central role in Hispanic culture, yet Hispanic parents will have great difficulty in teaching Spanish to their Deaf children, and their efforts will not be seconded by the school. Roberto Rivera, at the Metro Silent Club, reported that his mother spoke no English, his father only a little, and neither knew ASL. But Roberto's best languages were ASL and English. Spanish can be a barrier not only within the family, but also between the family and the school. The Hispanic Deaf pupil in the U.S. is inevitably engaged in an effort to master three languages and their expressive forms: the language of the home and the language of the school (neither of which is fully accessible), and the language of the DEAF–WORLD. Hispanic children who are immigrants to the U.S. will arrive with a significant disadvantage if they come from countries in which education is not available to many Deaf children or in which it is conducted orally.[62] Although hearing Hispanic children nationwide receive bilingual and bicultural education, they are usually deprived of that opportunity if they are Deaf, which is all the more regrettable since bilingual/bicultural education has much to offer ASL-speaking children (as we will argue in chapter 10).[63] Hispanic Deaf adults are also disadvantaged: interpreters, relay services, and appropriate captioning are very rare.[64] The National Hispanic Council of the Deaf, founded in 1992, has been laboring to promote the interests of this minority.

Terms like *Black* and *Hispanic* can mask the enormous diversity of the adults and children so designated. The term *Hispanic*, for example, groups individuals whose ancestors were born in the U.S. together with those who have immigrated recently. It combines people from homes where only English is spoken, and homes where one or another variety of Spanish is spoken. It pools people with cultural backgrounds as different as those of mainland Spain, Puerto Rico, and Venezuela. The category *Asian and Pacific Island* also exists more for bureaucratic reasons than by any logic. The Census Bureau acknowledges some seventeen different groups in this category: some are refugees from the Vietnam War; others come from centuries-old U.S. families. There has been a large influx of this disparate group in recent decades. In 1991, forty percent of immigrants were from Latin American countries and another forty percent from Asian / Pacific Island countries.[65] Many Deaf immigrants arriving on U.S. shores find that their signed language is utterly unknown in the U.S. DEAF–WORLD. Still others arrive without any signed language. Approximately four percent of Deaf schoolchildren in the U.S. come from the Asian and Pacific Island group. The first-ever Asian Deaf conference in the U.S. was held in San Francisco in 1994. At the second meeting in 1997, the National Asian Deaf Congress was founded.

Native American children are also a diverse and disadvantaged group. Half of them reside in rural areas. There are 278 reservations in the U.S. and 209 Alaska villages, but no two tribes have the same cultural characteristics, and many native languages are still in use. Nearly half of the children live at or below federal poverty levels. The difficulties in making language-appropriate and valid assessments of abilities and achievement, and in providing culturally sensitive educational practices, are enormous. Native American Deaf children who leave home to attend a residential school, as most do, must make difficult decisions about where and how to establish themselves after graduation: on the reservation with hearing Native American families and friends, in urban areas with the DEAF–WORLD, or in border towns with limited access to both groups. Native Americans have the highest birth rate of the groups discussed, so while their numbers in Deaf education are still small (an estimated six percent), they are projected to grow.[66] An organization of Native American Deaf people was founded in 1994 and held its first convention that year.

Gay and Lesbian Deaf people face several particular challenges within the DEAF–WORLD. Because the community is small, and because of the premium on plain talk in ASL, it may be more difficult for Deaf than for hearing Gays and Lesbians to keep their sexual orientation private if they choose to do so. If they openly seek a partner, they may find only a small number of people within the DEAF–WORLD eligible. This may make it more likely for Gay and Lesbian Deaf people than for other Deaf minorities to seek a partner outside the DEAF–WORLD. Nevertheless, at least one student of Deaf Gay culture contends that Deaf Gay males are Deaf first and Gay second.[67] In the wake of Gay liberation following the Stonewall riot of 1969 (incited by an unprovoked police raid on the Stonewall, a New York City bar frequented by Gays), an international organization of Deaf Gays and Lesbians, the Rainbow Alliance of the Deaf, was founded; it has chapters in many states and provinces in North America. Deaf Gay and Lesbian people have been empowered in recent decades as never before. The first social service program in the U.S. to focus on the needs of Gay and Lesbian Deaf people opened in 1992 in San Francisco. The Deaf Gay and Lesbian Coalition (DGLC) provides peer counseling, support groups, community education, a hotline, workshops and more. Its clientele has grown exponentially.[68] In the words of a recent anthology of Deaf Gay and Lesbian literature: "Oh, it is such a joy to be able to see each other's faces without having to strain our eyes in the dark."[69]

Estimates of the number of people in the U.S. who are both Deaf and Blind vary widely; a medical source gives 16,000; a Department of Education survey estimates 42,000 by the most exclusive definition, 425,000 with a criterion of severely limited use of one sense and no use of the other.[70] The number of Deaf-Blind people in the DEAF–WORLD has not been estimated. Many of these started life as sighted Deaf people, learned ASL, became acculturated to the DEAF–WORLD, and then gradually lost some or all vision. There are numerous systems of communication in use among people with severely limited sight and hearing, but signed language is favored by those in the DEAF–WORLD. When conversing in ASL, persons with restricted visual fields (tunnel vision) prefer to stand back from their interlocutor in order to see more of the signer's face and hands and may ask the signer to restrict the signing space. For the same purpose, they may rest their hands lightly on the signer's wrists, guiding them (this is called *tracking*). With more restricted vision, Deaf-Blind people will commonly use touch to "read" the ASL, placing their hands over those of their interlocutor. The change in ASL modality, from visual to tactile sign, affects its production, since information on the face and subtle differences in the use of space are not accessible, while tension in the speaker's hands can be detected. Modifications when producing tactual ASL include choosing one sign rather than another based on its tactile properties, and elaborating the production of a sign so that it is more readily perceived.

Interpreters serving Deaf-Blind clients provide different kinds of information than those serving Deaf clients. For example, they will describe who is present, what of significance is happening in the room, the speaker's facial expressions, and so forth. Support service providers (SSPs) also play an important role in the lives of Deaf-Blind people, serving as guides, reading mail and other text, and in various ways facilitating their clients' participation in community life.

The capacity of Deaf-Blind people for education and professional careers is more recognized today than ever before, but they are still excluded needlessly from many kinds of employment. More than one hundred Deaf-Blind Americans have earned college degrees and several have gone on to obtain doctorates.[71] The American Association of the Deaf-Blind (600 members) promotes the interests of this minority. At the last biennial convention of the association in 1994, there were some 250 Deaf-Blind people and 400 people working as interpreters and SSPs.

As with the other "double minorities" within the DEAF–WORLD, this one has several unique features. Deaf-Blind people, like Deaf people, do not need interpreters in one-to-one conversations if both parties know ASL. However, in a group setting, communication among Deaf-Blind people requires several interpreters. For example, at a recent meeting of the Boston Deaf-Blind club Contact, the club president spoke from the stage while a score of interpreters, mostly Deaf, "relayed" her signing to their Deaf-Blind clients, who sat beside them. This reliance on interpreters means that Deaf-Blind people must take special measures not to miss out on incidental information more readily accessible to others. Sadly, many Deaf-Blind people report that as their vision diminished, so did their contact with Deaf people, who turned away, even at the Deaf club.[72] Of course, transportation and employment also pose special obstacles. Nevertheless, wherever there are sizable numbers of Deaf-Blind people and support services such as transportation and SSPs, Deaf-Blind people commonly lead rich and rewarding lives. Computer technology, electronic bulletin boards and the Internet are also connecting Deaf-Blind people to one another and to the rest of society as never before.

Another minority within the Deaf community is that comprised of people with disabilities.[73] A 1982 survey of Deaf schoolchildren found that thirty percent had at least one such disability. However, available estimates of prevalence are untrustworthy, because they include not only criterion-based disabilities such as motor impairment and mental retardation, but also several categories of disability for which there are no objective criteria for membership. These categories that are not criterion-based include *learning disabled* and *emotionally disturbed*; they accounted for fourteen percent in the survey.[74] In the years 1964–1965, a worldwide rubella epidemic caused the birth rate of Deaf infants to double and also brought about a marked increase in the number of Deaf children born with impairments such as blindness and mental retardation. The "rubella bulge" reached the schools toward the end of the decade, resulting in expanded programming to meet the needs of this special population. Mental retardation and visual and motor impairments may interfere with the Deaf child's ability to acquire signed language and they pose additional educational challenges. Such children perform well below their Deaf peers without disabilities.[75] At the end of their schooling, Deaf students with disabilities face limited employment opportunities. On a more positive note, the disability rights movement in the U.S. and around the world has contributed to improving conditions for people with disabilities.

Members of the DEAF–WORLD are living longer in the U.S. while, as we have mentioned, the younger generations take less of an interest in the Deaf club. In other words, many Deaf clubs are "graying." This creates some stresses. For example, the classic flight of stairs leading up to the Deaf club, once a symbol of the club's special status as "a place apart," has become, in Boston in any event, an obstacle to the older members. Younger and older members of the club may have somewhat different priorities when it comes to, for example, athletics. They also tend to have different backgrounds. Most older Deaf men learned trades in school and had difficulty finding jobs other than in areas such as printing and carpentry. Many older Deaf women were primarily homemakers, although some took jobs related to work like sewing. Life in industry with few or no Deaf co-workers put a premium on the easy sociability of the Deaf club. Younger Deaf men and women, however, frequently have had more educational opportunity; there is, indeed, a Deaf professional middle class in the United States. In addition to the impact of the simple changing of generations, these social differences are associated with differences in interests, resources, and language use.

Nevertheless, the bonds of membership in the DEAF-WORLD are much stronger than these age differences. Friendships maintained at the club reduce social isolation for elderly Deaf people and such friendships may also help them cope with practical problems such as transportation. Then, too, the culture has always accorded special respect to its older members. They frequently have the longest records of activism in behalf of the community and they are repositories of its history. At the centennial convention of the National Association of the Deaf in 1980, a Deaf senior citizens section was formed. It was not until 1992, however, that the first national conference of Deaf senior citizens was convened. Following the second such conference, two years later, the National Association of Deaf Senior Citizens was established.

Another important minority group within the DEAF-WORLD are codas, hearing people who are children of Deaf adults. When they are quite young, codas in the U.S. commonly learn two languages and two cultures: those of the DEAF-WORLD and those of the larger hearing society that surrounds it. Thus they commonly become signed language interpreters and cultural mediators while they are still children. However, perhaps an equal number of codas do not learn ASL, many because their Deaf parents were falsely told that using ASL inhibits learning English.

Birth order and gender play a large role in the learning of ASL by hearing family members. Typically, the oldest child will learn ASL. If the oldest child is a female, she almost assuredly will, for she will be assigned many duties mediating between Deaf and hearing cultures. However, sometimes her siblings do not learn ASL very well. In some ways, they are like a Deaf child in a hearing family, because they grow up without fully understanding their parents' culture, and they must rely on others to communicate with their parents substantively. As adults, such codas function almost totally like hearing people, even though they come from a Deaf family. Many lead lives completely separate from their parents, and they never share in the culture of the DEAF-WORLD.

Most codas who learn ASL when quite young spend some time every day mediating issues between Deaf and hearing cultures. Most of these issues arise from the mutual ignorance of hearing and Deaf people concerning one another's cultures.[76] Unfortunately, most Deaf parents have nowhere to turn to learn all the rules of the hearing culture that they sometimes need to know, and there is no place hearing people can commonly turn to get accurate information regarding the DEAF–WORLD. Codas are recurrently put in the position of explaining both worlds to members of each. Almost all codas perform this function without any training except life's experiences. Those experiences of cross-cultural mediation can be rewarding, but frequently they are hurtful because of the prevailing negative views about Deaf people, the coda's parents, which are held by hearing people.

Deaf parents may ask their hearing children about the hearing world, how hearing people live, about sounds, and about English. Hearing friends will ask corresponding questions about the DEAF–WORLD. How do Deaf people use the phone? Can they drive? Since codas commonly serve, then, as a critical link to the alien hearing culture, a source of information for making decisions, and a spokesperson for the family, some grow up feeling they have been deprived of their childhood. On the other hand, they grow up with a command of the languages and cultural knowledge of two worlds, as Bob has done, and they frequently choose careers that build on those strengths.[77]

In a sense, the coda is "almost Deaf." Codas possess the cultural part of being Deaf, including DEAF–WORLD Knowledge, but they lack the physical difference and hence the experiences associated with it, experiences such as being stigmatized as deviant and attending a school for the Deaf. In effect, they are positioned between two cultures with behaviors learned from both. Deaf people's ambivalence on codas' standing in the DEAF–WORLD (and codas' own ambivalence, for that matter) seems to reflect this ambiguity in many codas' life situations: they've got the culture, but they do not have the constitution. Some codas say they feel shut out from the DEAF–WORLD, while at the same time feeling somewhat alien in hearing society. Recent decades seem to have been empowering for codas, as for other minorities in the DEAF–WORLD. They have written a spate of autobiographies to explain their unique situation to themselves and others. In 1983, codas founded a national organization, called CODA, that brings them together for mutual reflection and support; about six years ago, the organization opened its ranks to codas around the world.[78]

We have been examining what might be called horizontal diversity in the DEAF–WORLD. There is stratification as well. Individuals and groups differ in their standing. As we have seen, the DEAF–WORLD is not immune to racism, sexism, homophobia and other forms of discrimination. Deaf people have accused their own culture, which values unity and sees Deaf people as members of a family, of operating according to a "crab" theory, in which the group pulls down any of its members who crawl too high. Be that as it may, there are several ways in which members of the DEAF–WORLD can distinguish themselves and earn the respect and appreciation of their peers: we have spoken about the storyteller and Miss Deaf America; now let's turn to Deaf leaders.

Whether the minority leader be Martin Luther King, Caesar Chavez or Fred Schreiber, the late revered executive director of the National Association of the Deaf, the leader's traits throw much light on how the minority culture evaluates its members. A review of contemporary Deaf leaders in America would reveal that two relatively small groups within the DEAF–WORLD play a disproportionately large role in leading it. The first of these are leaders who were born hearing to hearing parents and became Deaf after learning to speak English. Such leaders are particularly to be found in roles and organizations that have extensive contact with the larger hearing society; we might call them *inter-cultural leaders*. Inference suggests that one of the goals of evaluation in the DEAF–WORLD has been to select Deaf leaders who will be effective advocates for Deaf people vis-à-vis hearing people, and so it places weight on the leader's ability to speak and write English.

A second group in the DEAF–WORLD that is extensively represented in leadership roles are members with Deaf parents. These leaders are predominantly to be found in positions in which cultural knowledge of the DEAF–WORLD and fluency in ASL are particularly valuable. For example, they may work in a residential school for Deaf children, hold office in a Deaf club, or manage a Deaf athletic organization. We will call them *culturally centered* Deaf leaders; they are sometimes called *grass roots leaders*. The training ground for many of them has been positions of responsibility in the residential schools, like manager of the softball team. Their skills were further honed in the Deaf club, where they were identified as having the knowledge and skills to be leaders.

This schematic picture of leadership in the DEAF–WORLD focuses on cultural forces and thus leaves out what is most important about leaders, namely their individual traits such as charisma, skill in managing people, physical appearance, motivation and so forth. And of course, all kinds of Deaf leaders are found in all kinds of settings. Indeed, the distinction we have made between inter-cultural leaders and culturally centered leaders appears to be breaking down. Ever since the Gallaudet Revolution (though perhaps the forces were already in play before then), the culturally centered leaders have increasingly assumed responsibilities in both inter- and intra-cultural roles.

Considering all the powerful forces that bind Deaf people together in the DEAF–WORLD, from language, schools and sports, to organizations, arts and oppression, it is no surprise that well-acculturated Deaf men and women find great strength in their Deaf identity. As we examine the growing body of knowledge concerning Deaf people all around the globe, we find that they vary widely from one nation to the next in their ability to find that strength, to acquire a full language, a proud identity, a knowledge of Deaf heritage, and thus a gratifying place in Deaf as well as hearing society. Comparing conditions for Deaf people in a wide variety of hearing societies can help us to discover which conditions favor and which oppose the growth of strong DEAF–WORLDS and strong Deaf people. We turn to that comparison in the next chapter.

❦

Chapter 6

The World Deaf Scene

CONDITIONS for Deaf children and adults vary widely around the world, and this should not be surprising. Economically, some societies are predominantly agrarian, while others, benefiting from an industrial revolution nearly two centuries ago, are in the throes of a technological revolution. The cultures of the world's nations respond to diversity in general, and to Deaf people in particular, in very different ways, as do their laws. Then, too, many nations have been colonized, and their differing histories of colonization have left differing practices in their wake with regard to all minorities, including Deaf people. All these factors combine with geography to influence the ability of Deaf people to congregate, to forge a common language, to advocate for their own interests, and to participate in national political life.

Thus we can only sample the world Deaf scene in this chapter—all the more so as it has received very little comparative study. We begin with case studies of two European nations, France and Sweden, that contrast markedly in the place reserved in their societies for the DEAF-WORLD. Then we venture some generalizations about the conditions of Deaf people in the "first world." Next, we turn to two developing nations in Africa, Kenya and Burundi, for contrastive case studies. Finally, we report some findings of a 1988 survey on Deaf people in the "third world."

The First World

France

France is an obligatory stop on any worldwide tour of the DEAF–WORLD. France was the cradle of Western Deaf education. More signed languages in the Western world today, including ASL, trace their roots to French signed language (LSF) than to any other.[1] And it was a Deaf Frenchman, Laurent Clerc, who established (with Thomas Gallaudet) Deaf education in the United States and built a nationwide network of residential schools that has made the American DEAF–WORLD what it is today.

As we have seen, the first public school for the Deaf in history, and the inspiration and model for hundreds soon to follow, was established in Paris in the 1760s by the abbé de l'Epée. The school created educated leaders among the Deaf, instilling pride in themselves and their language, as well as giving them an elevated vision of what the Deaf could become. It earned for its founder the gratitude of Deaf people down to the present. In December 1789, as Epée lay dying, a delegation from the legislature of the new French Republic joined the pupils at his bedside to tell him that his most fervent wish, the certain continuation of his school, was assured; it was proclaimed a national institution. This epochal moment in Western Deaf history was painted by French Deaf artist Frédéric Peyson (1807-1877), a student of Ingrès, and was displayed at the Paris *Salon des Beaux-Arts* in 1839.

The first generation European schools gave birth, in turn, to many more. In France, as schools proliferated, LSF became the predominant language among the pupils and Deaf faculty, although Signed French was often used in the classroom. LSF and Signed French were constantly under attack and frequently banned in favor of the exclusive use of French.[2] From its birth in 1789, the new nation felt threatened by the diversity of languages within its borders, all the more so as some of these languages, such as German, were spoken across its borders by its enemies. The legislature created primary schools where all children would learn French, and only French would be used in instruction.[3] From time to time renewed efforts had to be made, however, to discourage the use of minority languages in the schools.

Beginning in the 1830s, signed and spoken French fell largely into disuse in the French schools for the Deaf, which increasingly relied on LSF for instruction. Then came the Congress of Milan, attended by a large French delegation, and its infamous resolutions. The French government, complying like all others with the Milan resolutions, banished LSF from public education of its Deaf children and fired all Deaf teachers, on the grounds that they would be likely to use LSF.

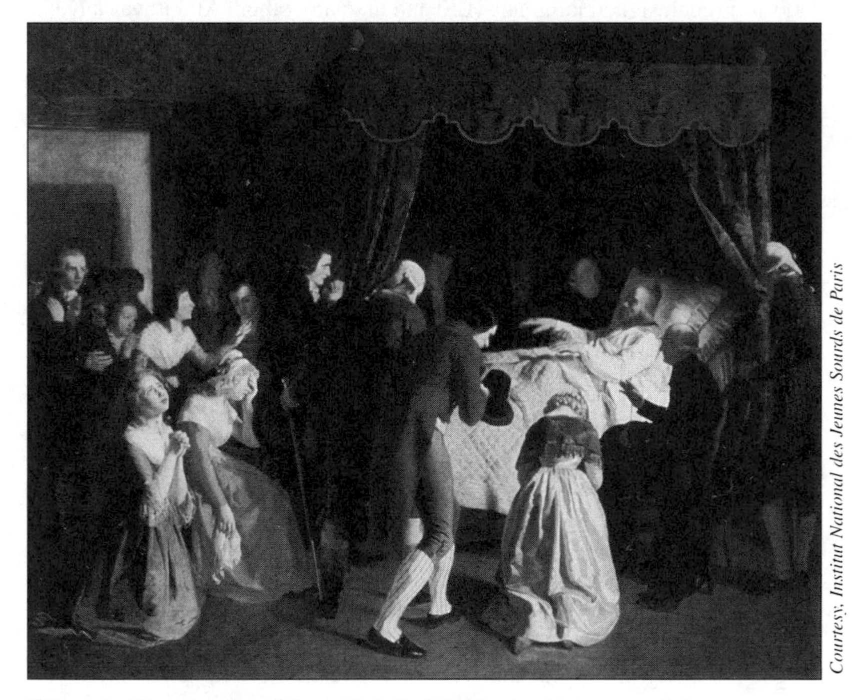

Courtesy, Institut National des Jeunes Sourds de Paris

Fig. 6-1. **The Death of the abbé de l'Epée, by F. Peyson (1839)**

"No more Laurent Clercs," lamented the director of the Paris school in a ceremony of adieu to the Deaf teachers, "No more Berthiers . . . The complete disappearance of mime has yet other sadnesses in store for us. We will have to discharge several teachers, as devoted as they are distinguished, whose only fault is to be deaf. It is not without great heartache—and I speak for all the institution—that we see step down from their chairs men like Dusuzeau [science teacher and Deaf leader], Tessières [author of the national curriculum for Deaf pupils], and Théobald [history teacher and Deaf leader], like M. Tronc, our devoted writing teacher, like M. Simon, our excellent deputy headmaster. I know, dear colleagues, with what selflessness you accede to this difficult sacrifice. You recognize that the welfare of the pupils is at stake and therefore you raise not a word of complaint in these painful circumstances . . ."[4]

Shortly thereafter, the government banished all minority languages (among them Basque, Breton, Occitan and LSF) from all its schools, both hearing and Deaf, decreeing the schools free, monolingually Francophone, and compulsory until age thirteen.

During the century that elapsed between the founding of Epée's school and the banishment of LSF, a formally structured Deaf society had developed in Paris and in many provincial cities. The earliest Deaf association, founded in 1834 by a towering intellectual in French Deaf history, Ferdinand Berthier (see box on p. 178), provided mutual aid, and an athletic, cultural and leisure program to its adult Deaf members.[5] In the years following the Milan Congress, additional Deaf organizations sprang up, as did numerous newspapers published by and for Deaf people. Although Deaf adults could no longer work in education, many found employment in printing, and there were numerous outstanding Deaf artists and sculptors, many of whose works were displayed at the prestigious annual *Salon* exhibits of French art, presented by the French Academy. Deaf leaders were active politically in securing civil rights for Deaf people, such as the right to marriage and to an education, and in protesting the hearing hegemony of Deaf education. This activism was reflected in three international congresses on the Deaf held in Paris around the turn of the century.[6]

By the end of the nineteenth century, the French colonial adventure had subjugated vast regions of Africa and Asia and imposed spoken French as the official language, particularly in the schools. Although most former French colonies had gained their independence by the 1960s, French activism aimed at promulgating the French language continues to this day. There is, indeed, a government high commission for the purpose. The colonial and neocolonial argument that the French make for their language is two-pronged. First, French is one of the world's great languages, with resources in grammar, vocabulary and texts that can enable people in developing nations to gain access to the world's store of knowledge, its corridors of power, and its boardrooms of commerce. Second, the local languages cannot fulfill these functions.

Ferdinand Berthier (1803 - 1886)

Ferdinand Berthier was born Deaf of hearing parents in Macon, France, in 1803. He attended the National Institution for Deaf-Mutes, the successor to the school founded by the abbé de l'Epée. Berthier was considered the most capable student in the school so, after graduation, he was invited to stay on as monitor at sixteen, teaching assistant at twenty-one, teacher at twenty-six, and then head teacher. Berthier learned to read French, Latin and Greek, but he preferred his signed language. "How few men," he wrote, "have deeply studied the immense resources hidden in this universal idiom, so clear, so positive, so reliable." During his long career, Berthier published numerous articles and books recording the struggle and advancing the welfare of the Deaf. His works include voluminous biographies of the abbé de l'Epée and his successor, the abbé Sicard; biographical sketches of Jean Massieu and Laurent Clerc; a book explaining the Napoleonic code to the Deaf; and numerous encyclopedia entries and newspaper articles. To enhance the lives of Deaf people through legal reform, education and fund-raising, Berthier created the first known social organization of the Deaf. In 1834, he gathered ten other Deaf leaders at his home and founded the *Comité des Sourds-Muets* (Deaf-Mute Committee), which launched annual banquets to celebrate the birth date of the abbé de l'Epée. In 1838, the group was renamed, to reflect its expanded functions, the *Central Society for the Assistance and Education of Deaf-Mutes*. Berthier was also vice-president of the first welfare organization for the Deaf and a member of literary and historical societies. For several decades he addressed a stream of letters to the legislature protesting laws unfair to Deaf people. When the Deaf in France were finally allowed to vote, in 1848, they put forth Berthier, unsuccessfully, for a seat in the National Assembly. Berthier was awarded the Legion of Honor, which had never before been conferred on any Deaf person. He lived to see all Deaf teachers in France fired after the 1880 Congress of Milan advocated pure oralism. He died in 1886.

Using the same lines of argument, French educators of the Deaf contend that the world will never learn signed language and that LSF can never fulfill the functions of French. (We will present the case for using signed language in Deaf education in part 2.) In a remark reminiscent of Napoleon's exclamation to abbé Sicard, that signed language had only nouns and adjectives, a modern French educator has written of LSF: "Mimic [*sic*] grammar is characterized above all by simplifications. No articles; adverbs and adjectives are indistinguishable."[7] In view of the slice of cultural and political history traced here, it is hardly any wonder that French administration and law consider LSF speakers, most of whose parents are monoculturally French, not as a linguistic minority, but rather as French-speaking citizens with a disability. Nor is it any wonder that hearing parents of Deaf children, aggressively working through their own national organization, have advocated spoken French "at all costs and in all cases."[8]

In recent decades, however, there have been some developments favoring a renewed role for LSF in the lives of France's Deaf people. French Deaf leaders at the 1975 Congress of the World Federation of the Deaf, held in Washington, DC, were impressed with the place that had been made for ASL in American society and the large number of American Deaf presenters. In the same year, French national television started a weekly program aimed at Deaf and hard-of-hearing people that was interpreted into signed language. The Confédération Nationale des Sourds de France (the French counterpart of the NAD) launched a study of Deaf communication and of the merits of the American system of signing and speaking simultaneously in the classroom.

In 1976, French sociologist Bernard Mottez and American sociolinguist Harry Markowicz undertook a study of the growing Deaf movement. A year later these scholar-activists began a graduate seminar on the Deaf community and a series of public lectures by American Deaf scholars invited to Paris. They also began publishing a hard-hitting underground newspaper that focused on the Deaf community and its language. During this period the International Visual Theater, with an all-Deaf cast led by American Deaf artist Alfredo Corrado, was founded in Paris. The group presented avant-garde plays in LSF on themes in Deaf culture. The high visibility of the theater group inspired respect for LSF among both Deaf and hearing audiences. In response to the growing demand for instruction in LSF, the interpreter for the troupe, Billy Moody (an American, since there were then no full-time professional interpreters in France), trained troupe members as teachers and established LSF classes for parents and professional people. The Deaf theater became a training ground for activism as well as acting. Four summer institutes at Gallaudet University brought some thirty French parents, professionals, and Deaf people each year face-to-face with American hearing and Deaf scholars investigating ASL, with politically active Deaf groups such as Deafpride, and with the American Civil Rights movement.[9]

On returning to France, one group of Deaf participants and hearing allies worked to reclaim French Deaf history and to investigate LSF. The Academy of French Sign Language was established at the Paris National Institute for Young Deaf People (successor to Epée's school); an LSF dictionary was compiled, and classes started to teach LSF. Other graduates of the Gallaudet summer institutes launched a nationwide association committed to the bilingual education of Deaf children, known as 2LPE *(Deux Langues pour Une Education*—"Two Languages, One Education"), which had its own magazine and conducted summer institutes based on the Gallaudet model. At these institutes, parents and their Deaf children, interpreters, and Deaf people gathered for mutual instruction. Deaf Americans taught workshops there. The association also created bilingual classes for Deaf children, with Deaf teachers, in several cities. This gave rise, in turn, to regional groups engaged in applied research and development related to LSF.[10] A great many French Deaf people, however, gathered in their fraternal, political and athletic associations, viewed all these activities with skepticism. They accused the activists of promoting the exploitation of Deaf people by hearing people, and of seeking a position of superiority vis-à-vis the rest of the French DEAF-WORLD.[11]

In 1985, events at a residential school for Deaf children in a provincial city brought the growing struggle between advocates of LSF and those of spoken French to national attention. A small number of hearing teachers and Deaf adults at the school staged a hunger strike, well-covered by the media, to demand the inclusion of LSF and Deaf teachers. A call to Deaf people and their friends a year later, to rally at the Bastille on behalf of official recognition of LSF, resulted in a media event in which three to five thousand people, including legislators and parents, marched through the city to the offices of the prime minister. The march not only enlightened millions of French people but also breathed pride, vigor, and a sense of power into the Deaf community of France. Among events reaching the general public, the widely attended play *Les Enfants du Silence* (the French version of *Children of a Lesser God*), had a significant role in awakening French society to the linguistic minority in its midst. Several major books on French Sign Language and the French Deaf community, as well as a splendid journal of French Deaf history, have appeared since the 1970s.[12] As part of the bicentennial of the French Revolution, a magnificent panorama of French Deaf history was prepared and placed on display in the Sorbonne.[13] An international conference on signed languages, in Poitiers in July, 1990, drew inspiration from the 1989 international Deaf culture conference, Deaf Way, in Washington, DC. In many respects the Poitiers meeting was also a political gathering to chart a course for reform. In 1991, bilingual education for Deaf children (French and LSF) was approved by the French Parliament. The following year, the first European Conference on Deaf History was convened by French Deaf organizations in Rodez. Then, in 1993, *Les Enfants du Silence* began a second run, starring Deaf actress Emmanuelle Laborit, who, when she was seven, attended the Gallaudet summer institute with her parents. Ms. Laborit is the most visible of the Deaf actors trained at the International Visual Theatre, a media star in constant demand with a best-selling autobiography. Other Deaf actors are also playing in hearing theaters around the country as well as in International Visual Theatre productions.

The present situation of the DEAF–WORLD in France is both good and bad. Definitely bad is the resistance of French society to accepting the DEAF–WORLD. In the words of one Deaf leader: "[There is a] mental block vis-à-vis the language and culture of the Deaf in institutions charged with serving them."[14] Those institutions are directed and staffed, with rare exception, by hearing people whose attitude toward the Deaf is commonly paternalist and intolerant of their language. French Deaf education is, for the most part, under the auspices of the Ministry of Health. There is still no state-sponsored teaching of LSF; most hearing teachers of Deaf children do not know the language.[15] There are no degree-granting programs for educating interpreters, and interpreters are not available to allow Deaf children to attend programs designed for hearing students. Public schools cannot employ Deaf teachers. Most Deaf children are in classes where spoken French is used and mainstreaming is strongly promoted.[16]

(Language policy and educational placement in U.S. Deaf education are discussed in part 2.) Deaf students in France rarely receive the regular high school degree; therefore, they rarely go on to college, although free access for hearing students to the French university is traditional.[17] There seems to be an implicit understanding that the appropriate calling for Deaf people is the manual trades, although those trades are dying in French society.

On the positive side, however, Deaf activism in support of LSF, and the pioneering bilingual education classes for Deaf children, have led to the passage of a law that allows parents of Deaf children to choose to have their children educated with both LSF and French, as an alternative to spoken French alone. Some French universities have begun providing basic services for Deaf students so that they are not effectively locked out.[18] Deaf people are increasingly providing professional services to Deaf people, as mental health workers, as museum tour guides and instructors, as teacher's aides and in private schools, as teachers, and as members of new interpreter organizations.[19] Moreover, Deaf leaders have been actively advancing the field of Deaf history in France.[20] However, French Deaf people have, for the most part, persevered in these professions without the formal recognition and remuneration that professional diplomas provide. In short, views of Deaf people and their language are becoming more positive, yet very slowly, and Deaf people are starting to gain access, but at the bottom. The evidence, then, that French Deaf people are discriminated against in education, employment and political life must be judged in the context of these positive developments in France in recent decades.

French Deaf history, in the context of the larger society, reminds us that the situation of Deaf peoples' language and community normally reflects the enveloping nation's policies with respect to minority languages and communities. A society that prides itself on a single language and culture seems less likely to recognize its DEAF–WORLD as a language minority and more likely to see all Deaf people in a single light, fundamentally as disabled hearing people.

A pluralistic society is less likely to cast difference as deviance; it has models in other language minorities for its understanding of culturally Deaf people. If we contrast French and American views of minorities in general, we can see the roots of their differing perspectives of Deaf people. In the French view, a democracy without institutionalized cultural distinctions is more just; many Americans also hold this view and claim, for example, that fair laws are "color-blind." For the French, to give everyone equal educational opportunity is to give each person equal access, in principle, to schools conducted in French. Not surprisingly, in view of its history, U.S. society is, on the other hand, more pluralist and more ready to institutionalize the wishes of the minorities. Language minorities generally put the preservation of their language high in their priorities. Acting through the courts and through law-making bodies, those minorities, such as Hispanic and Asian Americans, have won the right to instruction using their languages in U.S. schools.

The difference in pluralism between the United States and France is not so much in demographics as in the pluralism of government structures. France is, after all, a pluralistic society; numerous French citizens speak as their primary language Arabic, Turkish, Vietnamese, and LSF, to mention just a few languages. French people differ in their regional affiliations, cultural origin, social class, and political parties. However, until recently in France, ethnic groups did not intervene as such in French political life. That is changing. Perhaps the passage of the law granting parents of Deaf children a language choice reflects this growing tolerance of cultural diversity. Certainly the few experimental bilingual programs in Deaf schools still in operation is a positive sign. In the next few years, the cultural construction of Deaf people may well blossom in France, not merely reducing the contrast with the U.S., but implementing the aspirations of culturally Deaf people in entirely novel ways.[21] (In part 2 we discuss the issue of bilingual and bicultural education of Deaf children in the U.S., on the model of that accorded other language minorities.)

Sweden

Sweden is markedly different from France in its embrace of cultural pluralism in general and of Deaf culture in particular. The government has a policy of preserving minority languages and cultures. For example, all children whose parents speak a home language other than Swedish are given instruction in that home language each week and may be given instruction through that language in various academic subjects. In matters that affect minorities, the Swedish government deals preferentially with formal representative organizations from those minorities. Sweden has a population of nearly nine million, of whom roughly 9,000 are Deaf. Of these, approximately 550 are school age.[22] In the first half of this century, Sweden, like most other European countries, allowed only the spoken and written national language to be used in Deaf education. In 1969, free interpreter services were recognized as a right of Deaf people and an interpreter training program was established, conducted by the Swedish Federation of the Deaf (*Sveriges Dövas Riksförbund*, SDR).

In 1981, as a result of activism by SDR, by the association of parents of Deaf children, and by linguists at the University of Stockholm, Swedish Sign Language (SSL) was formally recognized as one of the nation's minority languages, and bilingual education was instituted in the nation's schools for Deaf children. The parliamentary declaration stated: "The profoundly deaf, to function among themselves and in society, have to be bilingual . . . to be fluent in their visual/gestural Sign Language and be fluent in the language that society surrounds them with: Swedish." Swedish Deaf leader and University of Stockholm Professor Lars Wallin comments: "The bill was a confirmation of our language situation. The Deaf community is bilingual." This is apparent from examining the work of the Deaf clubs: newspapers, minutes, letters to authorities and TTY communication are all in Swedish and have long been so.

Two years later, a new curriculum for the education of Deaf and hard-of-hearing children was issued; it provided that Swedish and Swedish Sign Language should be used as languages of instruction and that pupils must be given opportunities to develop as bilingual individuals. Subsequently, a knowledge of Swedish Sign Language was added to admission requirements for educational programs preparing teachers of the Deaf. Thus, the knowledge that Deaf people have concerning their language and culture is now widely respected and seen as essential to the successful education and psychological development of Deaf children. The schools have been hiring Deaf teachers and other Deaf staff members in large numbers, though the effects of banning them for many decades cannot be quickly undone. After ten years, the fraction of the faculty that is Deaf now ranges in various schools from one-fifth to two-thirds. Swedish is taught as a second language, using students' Swedish Sign Language as the vehicle for this instruction, and there are courses in the history, language, and culture of the Swedish Deaf community. The SDR also supports the right to speech training for those children able to profit, especially the hard-of-hearing.

Because many Deaf children, especially those from hearing homes in sparsely populated areas, learn SSL relatively late, and because the language is not used uniformly in schools due to a shortage of Deaf teachers and hearing teachers fluent in SSL, Deaf education in Sweden is not yet a true test of bilingual principles, although it may become one before long. Nevertheless, teachers who have been around for a while report informally dramatic improvements in academic achievement, and there are some research results that support their position. Tests of Swedish and of mathematics administered to eighth-grade Deaf children during the old oralist regime in Sweden were administered again in the late 1980s; the latter group outperformed the earlier one by a large margin, especially in Swedish proficiency.[23] The first Deaf students in bilingual classes in Sweden (and Denmark) graduated high school with reading and mathematics achievement levels comparable to those of hearing peers.[24]

A major outreach program is bringing SSL and Deaf adults into the lives of hearing families with Deaf children, and it is bringing those hearing families together for mutual support as well. There are special preschools, Deaf home visitors, and short-term live-in arrangements. The nation's Deaf clubs host SSL classes and parents' meetings. All this has led to a huge improvement, according to teachers, psychologists and speech therapists interviewed, in the concept mastery and signed language fluency that Deaf children now possess on entering school at age seven.[25] The success of the present system in Sweden, according to Lars Wallin, is the product of collaboration between the SDR, the association of parents of Deaf children, and scholars who have investigated SSL and its community of users. Working together, they have put a stop to depriving Deaf children of language, they have forged bilingual education, and they have blocked mainstreaming. In fact, there is no support for the mainstreaming of Deaf children in Sweden today.

Deaf adults in Sweden also benefit from the Deaf-culture-friendly environment. "From having lived on the outskirts of society," Lars Wallin writes, "in Deaf clubs that were always our safe havens, we are now stepping out into society, prouder than ever. . . ." [26] There are forty-seven Deaf clubs that are the foundation for the national organization, SDR. SDR counts an astonishing sixty-five percent of the Deaf population in its membership. As in the U.S., the Deaf clubs offer lectures, films and videos, and social events. Some clubs own resort facilities providing boating, swimming and other recreation. In addition, some offer courses in SSL, and the Stockholm Deaf Club also teaches ASL and nine other subjects in evening classes. Some idea of the cultural richness available to Deaf adults may be had by examining the fifteen organizations for Deaf people that meet at the Stockholm Deaf Club. There are four clubs with recreational themes: sports, fishing, bridge, chess. The sports club itself has fourteen sections, ranging from bowling to volleyball. Significantly, the Swedish National Athletic Association of the Deaf, which regroups Deaf teams sponsored by local clubs throughout Sweden, is seeking to withdraw from a disability coalition and gain entrance to the Swedish Confederation of Sports. In general, members of the Swedish DEAF–WORLD do not see themselves as having a disability.[27] Also meeting at the Stockholm Deaf Club are three clubs with cultural foci: folk dance, theater, and art. In addition, there are seven special-interest groups: youth, parents, retired persons, women's, deafened adults, international, and suburban.[28]

Swedish society tends to be formal, centralized, and bureaucratic. This helps to ensure that initiatives concerning Deaf children and adults involve the SDR, which is the official and centralized organization of Deaf people. The SDR is concerned with all facets of the lives of Deaf children and adults. It is a kind of DEAF–WORLD parliament, in which issues debated in local Deaf clubs are brought to a national level for discussion and action. It is concerned with education, from pre-school through primary and secondary, and into continuing education for adults. One of the SDR goals was to encourage the establishment of a professorship in Swedish Sign Language in the Department of Linguistics at the University of Stockholm, a position Wallin now holds. The SDR is involved in teacher education. In the past, programs preparing teachers of the Deaf discriminated against Deaf applicants for admission: they took no account of their fluency in SSL and their knowledge of Deaf culture, and they required five years experience teaching hearing children. With reforms promoted by SDR, not only is the study of SSL prerequisite for qualifying as a teacher of Deaf children, as we said, but also Deaf students can become teachers of the Deaf without first teaching hearing children. SDR has been involved as well in interpreter education, child care, health care and employment, recreation, services for the elderly and people with disabilities, audiology centers, provision of psychological and other social services, development of media and technology, national newscasts interpreted into SSL, research on the signed language, and Deaf theater. There are an estimated twenty Deaf cultural workers in Sweden who produce cultural events, including thirty television programs, eight publications, and two plays each year.[29] SDR has its own TV production unit, which sells television programming on Deaf themes to the Swedish Broadcasting Company and has been active in improving the lot of Deaf people in developing nations, particularly Nepal and Kenya.

Patterns in the developed nations

The signed languages of Deaf communities in Europe are continuing to receive extensive scholarly investigation by hearing and by Deaf scholars.[30] Reports of this research are appearing in a variety of journals and books, many of them in the U.S. journal *Sign Language Studies*, which has been published quarterly since 1972. The International Sign Linguistics Association was formed in 1986 and publishes a newsletter, *Signpost*. An international workshop for Deaf researchers focusing on signed language and Deaf culture was held in Bristol in 1985, then biennially in other European cities. Participation is restricted to Deaf scholars.

Signed languages are receiving greater social acceptance as well. In 1988, the European Parliament voted a motion urging all member states to promote and preserve their signed languages.[31] These developments, however, are recent. Most Deaf adults in Europe today were educated orally, and oral education remains widespread. However, three new trends (discussed in detail in part 2) are making inroads. These are: Total Communication (*TC* for short), which in practice entails speaking and signing at the same time, with the order of the signs following the order of the spoken words; bilingual/bicultural education; and mainstreaming. Deaf education in Europe continues to prepare most Deaf students for non-professional jobs. Deaf adults are not so much unemployed as underemployed, segregated into trades such as carpentry, printing, leather work, baking, tailoring, and dress-making. National Deaf associations tend to be active, abetted by the European Union of the Deaf (the regional secretariat of the World Federation of the Deaf). In some countries Deaf adults are hired as teachers or teachers aides. In general, however, Deaf people are excluded from decision-making about the lives of Deaf people.[32] This problem is aggravated by a dire shortage of interpreters.

A very significant force on the world Deaf scene has been the World Federation of the Deaf, or the *WFD*.[33] The WFD grew out of the international congresses of Deaf people late in the nineteenth century, which were organized in part to defend Deaf language and culture in the aftermath of the Congress of Milan. Perhaps it was especially fitting, then, that the Italian Deaf Association took the initiative to unite the national Deaf associations at a Rome congress in 1951. The WFD General Assembly is a law-making body comprised of two Deaf delegates from every national Deaf association. The General Assembly convenes every four years to elect members to the WFD Board and to adopt policies and programs.

The WFD has standing commissions that focus on developments in fields such as audiology, education, psychology, signed language, interpreting, and Deaf culture. The commissions are the site of formal presentations at the WFD congresses, and they make recommendations and propose resolutions based on those formal papers and their discussion. The eleventh Congress of the WFD, held in Vienna in 1995, with some seven thousand participants from more than seventy-five countries, elected its first woman president, the former general secretary, Liisa Kauppinen. Of the approximately 112 national Deaf associations in the WFD, European organizations make up forty percent, while African, Asian and South American organizations comprise only seventeen percent. Table 6-1 gives some characteristics of national organizations of the Deaf in nine European countries and the U.S. in 1989.[34]

The National Association of the Deaf in the U.S. is probably the oldest nationwide Deaf organization in the world. Of the organizations listed in Table 6-1, the British Deaf Association, which was modeled after the NAD, is the second oldest. The Nazi regime forced the German federation to close and a new one was established in 1950. Some Communist governments forced Deaf and hard-of-hearing persons to form a single organization, but these separated anew in several countries after the

Communist collapse. Percent participation is particularly high in some formerly communist countries, which require membership to receive government benefits. The high level of participation in Sweden has already been mentioned; rates are similar in Spain and Denmark. Former WFD president and sociologist Yerker Andersson attributes the high percentages to the direct involvement of local Deaf clubs in the management of their national federation. In the U.S., the NAD, with an estimated fifteen percent membership size, is not an organization of Deaf clubs, but rather an organization of state associations of the Deaf. In 1994, the British Deaf Association changed its structure from one with eight regional branches representing local organizations, to one representing individuals. This appears to have had a disastrous effect on membership, which in a single year declined to three percent of the British Deaf population.

National organization of the Deaf	Year established	Membership size (% of Deaf population)	No. of local organizations
Belgian	1977	23	20
British	1890	16	224
Czech R./Slovakia	1952	65	2,000
Danish	1935	60	20
Dutch	1955	21	13
German (West)	1950	41	236
Polish	1922	78	153
Spanish	1936	55	75
Swedish	1922	59	40
United States	1880	15	150

Table 6-1. **National Organizations of the Deaf in Nine European Countries and the U.S.** *(Adapted from Andersson, 1994a.)*

In recent years, the WFD has emphasized outreach to developing nations, whose Deaf citizens comprise eighty percent of the Deaf people in the world. The WFD has created regional secretariats in an effort to better serve Deaf people in those nations. Before turning to the results of the 1988 WFD survey of the conditions of Deaf people in the developing nations, we consider two case histories.

VISITS TO TWO DEVELOPING NATIONS

Reliable information about the DEAF-WORLD in developing nations is generally hard to come by. There are few, if any, relevant surveys, and the historical record is even scantier. One of us (Harlan) traveled to Kenya and Burundi to gather information firsthand.

Kenya

There are some twenty million Kenyans in a country the size of Texas; a fifth of them are Kikuyus, but there are a half-dozen other prominent ethnic groups. Deaf children taught in English are often working in their fourth language, having previously learned their tribal language, Swahili (like English, a national language), and the signed language of the DEAF-WORLD.

Nine out of ten hearing children go to primary school in Kenya, although attendance is not compulsory. Teachers are supplied and paid by the government but each community must construct, furnish, and maintain its own school.

Among Kenya's children of school age, two per 1,000 are Deaf. There are seventeen residential schools for Deaf children and one for Deaf-Blind children; these are all elementary schools. There is also one high school, and five self-contained classes in schools for hearing children. Some two thousand Deaf children are taught by about two hundred teachers, half of them with special training. The Ministry of Basic Education conducts a two-year training course for teachers of the Deaf, and an inspectorate monitors their performance in the classroom. There is a Kenya Institute of Special Education, which trains about one hundred teachers of special education at a time in a three-year program. A teacher's certificate and three years' experience are required for admission, so Deaf people are clearly excluded from the profession of teaching Deaf children. The Institute is also concerned with assessment, documentation, research, teaching aids, correspondence courses, and in-service training.

Teachers trained in educational diagnosis are given a reduced classroom schedule so they can work in one of seventeen assessment centers where parents bring their children with handicaps. There, audiologists measure hearing loss, and the centers arrange for pupils to transfer from regular to special schools as appropriate.

Schools for the Deaf have the same curriculum and use the same examinations as regular schools, but their method and pace are different. Until recently, that method was modeled after that used in Great Britain, the former colonial power, with a strong emphasis on speaking and lipreading English. As Great Britain (like the United States) has increasingly integrated Deaf children into the local public schools, so, too, the emphasis in Kenya lately has been on mainstreaming those children who, it is believed, can study in an ordinary classroom if special services are provided.

The performance of Deaf children on national examinations revealed, however, that they were not making satisfactory progress in school; this led some teachers and officials to advocate the use of signed language in Deaf education, at least on an experimental basis. The Kenyan National Association of the Deaf has published a dictionary of signs. It is not clear whether a single signed language is in general use, or whether there are several distinct signed languages in use among the numerous tribes in Kenya. Believing that Deaf education faces a serious problem of standardized usage, a Deaf member of the Kenya Institute of Special Education supplemented a basic list of Kenyan signs with others from ASL; the wisdom of this practice has been hotly disputed. These materials were then put to work at a new residential school, the Machakos School, using both sign and speech in instruction.

While the Institute of Special Education was created with the help of Danish funds and experts, the Machakos School was established with help from Sweden. On a tour of several Kenyan Deaf schools, we drove to the Machakos School in the company of a government inspector of Deaf education. At the school, a large field of red clay is encircled by a half-dozen one-story concrete buildings, their whitewashed facades glistening in the equatorial sun. One of the 120 pupils, a slim, smiling girl of nine or ten, clad in a blue uniform, led the inspector and visitor to the airy dormitory with its rows of double-decker beds, then to the washroom building, where a dozen spigots emptied into a metal trough, and finally to one of the classrooms with its posters and maps and little wooden tables and chairs. The teachers live on the grounds in spartan one-bedroom homes arrayed behind a screen of bushes. The inspector explained that the annual cost per pupil to operate such a school is the equivalent of two hundred fifty U.S. dollars. At the Machakos School, instruction was conducted in spoken English, with each word accompanied by a sign. Many of the signs had to be taught to the children. The teachers apparently did not know Kenyan Sign Language.

Three of Kenya's seventeen residential schools for the Deaf are vocational. Students are frequently transferred among the schools, the more so as each has its own vocational specialty. In addition, graduates of the schools have been mingling for some three decades now in cities such as Nairobi, where there are reportedly several hundred Deaf adults. At the Kambui school, three long-time residents encountered in the carpentry shop took evident pride in their woodworking equipment and products; the bedframes, cabinets and other furniture were skillfully made. The students must pass national trade exams, and several, beaming, presented their journeyman's papers.

Compared to other developing nations, Deaf people have some significant advantages in Kenya: There are enthusiastic and well-informed officials and teachers; an inspectorate for monitoring and improving classroom practices; uniform national exams to evaluate the system's successes and failures; and a dynamic parents' association which constructs schools, founds clinics, gathers data, raises funds, and meets the boarding expenses of about half of all the Deaf children educated in Kenya. At the same time, in Deaf education as in many other sectors of Kenyan life, the country, which became a republic in 1963, has yet to shed its onerous legacy of colonialism. Oralist educational practices imported from Great Britain were particularly unsuitable in Kenya, where there are few hearing aids, no classroom amplifiers, and no single oral language of broad communication that is the children's first language. The systematic introduction of signs from ASL has also met with protests of linguistic imperialism from Africans and Europeans.

Burundi

Burundi has one-fourth the population of Kenya crowded into a twentieth of the space. Virtually all the adult population of five million is engaged in subsistence agriculture on scattered family plots in the highlands. The cities are few and small, and travel among them has been slight. Under these conditions, Deaf children and adults seem to be rather isolated from one another. In visiting homes with a Deaf child, we came upon complex systems of manual communication that had evolved in individual families with several Deaf members, but found no evidence of a manual language of broader communication, and therefore no self-instructing pool of signed language users.

There are two major ethnic groups in Burundi, the Hutus (85%) and the Tutsis (14%), with a common language, Kirundi, and a second official language, French. Less than a quarter of the adult population is literate, and about one child in three is enrolled in primary school. There are an estimated four thousand Deaf children of school age, but there is no system of Deaf education, and Deaf children are also unwelcome in hearing schools. With very rare exceptions, Deaf children are thus uneducated and believed ineducable. Deaf people are not designated by their names in Burundian society, but rather by a common designation, *nyamuragi*. This word is related to the word for children who are mentally retarded and might be translated *Dumbo* or *Deafie*.

A few years ago, a Burundian psychologist, Assumpta Naniwe, interviewed a dozen parents of Deaf children in Burundi. The interviews were conducted in Kirundi, tape recorded, transcribed, and translated into French. A content analysis reveals the perception of Deaf people by hearing adults who are unable to communicate with them. It shows the highly restricted social roles assigned to Deaf people in such a hearing society, and explains the significance of the discovery of Deafness for the family and the family's ultimate adaptation. In addition, there are two church-related schools for Deaf children, and these signing micro-societies are changing hearing peoples' perception of Deaf people and Deaf peoples' perceptions of themselves. The following are two representative interviews, translated from the French, which was in turn a translation from Kirundi, and abridged.

Interview with the mother of Cécile. Cécile, known as 'Deafie', is a Deaf woman thirty-three years old. The fifth child in a family of nine children, she is the only Deaf person in the family.

Assumpta Naniwe: I would like us to talk about Deafness, your Deaf child, and your relations with her.

Mother of Cécile: When you see a Deaf person walking down the street, you think he is perfectly normal, someone like every one else, but . . . in fact he has no intelligence whatever. You have to feed him, supply all his wants, dress him . . . In fact, you have to do everything for him.

AN: You say that the Deaf person is a being without intelligence?

M: Alas, yes. Do you think I consider my Deaf daughter to be like all my other children? A child whom you can't rely on, who relies on other people for everything? . . . The other women her age have three or four or even five children and she, what is she? She's always trailing around behind me, she never got married, she can never get married . . . But you know, it's not that she doesn't want to. I've done everything on earth to stop her running after men. You know, men only think about having a good time [with her], none of them considered marrying her. You understand, Deafie doesn't know what it means to have children out of wedlock so it's I who must think of these things for her.

AN: Have you considered explaining the birds and the bees to her?

M: How am I supposed to talk to someone who doesn't speak? Tell me how I'm supposed to explain all that to someone who seemingly lives in another world? It's hard enough as it is with someone normal, those who have a language as we do, to whom you can say, this is not good, this is very bad, this is good . . . and who manage anyway to get into trouble. So when it comes to a being without ears, without intelligence . . . [When she was a child] I gave her little tasks, like cooking, sweeping, getting water from the well. You could never rely on her, but since I had other children I could ask them to keep an eye on her. When she was quite young it was easy, but now she does as she pleases. If she gets up in the morning in a good mood, she takes the broom and cleans the house, fetches water, prepares the meal. At such times I don't say a word for fear she may change her mind. But another day she can be in a bad mood, remain in bed, or sit in front of the house and do nothing . . . After her younger sisters got married, she realized that she would never leave our home. She explains in her own particular gestures that everyone has found a husband, has had children, but she, she will always remain at home. All I have is problems with her; bringing up a child who can never turn out good, who can never fit in—that's truly a waste of time.

AN: You say that she doesn't fit in?

M: Who can befriend a Deaf woman? People see her, take pity on her, and that's it. She's her mother's baby, and as long as I live, I will take care of her, and when I'm no longer around, the family will look after her . . . but I'm quite concerned about her future.

Interview with the mother of Vincent. Vincent is the oldest child of four; he is thirteen and in the third grade of the church-sponsored school for Deaf children. He is the only Deaf person in his family.

Mother of Vincent: I myself feel that every Deaf person should have some kind of work he can do, a profession, and I'm sure that even if he is Deaf he can do his work well. For example, that child there (pointing to her Deaf son) took it in his head once to sell peanuts and I let him do it because . . . once he gets an idea in his head, Vincent doesn't let anyone tell him otherwise. I was afraid because I thought he'd never succeed in doing it. But he stuck to it and he makes a lot of money with it . . . If other people understood that he can do as they do, if people would give him work, Vincent could do all right in life.

AN: You mentioned that other people don't let him do as he wishes. Who are these other people?

M: Everyone. Starting with me. It's not because I don't love him, it's because I'm afraid of what can happen to him. Look, when you can't communicate with him, it's hard to know exactly what you're supposed to do. When Vincent wants to sell things, I'm afraid. I'm worried that he won't know how to count his money, that some robbers will come along and cheat him of everything he's got or attack him and steal all his money. . . . There are lots of things that can eat away at the heart of a mother who knows her child's problems. Whereas other people, they simply underestimate him, they take him for an idiot. Even though, as I've told you, he is a good work-er, I'm sure that when the day comes that he tries to find a job as a mason no one will bother with him because every-one thinks he is incompetent.

AN: Even though you tell me that he has a nice little peanut business?

M: (*Laughs heartily*)Well, this Deaf little fellow knows his busi-ness well and he knows what he wants. For, as I have already told you, when he decides to do something, he does it or, if he can't, he has fits of anger that everyone in the family dreads. Actually, he is known in these parts as a brawler and I think no one dares touch him for fear of being flattened . . . I think that's why his little business is working out okay. Everyone's afraid of him.

AN: You don't think people will cheat him?

M: Ahh . . . Cheat him! Don't worry about it; ever since he start-ed school he knows how to count. He knows the difference between a hundred-franc note and a thousand-franc note. He's quite familiar with the value of money. It was from that moment that he began to do business. It's three years now that he has been going to school, and I have the impression that he's learned a lot. Don't ask me what, because I'm illit-erate, I don't understand a word of all that they write, but I notice that he has changed his ways a lot. He's learned to read, to count, to speak with gestures. I don't understand those gestures, but when he's with his schoolmates, they communicate with their eyes, their arms, their mouths. It's quite intriguing, but no one else understands them. When you come down to it, that's the only situation in which I see

> Vincent really come alive—he makes fun, tells stories, you can hear him laugh, whereas with the rest of us, and his sis ters and brothers, all you hear are slaps echoing. Sometimes I wonder what will become of him when he grows up, with that temper of his.

Clearly, Vincent will have a better life than the Deaf woman, Cécile, from the generation before him, because Vincent has been going to school, he has found people with whom he can communicate, and his signed language is allowing him to learn such basics as buying and selling with money.

The full set of interviews with parents of Deaf children, including this pair, makes clear that a breakdown in communication with Deaf people fosters the belief that they are mentally retarded. As a result, they are looked down upon, assigned modest social roles, and largely excluded from education. These conditions, in turn, reinforce the belief that they are mentally retarded.

For all cultures, we may distinguish five types of instruction, depending on the source of the instructive messages, which shape the child into an informed adult. These are self-instruction, peer instruction, parental teaching, community teaching, and formal instruction. Many children, hearing and Deaf, do not receive the last of these, formal instruction, either because they simply do not have physical access to it or because they do not have linguistic access to it, since that instruction is conducted in a language they do not know and cannot understand. A child without formal instruction frequently grows up to become an economically disadvantaged adult, but not one who is perceived as mentally retarded. Such a child still receives informal instruction from friends, parents and relatives, and neighbors. With talent and luck, the child may become a leader in the hearing or Deaf communities.

Consider, however, the plight of a child who does not go to school, who is separated from the peers with whom communication is possible, and who cannot communicate with parents or neighbors. That child grows into adulthood with self-instruction as his or her only resource. It is no surprise that such a person is often seen as mentally retarded and assigned social roles accordingly.

If one examines the complete interviews with the mothers of 'Deafie' and Vincent, as well as the others in the set, it becomes clear that the parents of Deaf children in Burundi most often see their children as, fundamentally, stupid and angry. What are the possible lives imagined and allowed for Deaf people in a society that views them as stupid and angry? The perception shapes the reality and the reality reinforces the perception. For example, Deaf women are not marriageable in Burundi; hence they do not have the opportunity to perform certain key roles of womanhood. And if a husband will not shelter them, then they must remain with their parents all their lives. Deaf girls, then, are cast in the role of perpetual children, but children whose labor is demanded.

Most of the parents have established some rudimentary communication with their Deaf children, but it is so limited that the parents cannot gauge their intelligence, much less instruct them as they do their hearing children. It is remarkable that the solution to their terrible predicament—their inability to communicate with their child—is, in some cases, right under their noses. Like Vincent's mother, they see their Deaf child communicate with other Deaf children, yet they do not see the possibility of exploiting that avenue themselves.

Harlan's visit to Burundi

It was the rainy season when we arrived in Burundi; the tropical vegetation was green and lush, the clay roads rutted and muddy. We drove to a suburb of the capital, where a church-sponsored school for Deaf children is located. Since very few Burundians know English and fewer still have been to America, we were astonished to see teachers at the school using signs from ASL—in French word order!

The director explained that he and one of the other teachers had received a three-month training course in Nigeria, conducted by Andrew Foster, a Deaf Black American and graduate of Gallaudet University (see box). The school offered four grades (first, and third through fifth), but the one-room chapel that served as a school could only accommodate two classes at a time (a burlap curtain was hung down the middle), so each met for a half-day. (More recently, the school has expanded and is housed in several concrete buildings.) The youngest children, seven to eight, learn math and written French (although some people contend that Kirundi should be taught first, as in the hearing schools). In later grades, natural and physical sciences are added, and in the last, history and geography.

Andrew Foster (1925 – 1988)

Andrew Jackson Foster is known as the father of Deaf education in Africa, where he and his disciples founded thirteen schools for the Deaf in as many countries. He was the first Black person to graduate from Gallaudet. Born in Birmingham, Alabama, in 1925, Foster became Deaf at eleven and attended the Alabama School for the Deaf. He worked his way through high school, taking a correspondence course to earn his diploma. He entered Gallaudet College in 1951 and graduated three years later. Foster went on to earn master's degrees in special education and in missionary work. He founded the Christian Mission for Deaf Africans in 1956 and three years later went to Ghana to begin bringing the gospel and education into the lives of Africa's Deaf people. Foster personally founded schools for Deaf children in Nigeria, Ghana, and the Ivory Coast. From his base in Ibadan, Nigeria, he taught seven-week courses in ASL vocabulary to future teachers of the Deaf from numerous African nations, all of which were former British and French colonies. Many hearing and Deaf adults learned ASL signs from Foster and returned to their countries to teach Deaf children.

While Dr. Foster's memory is revered by many in Africa and America, he has his detractors as well. They point out that because Foster's disciples propagated signs from ASL, which were used in the classroom simultaneously with spoken English or French, the children's home languages, as well as the indigenous national language and signed language, had no place in the embryonic schools for the Deaf. However, as Deaf communities develop around these schools, the Deaf children are increasingly gaining access to a natural signed language and there is growing interest in capitalizing on that language fluency.

Andrew Foster's very presence changed African's beliefs about the potential of Deaf people, and he led various religious organizations working in Africa to make a place for Deaf people in their ministry. In 1970 Gallaudet conferred on Foster the doctorate in humane letters. In 1988, when he was in his sixties, still tirelessly traveling from one African country to another to administer schools and missions and to persuade governments, Andrew Foster died; his twin-engine plane crashed in Central Africa during a routine visit to one of the Deaf schools he had helped to found.

(Based on biographical sketches by Peter Mbu of Gallaudet University, and by Hairston & Smith, 1983)

We attended several classes, beginning with geography. The children knew the locations and names of neighboring states and fingerspelled them rapidly. We asked to meet a child who was clearly following every move and whose hand was often raised first; it was ten-year-old Claudine Umuvyeyi, from a family with five children: two teenage brothers, an older sister and a younger brother—four of them Deaf.

Claudine agreed to serve as informant and we adjourned to her home. Her mother explained that her fifth child was losing his hearing, yet he, like the other children when their Deafness was discovered, had not been seriously ill. She had noticed with her first child that by the age of two she still was not speaking as other children would, so she tested her hearing with various kinds of noises and came to the sad and unexpected conclusion (her husband and all relatives were hearing) that her child was Deaf. Her second child spoke fluently by age two, but shortly thereafter stopped responding to sound and gradually his speech disappeared. The mother was despairing.

In time, however, and especially with the advent of two more Deaf children, a manual language grew up in the home. The mother could understand all that her children said to her in this language, including their complaints, requests, and reports, and they could understand all she said to them. So in the end she adjusted to the situation, although the father, who never learned the home sign, never did.

On request, Mrs. Umuvyeyi told her daughter to go and see if the beans she had put on the fire to cook were tender. Claudine left immediately and returned a moment later, her hands flying. "They're not ready yet," her mother translated. We asked one of the teenage brothers to describe selected pictures to the other in their home signed language (since they hadn't been to school, they didn't know signs from ASL), which he did readily, using different signs and sign orderings than had our informants in Kenya. We asked them about their friends. They were mostly Deaf people from the city. Perhaps a dozen. They had picked up the Umuvyeyi family's signed language, though of course they were not as fluent as their hosts.

The brothers had a question to put to us (through Claudine): What trades did Deaf people practice in America? We listed a few, and said that some went on to university; the young men's eyes were filled with wonder. They themselves work as assistants to a tailor in the city. "Who exploits them," added the father, who had meanwhile returned home from his job as a typist. We complimented him on his family: two employed sons, his youngest daughter in school, his oldest, Christine, employed at a shelter for the handicapped. "Five Deaf children," he said. "Some days I really wonder. Why me?" He paused. "What is to become of them? Will Christine be able to marry? Claudine should go on in school, but after the fifth grade there are no more classes."

Another day we made an excursion to the interior city of Gitega, where there is a small school for Deaf children conducted by the Catholic archdiocese. We were ushered along garden paths, past breathtaking vistas, a little way down the mountainside to a brick building where the school was held. Its director had attended a teacher's institute at Gallaudet University the summer before. She explained that the school drew twenty-five day students and ten residents from the surrounding area, and she described its philosophy, which placed a decided emphasis on speaking and lipreading Kirundi, although signs were used in the classes. We had seen many of the signs before in the school in the capital: some were from ASL; others were based on gestures accompanying spoken Kirundi; still other resemblances, we were told, were due to cross-pollination between the two schools.

Following our visit, a hearing high school principal, together with Claudine and one of her schoolmates, were invited to America to continue their schooling. On graduating from the Model Secondary School at Gallaudet University, Claudine returned to Burundi and took up the profession of teaching Deaf children. Her reports were similar to those of her counterparts in many lands: she felt gratified by her important work and her pupils' progress, but isolated and frustrated by the lack of interpreters.*

---

* In the wake of the 1994 genocide in neighboring Rwanda and related bloodshed domestically, education in Burundi came to a near standstill. The high school principal and Claudine and her family fled. Claudine's former schoolmate remained in an American school for the Deaf.

Patterns in the developing nations

The fact that the vast majority of Deaf people in the world live in the developing nations underscores the importance of gaining a general understanding of the common problems Deaf people face in those countries, despite significant differences from one country to the next. With that in mind, in 1991 the World Federation of the Deaf published the results of a survey of Deaf people in the developing world.[35] The organization queried a variety of sources (national Deaf organizations, charities, schools, etc.) in ninety-seven countries not in North America, Europe or Australia, and excluding Japan, New Zealand and South Africa.

The 1991 WFD survey showed that unemployment among Deaf people is three times higher than the national average in the developing world. Nearly half the respondents reported major discrimination against Deaf people in employment. There is widespread lack of vocational training and there is often legal discrimination against Deaf people, for example, prohibiting them from obtaining a driver's license (twenty-six countries). Deaf adults commonly live in poverty and without any contact with Deaf children. Nearly half the countries have no interpreters whatsoever, and those that do commonly have only one or two for the entire nation.

Living conditions for Deaf people in the developing nations frequently involve violations of the Universal Declaration of Human Rights. Deaf people are deprived of the right to vote, to marry a Deaf person or to marry at all, or to establish a club or other organization. There are seventeen countries in which Deaf people do not gather formally at all; hence there is no national Deaf organization. In the remainder, they gather notably in clubs and churches. On a brighter note, there are Deaf sports in two-thirds of the countries and cultural events in half. These include theater, mime, magic, and dance.

Questions about signed language in the WFD survey of developing countries revealed how widespread were several of the practices we described in Burundi. Families with several Deaf members develop home sign. Schools foster the development of the signed language by bringing Deaf people together, many of whom have distinctive signing practices learned at home. Signs from foreign signed languages are introduced into the community by teachers trained abroad, by missionaries, and by Deaf people educated in other countries. Increasingly, Deaf communities in the developing nations, encouraged by UNESCO and the WFD, have undertaken the systematic description and analysis of their indigenous signed languages, much as the French Deaf community did in the 1970s. And WFD policy on the use of national signed languages is clear: indigenous signed languages should be given priority over the importation of foreign signed languages such as ASL or Swedish Sign Language.

Answers to survey questions about education revealed that Deaf education had begun only recently in most developing countries and commonly was initiated by religious groups. Only one Deaf child in five attends school in the developing nations, although nine out of ten hearing children do. About half the respondents said that their countries, like Burundi, do not provide for the education of Deaf children. There is little or no high school education for Deaf people and no college education. Deaf teachers are employed in about half the countries surveyed, and some form of signed language is used in forty percent of all classes. However, teachers are not trained in the national signed language in most developing countries.

About half the developing countries that do have Deaf education cleave, like Kenya, to an oralist philosophy imported from the former colonizing power, usually Great Britain or France. A 1972 report, Special Education in the Developing Countries of the [British] Commonwealth, illustrates the ideas about Deaf people promulgated in the former colonies. The report states that Deaf children "cannot think in words, so their mental growth is severely retarded." It laments that "pupils are taught by the outdated sign language system," in some countries, and that "hearing-impaired staff are found working with Deaf children although experience in the more developed countries has indicated that Deaf people cannot be trained to a satisfactory standard as teachers of the deaf."[36]

In 1985, UNESCO undertook to discredit this view of Deaf education, inviting experts from more than a dozen countries to convene and advise it on the different approaches to educating Deaf children. Their report affirms that Deaf people have the same intellectual capacities as hearing people, and that Deaf adults have an important role to play in the socialization and education of Deaf children. Although Deaf schoolchildren worldwide are not allowed to use their most fluent language, the signed language of the Deaf community in their country, the UNESCO consultants assert that signed languages ought to be accorded the same standing as oral languages, and they reject the old idea that signed language interferes with learning the national language.[37]

Complementary information about the role of signed language in Deaf education around the world comes from a 1993 WFD survey with forty-two nations responding. Most member countries had a period when the signed language of their DEAF–WORLD was prohibited, as in Kenya, but most report now that some form of signing is used in their schools. However, it is rarely the natural language of the local DEAF–WORLD (or, indeed, any DEAF–WORLD), but rather one of the invented systems for coding English or French on the hands. Only twelve nations report that the signed language of the DEAF–WORLD has official recognition in their country. Over half of the member countries report little or no signed language instruction in their nation. In those countries where instruction in signed language is offered, Deaf children's parents and teachers, who need to know the language, commonly do not enroll, and the instructors are frequently not fluent in the language. Half the responding countries do not require that a Deaf person on trial be provided with a signed-language interpreter. Most countries have some interpreters, although five said they have none at all. However, more than half do not have an organization of interpreters, nor do they require that interpreters be provided for Deaf persons seeking access to education, government services and the like. Finally, the survey showed that signed language rarely appears in the media, and there is rarely any provision for preserving signed-language literature on film or videotape.[38]

ASSIMILATIVE SOCIETIES AROUND THE WORLD[39]

In geographically isolated places around the world, such as islands, forests, or mountainous regions, there are, or were, communities with strikingly high percentages of Deaf members. Some of these communities have vanished and some are still thriving, but all teach us some important lessons about the DEAF–WORLD. Examples of these signing communities are Chilmark on the island of Martha's Vineyard, Massachusetts; a Yucatec Mayan village, Mexico; Adamorobe village, Ghana; Providence Island, Colombia; and Urubu, Brazil.[40]

Anthropologist Nora Groce traced the genealogies of the Deaf people of Martha's Vineyard back to common English ancestors from an area in the county of Kent called *the Weald*.[41] It was a land-locked, sheep-raising region whose people married within their own villages or nearby villages, so that most people in a small area were related to one another. Hence, they shared some of the same genes. Anecdotal evidence suggests that a Deaf community existed in the Weald in the seventeenth century. Some people in Kent were Puritans who settled in southern Massachusetts. Joined by further arrivals from Kent, many of whom carried a recessive gene for Deafness, several families moved to Martha's Vineyard and to the remote hills of Chilmark by the late 1600s.

With isolated villages, the pattern of marrying people within walking distance of one's own home continued, just as it had in Kent. In nineteenth-century America, the incidence of hereditary Deafness was estimated to be one out of 5,728. On Martha's Vineyard the incidence was one out of 155; in the town of Chilmark it was one out of 25, and in one area of Chilmark, one out of 4 people was born Deaf during this time.

By interviewing the last and quite elderly people, all hearing, who had a direct memory of the Martha's Vineyard signing community, scholars have learned about the townspeople's attitudes toward all the Deaf people who commingled and intermarried with them. Essentially, they felt that some people were right-handed, some left-handed, some were hearing, and some Deaf. Though there were marriages where both husband and wife were Deaf, most Deaf people married hearing people, all of whom knew the signed language. The Deaf were full participants in town politics. Though none are known to have served as selectmen, they did serve on committees and hold other elected offices.

Recounts one informant: "[The store] was the meeting place for everyone, the Deaf and dumb as well as the, ah . . . those who could talk. And of course everybody used the signed language, and they'd be making the signs in the signed language and there'd be complete silence in there, even those who could talk would be silent. Although those who could talk usually expressed the words with their mouths while they were making the signs . . ."

Hearing adults used signed language among themselves. Often they used signs when they were too far away to hear each other. Fishermen out on the ocean, for example, would sign between boats, or from ship to shore, which was of great benefit in the time before radios. People were described using spy glasses to see the signs of a neighbor across the way, taking turns signing and looking in the days before telephones. The Deaf and the hearing were equally adept at this long-distance communication.

During boring town meetings, people would sign across the room to each other, thus making good use of their time! They didn't mind that everyone could understand what they were saying, and since they weren't technically interrupting the meeting, which was being conducted in speech, they got away with it.

The Deaf as a group were remembered as being very well-educated for their era. Informants indicated that Deaf children received their early education at home. Between the ages of ten and twenty, they attended the American Asylum in Hartford for a course of five to seven years. This was at a time when many hearing children in town attended school for only two or three years. When Deaf children went from the Vineyard to Hartford, they brought their signed language with them, of course, and this apparently had a large impact on the ASL that was forming. One study found that Martha's Vineyard Sign Language had twenty-two percent cognates with ASL. It also had forty percent cognates with British Sign Language, which gives an indication of its origins.

Improved transportation and marriage with off-islanders ultimately led to the demise of the Deaf society. By 1952, there were no Deaf people living in Chilmark.

Communities like the one on Martha's Vineyard have been termed *assimilating*.[42] Since both Deaf and hearing people learn the signed language, Deaf people are assimilated into the larger hearing society. Deaf Yucatec Mayan villagers, for example, are reported to identify first with their family, then with their village, and third with the Mayan society. They had never thought of singling themselves out as a group until an American researcher invited them as a group to a party.[43] For a community to be assimilative, three ingredients appear to be essential: several generations of Deaf people (which assures the transmission of language and culture); a relatively high incidence of Deaf people (which motivates hearing people to learn the signed language); and geographic isolation encouraging intermarriage (which perpetuates the Deaf population) and face-to-face communication.

International Sign

Extensive contact among Deaf people from different nations probably dates from the first International Congresses of the Deaf, beginning in Paris in 1889. The first international Deaf organization, now known as the International Committee for Deaf Sports, was established in 1924 to host the quadrennial World Games for the Deaf (see p. 132). Today, more than fifty nations send players and spectators to the summer and winter world games. As we have seen, the World Federation of the Deaf has held its quadrennial international congresses, at which member states are represented, since 1951. Deaf scholars also gather at the International Workshops for Deaf Researchers, mentioned above, and at international and regional congresses on signed language, Deaf history, and other disciplines.

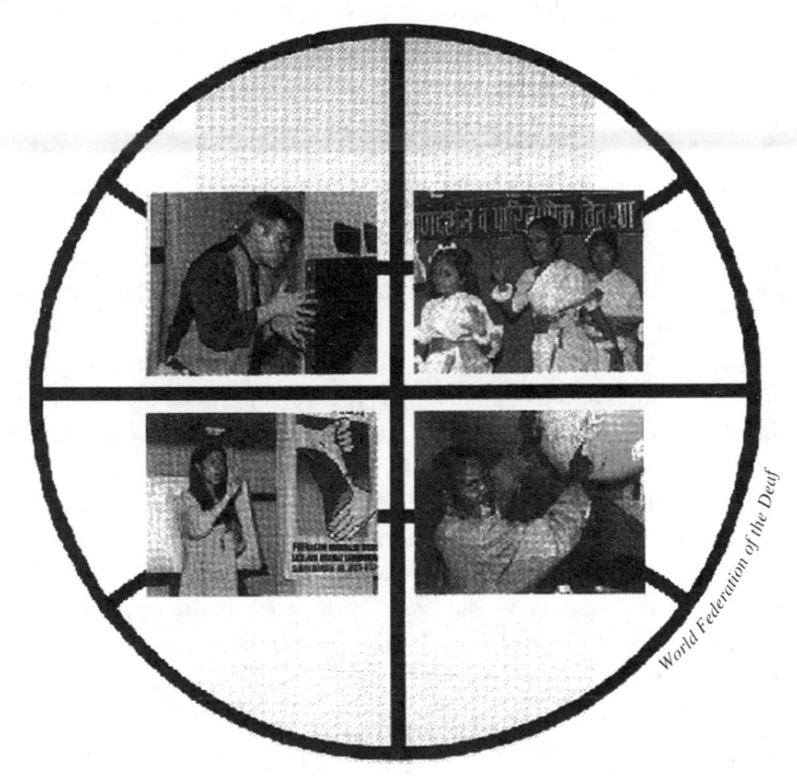

Fig. 6-2 **Speakers at regional meetings of the World Federation of the Deaf**

Partly as a result of international organizations such as these, contacts among Deaf people from different lands have proliferated in recent years, and a contact language known as *International Sign* has developed spontaneously, allowing speakers of mutually unintelligible signed languages to communicate. Increasingly at international meetings of Deaf people, speeches are interpreted not only into the signed language of the host country and sometimes into ASL, but also into International Sign. At WFD congresses, for example, Deaf participants from developing countries are frequently unaccompanied by interpreters of their signed languages. The vocabulary used in such contact situations is quite restricted: it consists mostly of nouns and verbs, with a few adjectives and adverbs; however, this depends on the creativity and experience of the signers. Vocabulary comes from three sources: the national signed languages of the interlocutors; mime; and a limited number of signs that have been adopted informally over the years as a standardized International Sign vocabulary.

In the 1970s the WFD led an effort to expand and standardize the vocabulary of International Sign. Three books were published presenting a total of nearly fifteen hundred signs selected from various signed languages. The first two books were inspired by the goal of a shared international language; the third, *Gestuno*, sought to facilitate communication at international meetings (just as Esperanto had been proposed as a standardized spoken language to facilitate international communication). The impact of this standardization effort on contemporary International Sign practiced in formal and informal situations has been limited. The grammatical structures of International Sign are surprisingly complex for a pidgin, although all are familiar to the student of various signed languages. Subjects and objects are placed in space and verbs are made to agree with those locations. Verbs are generally inflected for temporal aspect (e.g., continuous, habitual) and number (e.g., plural). Facial expression is used in questions and negation. There are several other negation markers (such as "finger wag," "palm up," and "zero") whose use is strictly determined by the structure of the sentence.[44] There may well be something universal about these features that makes them suitable for inclusion in International Sign. Consider verb agreement, for example: movement of the verb, from the location where the agent of the action has been placed to the location where the recipient of the action has been placed, may have transparent meaning to any observer. Indeed, one survey of the grammars of a half-dozen signed languages found verb agreement in all of them.[45] On the other hand, it is possible that the International Sign that has developed in formal situations such as WFD congresses is based largely on contacts among speakers of European signed languages. Most of those languages are historically related and would be expected to have common structures that would serve well in a contact language.

Integration of Deaf People in Hearing Nations

Because each nation is unique in its composition and history and in the place it makes for minority language groups, Deaf people around the world are positioned in radically different ways within the larger hearing society. In all four of our case studies of the world Deaf scene, Deaf people might well be said to be integrated into hearing society. In France, Sweden, Kenya, and Burundi, Deaf people do not live apart from hearing society; rather they live in its midst. They build or buy houses, pay taxes, shop and work among hearing people. In this integration, the Deaf are unlike some other language minorities—the Amish in the U.S., for example. Yet what a difference there is between Deaf integration in Burundi, on the one hand, and Sweden on the other. In Burundi, because of geography, history and poverty, Deaf people are present in the midst of hearing people, yet they have very limited possibilities of communicating with them or, indeed, with other Deaf people. Moreover, they have an extremely small sphere of self-determination. We can call this social structure *integration with isolation*. In Sweden, on the other hand, Deaf people's integration is founded on their distinct culture, language, and ties to the Deaf–World. We can call this *integration with autonomy*. Using a metaphor, Ben explains why there is no paradox in founding integration on a basis of autonomy. In the sea of humanity there are many harbors; one of them is the Deaf–World. Deaf people go to the harbor to anchor their connections to one another. Every day they venture out into the sea to deal with everyday matters, like work and purchasing. Deaf people know they are built to travel the entire sea of humanity and that they have to venture forth in order to enjoy life more fully and reap its benefits. Yet every sailor knows there is a time when the ship must be anchored in a snug harbor, safe from the stormy seas of life. There is nothing better than to anchor one's ship in a familiar harbor, where fraternity and bonding are readily accessible.

Ben's metaphor is meant to convey that Deaf people want integration with autonomy. That kind of integration requires that Deaf children grow up with pride in themselves and their DEAF–WORLD, fluency in its language, and strong bonding with its members. Hearing people have always wanted to help Deaf people to integrate into the larger hearing society. They underestimate, however, the extent to which Deaf people are already integrated into everyday life, getting and spending their income. And hearing people aim to achieve integration for this minority by integrating Deaf children into hearing classrooms (see chapter 8), minimizing what sets the Deaf child apart—Deaf language and culture. In our view, a dubious strategy with any language minority (see chapter 10), this was bound to fail with Deaf children, who can never supplant their signed language with spoken language. What it actually amounts to is *integration with isolation.* The schools unwittingly blockade the snug harbor of the DEAF–WORLD, urging the child out to sea without its resources—its language, a sense of one's place in history, and the knowledge that one belongs to a culture that transcends the individual. Such schools launch the Deaf child without resources because they are designed by hearing people who do not really know the DEAF–WORLD, and who have hearing pupils primarily in mind.

When school days are over, the hearing-oriented and hearing-conducted agenda for Deaf children does not end. Having failed to educate autonomous young Deaf people, the society finds it necessary to offer numerous services to Deaf adults, many in the hope of alleviating disadvantages arising from their school years. These services, too, fall short of the mark, because they begin and end with the hearing world; there is little or no place for Deaf culture in them. Our journey into the DEAF–WORLD requires us, then, to take an unsettling voyage onto the rough seas that the larger hearing society has in store for Deaf children and adults. It is into these waters that we venture in part 2.

❧

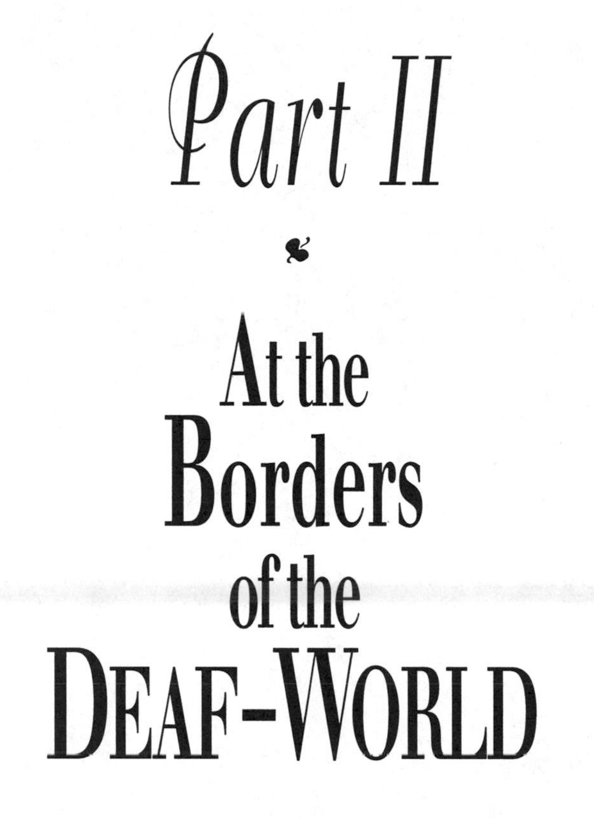

Part II

At the Borders of the DEAF-WORLD

Chapter 7

Disabling the Deaf-World

In the preceding chapters, we explored the meaning of DEAF–WORLD, including the centrality of the signed language of the Deaf in Deaf culture; the vital importance of organizations and educational institutions, especially residential schools for the Deaf, in the coalescing and maintenance of DEAF–WORLDS; the complex relationship between the DEAF–WORLD and the hearing world in which it is embedded; and to whose dictates it has historically been subject. We have also sampled some of the cross-cultural differences among DEAF–WORLDS. In this second part of our journey, we will focus on the interface between the two worlds in the U.S., in an area where the power of the hearing world has been most consistently exercised—the education of Deaf children.

As we saw in chapter 3, in the late nineteenth century, American Sign Language was banished from classrooms for the Deaf, and often, to the extent possible, banished from the schools themselves. From that point on, the language of instruction was to be English, and the focus and aim of all educational endeavor was that the Deaf should speak and understand speech. In the following chapters, and through the accounts of Jake, Henry, Roberto, and Laurel at the Metro Silent Club, whose story continues below, we shall explore in some detail how the obsessive concern with spoken English in Deaf education began to wane in the 1970s, though not with the result of restoring American Sign Language to its role as the language of instruction. What took the place of oralism as the dominant philosophy of Deaf education was Total Communication. In principle, subscribing to TC meant using all the means of communication with Deaf people at your disposal, including ASL, spoken and written English, fingerspelling, mime, etc. In practice, TC came to mean accompanying one's speech with a certain amount of signing.

We shall also see how the place of the residential schools in the education of Deaf children has been diminished under the influence of the movement to educate children with disabilities, to the extent possible, in ordinary public schools, and what this mainstreaming means to the DEAF-WORLD.

The phrase "children with disabilities" brings us to a controversy and conflict between the hearing world and the DEAF-WORLD that will concern us profoundly during the remainder of our journey. Baldly put, the hearing world sees the members of the DEAF-WORLD as disabled because they have limited hearing. The aim, by and large, of most of the hearing professionals who are their therapists and teachers, is to minimize their disability by the use of hearing aids, on the one hand, and by teaching them to speak, on the other. The members of the DEAF-WORLD, however, see themselves not as people with a disability, but as members of a language minority whose native language happens to be a signed language. This difference in perception has profound consequences, many of which we will observe in the chapters to come. Here, however, let us look at this business of spoken English, which, as we shall see, continues to be emphasized even in Total Communication programs, and especially in programs for young Deaf children.

Almost all the Deaf adults we know have gone through their formative years being taught speech, and they all (including the most skillful speakers) report that endeavoring to speak and in many cases to "hear" is very laborious and frustrating. It takes some more than eight years to finally get to the point where they can pronounce their name right. Ben didn't take that long, but to him it seemed like forever before his attempts at *Ben* didn't come out *Pat* or *Pen*. Even now, when he arrives at a restaurant and is asked for his name so the host can put it on the wait-list, it is not unusual to find that *Pat* has been written down instead of *Ben*—not to mention the occasion when one host put down Michael! Since *Ben* has one syllable, how this particular host heard two remains a mystery, though as Ben says, "if my name were Christopher, I probably would still be sitting in that speech therapist's chair today trying to get it right." Of course, now he can look back and joke about the experience. But when he was a child, going through the drills was a nightmare. You can see this struggle and pain in a French documentary film, *The Land of the Deaf*. When Ben saw this film, he found himself writhing in his seat, as if he were going through the oral drills of his school days all over again. He felt the anguish of the child as if it were his own, which in fact it was. Another account is given in *When the Mind Hears: A History of the Deaf*, where Harlan, guided by Laurent Clerc's autobiographical notes, portrays Clerc's efforts to learn to speak:

> The abbé would pull his chair up to my stool so close that our knees were touching and I could see the fine network of veins on his bulbous red-blue nose. He held my left hand firmly to his voice box and my right hand on my own throat, and glowered down at me through beady, rheumy eyes. Then his warm garlic-laden breath would wash over my head and fill my nostrils to suffocating. "Daaa," he wailed, exposing the wet, pink cavern of his mouth, his tongue obscenely writhing on its floor, barely contained by the picket of little brown and yellow teeth.
>
> "Taaa," he exploded and the glistening pendant of tissue in the back of his mouth flicked toward the roof, opening the floodgates to the miasma that rose from the roiling contents of his stomach below. "Taaa, daaa, teee, deee," he made me screech again and again, but contort my face as I would, fighting back the tears, search as I would desperately, in a panic, for the place in my mouth accurately to put my tongue, convulse as I would my breathing—I succeeded no better. One day he became so impatient he gave me a violent blow on the chin; I bit my tongue and dissolved in tears—the awful boundless grief of childhood, the careening through anguish of a frightened boy who had drunk more than his fill of disgust and frustration and knew he could not follow this false route any longer.[1]

And all this for what? Just so Ben can properly say *Ben*, and someday the host in a restaurant can write down his name right?

Many parents and teachers claim that their Deaf children and pupils need to be taught speech so that as adults they will not appear "disabled" and will be able to talk and mingle with hearing people on an equal basis. But in the view of the DEAF-WORLD, to be subjected to extensive speech therapy and remedial work is in itself a very disabling experience. Of course, being able to speak is a convenience, but to members of the DEAF-WORLD that is all it is—and it is much more of a convenience for the hearing than the Deaf. Parents are often told that their Deaf child should not learn American Sign Language early in life because signed language is easier to learn than speech, and if it is learned early, it will become a crutch and the child won't ever learn to speak. Johnny can always learn signed language later in life, Johnny's parents are told, after he has had a go at speech. People in the DEAF-WORLD know there is a penalty for delaying the acquisition of signed language: very few late learners possess native-like competency in ASL. And the scientific research supports this cultural tenet, as we saw in chapter 4.

Actually, the notion that signed language is easy is promoted by some Deaf people themselves, especially those who entered the DEAF-WORLD later in life. One such person claims it took only six months to learn signed language; another says it took her merely two. The truth is that in such a short period of time, Deaf people may be able to establish useful communication, but that does not mean they have attained competence in the language. The mistaken judgment of the fluency of short-term learners leads to another more serious mistake: ASL's detractors reason that if it is so easy to learn, it must be a simple language. However, learning ASL appears easy to Deaf people, even late learners, not because the language is simple, but because it is so *natural* for people whose lives revolve around vision. It is incomparably easier than struggling to learn a spoken language that one cannot hear.

Any first language should come to its learners naturally. When they have to struggle to acquire competency in it, then that language is not natural to them and the experience of trying to learn it turns into a disabling experience.

Deaf people are frequently reminded, growing up, that it is extremely important for them to use their voice, that relying on signed language alone is a mark of being a "loser." The distinguished writer David Wright, who lost his hearing when he was seven years old, contends that "the choice between defiance and playing victim is a central part of the Deaf experience." He equates defiance with struggling against the odds to overcome one's handicap and communicate orally, and playing victim with using signed language. The hearing world drills this notion into the Deaf from grade school through post-college career advancement seminars, until the Deaf themselves may come to believe it. It is based on trying to make Deaf people into hearing people, which they can never be. When Deaf people fail at the alien task, as they must, then they are considered to be in need of rehabilitation. Is it then really the case, as Wright would have it, that saying, *My name is Ben* (and having *Pat* written down) is an act of defiance? If Deaf people have been taught to use speech while growing up, then how are they defying anything if they are conforming to that teaching? To the contrary, the view among members of the DEAF–WORLD is increasingly that the use of signed language, and the declaration of adherence to the use of signed language, is the act of defiance. Those who comply with what they were taught—to value speech and English over ASL—are falling victim to the hearing world's designation of them as disabled. Many Deaf people want to be viewed as part of a linguistic minority and are defying the portrayal of them as people with disabilities.

We have seen and will continue to look at how the choice of spoken language as the language to be used with Deaf children can turn into a very disabling practice. However, there is an even more threatening development underway now in the education of the Deaf, another potentially disabling experience that Ben and the Deaf adults in the Metro Silent Club were spared. Like oralism, this movement is predicated on a rejection of the central fact of the Deaf child's life, the reality that he or she is Deaf. This drive, which began as early as the 1960s, then accelerated in the '70s with the passage of the Education for All Handicapped Children Act, aims to the extent possible to place all children considered to have disabilities, including the Deaf, in regular local schools. As we shall see in chapter 8, because there are so few Deaf children in any locale and age group, most such mainstreamed Deaf children find themselves with one or no other Deaf child in their class. While the members of the Metro Silent Club interviewed by Gloria have attended different kinds of schools, and some of them were at one time or another placed alone in classrooms filled with hearing students, they all nevertheless had a time in their life when they were in the company of other Deaf children. This is not the case for a significant number of Deaf children today. The consequences of this will be explored in chapter 8.

While you're reading the second part of the story of Gloria and the Metro Silent Club, keep in mind this issue of disability. Note that here in the club is one place where members of the DEAF–WORLD all feel equal, where no one and nothing suggests that they have a disability of any sort; where, indeed, there is only one "disabled" person in evidence: the hearing woman sitting at the table, who looks (and is) totally out of place.

AT THE METRO SILENT CLUB II

Gloria sat at the table while the others busily conversed for what seemed like eternity, before the interpreters finally returned from their short break. She was mightily relieved to see them. She had felt like she was drowning in the flurry of signed conversation, not understanding anything. When the others laughed, she wondered why they were laughing. When she noticed Laurel reacting to a comment of Henry's with a shocked look, she wondered what Henry could have said to cause this. After a while, she had settled for watching their faces and trying to follow the mood of the conversation. At times, she had found herself laughing along with them, and felt incredibly silly.

Now she glanced up at the interpreters and the group and was surprised to find that they were all looking at her expectantly. "I was just thinking," she said.

"What about?" asked Jake, eyeing her quizzically. And she thought, He already knows, they all do, because they've been there all their lives, except when they come here. Finally, she responded, "I was thinking about how out of place I felt just now. I mean, watching you talk, hearing you laugh, and being completely out of it. That's why you wanted to meet me here, isn't it?"

For once Jake looked nonplussed. Then he smiled. "You're being very blunt for a hearing person," he said. "Yes, that was it. I wanted you to glimpse what it was like for Roberto, Henry and Laurel when they were kids, not understanding, not being able to make themselves understood. I wanted you to see what it's often like for all of us when we are outside the DEAF–WORLD. People in the hearing world think of the DEAF–WORLD as a cultural ghetto. We think of it, you might say, as a place where we can understand the jokes."

"That's it," said Henry. "At home, dinner was absolutely the worst time; I couldn't understand the jokes. Everyone was laughing and I'd say, 'What's so funny?' and they'd sort of shrug it off and say 'Nothing.' I couldn't follow the conversations my parents and sister had either, though sometimes I could tell they were talking about me.

"Eventually, my mother learned fingerspelling, so she could communicate with me a little. To this day, that's how we communicate—fingerspelling and gesturing, and I can read her lips some of the time. All these years, my father has been mostly absent, he is even absent when he's around, you know what I mean? To this day when he wants to talk to me he just mumbles, which makes it impossible to lip-read, so we end up writing to each other. Prior to my placement at the day school, I vaguely recall that my mother and I used some home signs. It's funny, because back then my parents prohibited me from using signed language, but we developed those home signs just the same.

"I don't mean to imply I was always miserable. There were good times with my family, when we had trips together. But I didn't have much contact with the other children in the neighborhood. Either they were afraid to play with me or my mother was afraid to let me go out alone. It wasn't until I got to school and met some other Deaf kids that I had friends to hang around with, and then I could get the jokes."

"It's true," said Roberto. "You know, when someone tells a long joke and people are laughing throughout. Finally, you ask somebody in your family what was said, and they kind of tell it to you quickly, very condensed, and it isn't funny at all."

"It made me so mad growing up," Laurel added. "I mean, always being left out. It didn't have to be that way. But my parents felt that if I ever learned fifty signs I'd be contaminated. So I can say, I never relaxed.

Every sentence was an effort, all day long. At Gally—that's Gallaudet, Gloria—I had a friend from a hearing family just like mine, except everyone in her family knew how to sign. Everyone: parents, brothers, sisters, grandparents, aunts, uncles. It was amazing. So I could have been connected all along. The heartache was needless. It really made me furious. If I sound bitter, well, I am. Henry and Roberto were lucky by comparison. Their parents couldn't communicate with them either, but they didn't try to prevent them from communicating, or if they did, they didn't try very hard. Well, now I try and think positive. It happened late but it happened; at eighteen I started my life."

Gloria was both stunned and touched that Laurel felt able to be so open with her. Jake had a look of, You see? *written all over him. Henry and Roberto were nodding in agreement. "So each of you had to wait years before you could have a real conversation, except Jake, I guess. It seems so strange, not to understand just naturally."*

"The funny thing is," Jake said, "I understood things just naturally until I got to school. Every Deaf person has a school story. I'll tell you mine and then the others will tell you theirs. Okay?"

JAKE'S STORY

"I went to the same residential school that my parents went to. I clearly remember my first day at CSD, as we called it. I was about five years old when they dropped me off. I was taken to the primary department and to the dorm. My parents told me, 'This is where you will live while you go to school and get an education,' and they left me with this hearing 'house parent' who didn't know how to sign. It was a drastic change for me, coming from a home where everything was understood and signed language was used, and then finding this lady who gave instructions with her lipstick-smeared lips. I didn't understand her. All I knew was that whatever she was trying to say was coming from lips I couldn't help staring at in amazement. Why would anyone apply something so thick and so red? The dorm was empty and she pointed to another building across the yard and mouthed the word "Ssss kuh oooll," after which she took my hand and ushered me into the building she was pointing to. That's where my primary school education began. I remember that day vividly. It was the beginning of not understanding.

"At that school the method of teaching Deaf children was primarily oral in the elementary department. The teachers and dorm parents used nothing but the oral method to talk with us. The kids were signing to each other, but as I recall, I was one of only four in the entire primary department who could sign fluently at five years old. It turned out that the three other kids who could sign either had Deaf parents or older Deaf brothers or sisters in the same school. We would sign to each other and other kids would gather around us to observe our conversation, and soon they began to pick up signed language and were able to carry on a conversation in ASL. All through our elementary school years, wherever we were except class—in the dorms or on the playground—our primary way of communicating was in ASL.

"In the classroom the teachers would teach us how to read and write and do basic arithmetic, but most of the time was spent on practicing our speech drills. When a new subject was introduced, for example if we were learning about different colors, the teacher would stop midway in the instruction and make us articulate the colors: 'Orange, orange, orange,' over and over again until we all got it right. After about a week we probably covered four colors. In class we had to use headphones all day and they were goddamn uncomfortable—this huge black thing that pressed against your ears as if it wanted to compress your head.

"Throughout my elementary school years, my classmates and I remained together—except for one boy who was moved to a lower track. The school had several tracks for each grade: A was the highest, B next, and so on. Anyway, this boy was as smart as the rest of us but he couldn't speak at all, so they placed him in a lower track. One day, they passed out buttons to all the kids in the A and B tracks that read: I TALK. We were so proud to wear that button walking down the hall. I remember vividly passing that former classmate of mine, seeing him lined up with the other students in the D class. He was standing there looking at my button. He didn't have one because he didn't talk.

"There was one teacher in the elementary school who had an interesting way of teaching. Her name sign was N-ON-THE-CHEEK. *She was a skillful artist. When she taught us, she was able to use her drawings. I recall learning a lot from her because of the link between the drawings and the written word.*

"Basically, as we got older in the primary department, more and more kids were signing fluently in the dorm and would 'sneak' a signed conversation in class, in the hall or in the playground—whenever the teacher wasn't looking. All the teachers in that department were hearing and none of them signed, or if they knew signed language they never used it. It turned out that as kids, we depended on each other to understand and to transmit what was being said. One classmate was a good lipreader and we would count on him to repeat in signed language, when the teacher wasn't looking, what she had said. The school was strictly oral in the elementary department. But the older I got, the more signed language was used in class. In high school all teachers used some kind of signed language in class and I understood everything."

ROBERTO'S STORY

"I discovered other Deaf kids when I went off to preschool. It was a mainstreaming program in a hearing elementary school. My hearing brothers and sisters went to the same school, but I was assigned to part of the school for kids with special needs. I was put in a class with other Deaf students. That's what they call self-contained, *Gloria, a special class or section for Deaf kids in a regular school. From preschool up through second grade the class was mostly oral with a lot of emphasis on amplification. We wore big earphones a lot of the time. After that, it was TC, which involved the use of Signed English, you know, with made-up signs like IS, ING, NESS, etcetera, along with spoken English.* But the emphasis was still on speech and English grammar. I didn't understand much of it.*

"In third through fifth grade the teacher would make us go through various English drills. Each one had a different sentence pattern that we had to repeat over and over in order to memorize specific rules, like when to put an article before the noun, and which linking verb is appropriate for which situation. I remember one teacher had us act out what was written on the blackboard. She wrote 'Jeffrey is swimming'; she signed J-ON-CHEST

---

* As noted in chapter 2, Signed English is among the artificial signing systems we call MCE systems. We gloss the signs of such systems in capital letters.

IS SWIM ING. Jeffrey would have to stand up and pretend to be swimming. While he was still doing this, she would then write and sign, 'Heather is jumping,' and Heather had to jump up and down. Then while Jeffrey was swimming in the air and Heather was jumping, the teacher would write and sign, 'Adam is falling,' and make Adam fall down and get up just to fall over again, to keep the concept of falling down going. 'Chelsea is dreaming' meant Chelsea had to stare into space. Can you imagine if you were a visitor walking by this classroom? The impression you would get if you glanced into this room would be, 'Boy, there is a bunch of wackos in room thirty-five.'

"All three teachers we had knew signs, but only one could sign really well and could understand the kids. With the other two teachers, if we didn't want them to understand what we said, all we had to do was just shut off our voices and keep on signing.

"In elementary school we were mainstreamed with hearing kids in two situations: for gym, and if there was a general school activity. Then our teachers became our interpreters. Sometimes a teacher's aide would do it in place of the teacher. This pretty much continued into middle school. I would still hang out with my classmates all the time, though, even when we were in gym or in the lunch room.

"The older I got the more integrated I was. Most of my classmates from elementary school stayed in the self-contained class, but I was placed in hearing classes with an interpreter following me most of the day. I was in self-contained class for home room in the morning and English. I was integrated for math, science, history and shop. I remember in high school, the interpreter, who was also a tutor, was at times the only friend I had. I still socialized with my Deaf friends, but we were separated most of the time. The hearing kids were very cliquish. I was the odd one out, it wasn't 'cool' to hang around with someone like me. When I walked into a classroom, I would see groups of kids seated together. There were the cheerleader girls, who would sit near each other in one group. Another group would be Latinos, and another group would be jocks. I was never sure where I belonged. I wanted to join some of them, but never felt totally welcome, even among the Latinos, since I didn't know Spanish. I would walk into a classroom and scan the room, and when I found my interpreter over in the corner, I would be relieved and walk directly to her

and strike up a conversation until the teacher showed up. Now as I look back I think to myself, 'Gosh, the interpreter was my only friend.'"

LAUREL'S STORY

"I went to an oral school that was a residential school but with an oral-only philosophy. We had to communicate with each other and with the teachers and other staff orally. Any use of signs or gestures was forbidden. My experience in the early elementary years was like Jake's. But instead of phasing out into signed language, we stuck with oralism and auditory training throughout middle school. There was no high school. The concept was, quote unquote, 'you prepare the kids to learn how to hear, lip-read and speak until they are ready to be integrated into the hearing world.' It was set up as if we were expected to be integrated into a hearing high school in our town.

"We would have speech lessons in every class. If the teacher was introducing a new word in, for example, science, like, say 'conductor,' she would make us all pronounce it in succession: kon duk' tor. If one of us got it wrong, she made that person repeat it until it was right. The right pronunciation and the right stress.

They had a merit system where you earned points for not 'waving your hands' (that is, signing) for one week, for paying attention in class, for good behavior. We had an assembly on Fridays where they announced the names of those who had earned lots of points. If you were caught signing, points you had earned were taken away. Teachers or dorm parents would monitor this everywhere, in the dining room and even the playground. It was even monitored at home. My mother would punish me whenever I tried to use my hands to communicate.

When there were no adults around, if you were in a dorm room, for example, you could talk a little with gestures and some homemade signs. Not real language though, because signed language was considered bad for you, bad for your brains—it made you lazy and your speech skills would wither once you used signed language. That was what they told us. It was important to resist the urge to sign or use gestures. Teachers and dorm parents would say, 'Stop waving your hands around, it's not attractive.' A lot of us grew up believing this. I know some of my schoolmates today still refuse to learn signed language even though they are adults.

"After finishing middle school I was sent to a public high school near home. There were no interpreters. I was expected to lip-read and be able to participate. It was a nightmare for me. I barely survived. I remember being humiliated almost every day. Even though I played some sports, which were okay, I still would come home crying from frustration and embarrassment, and my mother would tell me, 'You have to face it. After all, this is a hearing world. This is what the world is like, you've got to live with it.' I remember thinking to myself, 'If this is what it's like, I don't want to live.' Little did I know that there was a wonderful DEAF–WORLD. I didn't get to know that until I went to Gallaudet. The school and my mother preached that being in the DEAF–WORLD retards your intelligence and limits your overall personal growth. I was deliberately kept away from it. We even went on a school trip to Washington, DC, and they never mentioned or showed us Gallaudet. I was kept in the dark about the history and culture of Deaf people. I found out about Gallaudet while I was discussing different options with my hearing high school counselor. She brought me to the library to examine materials about different colleges and universities. We happened on Gallaudet University. It was like a sign. Right there, I decided to enroll, against my mother's wishes. It did occur to me when I arrived at Gallaudet that what I had been warned about might be true and that I might be making a mistake. But I discovered there a totally accessible environment where everyone and everything, from signed language to captions, were designed for my eyes. For the first time in my life, I didn't feel left out. It was the opposite of what I had been told. In fact, I bloomed; I discovered myself. I finally saw myself as a Deaf person, rather than as a 'hearing-impaired person.'"

HENRY'S STORY

"If you look at all of them, Jake's, Roberto's and Laurel's experiences, and take a little bit of each of them, you can explain my experience, although I went to a day school where all the kids were Deaf or hard-of-hearing. There was no Deaf teacher, but there were several Deaf teacher's aides. My experience was much like Roberto's in that I would just go home after school. Although we did have varsity sports in high school, and I played baseball, I wasn't a starter. The school used TC with the kids. My

school had two different tracks: the hard-of-hearing track and the Deaf track. The hard-of-hearing track was primarily oral, and the Deaf track was TC. Sometimes biology class, for example, would have some hard-of-hearing students and some Deaf students in the same room. When that happened, the language of the classroom suddenly shifted to mostly oral. It seemed like the hard-of-hearing kids were the most important. Also, teachers wouldn't sign with each other, they tended to use speech with each other in front of the kids. When we asked them to sign they would say, 'it's a private matter.' But we Deaf kids would think to ourselves, If it's private, how come the hard-of-hearing kids are able to follow?

"Remember Roberto's story about the teacher teaching JUMP ING and all the structured lessons? Well we went through the same thing. I remember very well when I was young, around fifth grade, I went to the bathroom, and as I went down the hall I saw a clown in another classroom. I was so thrilled that I ran down the hall to my classroom and signed in ASL 'SAW THERE SAW THERE CLOWN, NOW!' My teacher stopped me and said, 'Sign that again using English.' So I signed, 'I SEE-past CLOWN *THERE OTHER CLASS THERE NOW!!' The teacher stopped me again and said, 'Say it right, say "I SEE-past A CLOWN,"' and I signed, 'I SEE A CLOWN.' And she said, 'You forgot the past tense, "SEE-past." Say it again, "I SEE-past A CLOWN."' Finally I signed it, 'I SEE-past A CLOWN,' and she praised me, saying, 'Wow, that is good, now use your voice.' When I saw the clown I was very excited. But after this exercise, I didn't care about it anymore.*

"In high school I became interested in drafting. Then I was placed in a vocational track with special emphasis in drafting and technical drawing. We had a good graphic arts teacher who was a child of Deaf parents. He would teach us about graphic designing and also about life in general. He would bring strange and amazing stories to class every day. He would pull stories from the newspaper and tell them to us. The stories were sometimes funny, sometimes serious, sometimes weird, but the bottom line was that he was teaching us that there was a life outside of school that was as crazy as could be, and that we were better off despite being Deaf, and that being Deaf was nothing compared to the stories he told us. I think it was he who got me interested in graphic arts and drafting. In fact, I think I decided to major in this vocation because of him. I think it

takes one teacher out of many to make an impact on our lives. Each of us has one teacher he or she can look back on and say, 'This person changed my life.' If I am right, it appears that the teacher who signs the best is the one who reaches us.

"In any case, it was that teacher who got me to go to NTID—that's the National Technical Institute for the Deaf, part of the Rochester Institute of Technology—and that's where I really discovered the DEAF–WORLD. For the first time in my life, I was able to participate in all kinds of activities with Deaf friends. Some of the Deaf students preferred to hang out with hearing students from RIT, but I would hang out with other Deaf people. So, sort of like Laurel, going away to college was coming home for me."

"We have to stop," Jake said. "The interpreters need a break, and so do I. I can sum it up this way. All these stories are different, but they're all the same.

"Except Jake, we all had to go in search of our place in the world, our community, even our language," Henry said. "Thing is, we found them."

"But it's not like we live in the DEAF–WORLD," Roberto said. "Every day we go out and work and shop and do everything in the hearing world. Work is in the hearing world. The schools are sort of in between. But when you really want to relax and be with your friends, people like yourself, then you come to the club, have a few beers, whatever."

"Now there's a good idea," said Jake. What would you like, Gloria?"

❧

Chapter 8

Educational Placement and the Deaf Child

WHAT if you were a child and you had to go to a school where you didn't understand the teacher in your classroom? At the very least, your access to the subject matter would be limited, dependent on what you could learn from texts.

But what if you couldn't read very well either? What if you were thirteen before you were able to understand print, and even then your comprehension was extremely limited? What if, on entering junior high school, you were reading at the third-grade level, which is the situation for the typical Deaf child?

What if you were unable to gain access to incidental information either, for example, conversations between teachers and other children or adults? What could you learn?

We may surmise from the accounts of Jack, Roberto, Henry and Laurel in the preceding chapter that this was the situation during the education of most members of the DEAF–WORLD alive today. As we shall see, it continues to be the situation for most of their Deaf children, as well as for the Deaf children of hearing parents (the vast majority of Deaf children, as we saw in chapter 2).

Suppose you were unable to understand even your peers, so that your only meaningful interactions at school took place between you and one other adult, your interpreter or teacher, who "filtered" all information from the environment for you. What would you learn then? How would your psychological and social development proceed? How could your teacher evaluate your progress?

As we shall see, young Deaf children often face educational environments like this. We will examine some of the forces that place these obstacles in the way of their education: the hearing parents' natural desire to have their children schooled close to home; the small numbers of Deaf children; the higher academic quality of many local schools compared to specialized programs; and especially, the dominant educational philosophy, which views Deaf children as children with a disability and has a single solution for virtually all categories of children with disabilities—inclusion in mainstream schools and programs.

Suppose that you are being tested and the measure of your success is contingent on your figuring out what the examiner wants you to do, because the person who is testing you is not proficient in your signed language. Maybe you have a minimal command of English. Your teacher is a native speaker of English and she knows one of the invented signing systems for representing English. When talking to you, she speaks and signs the signs of the MCE system at the same time. Research has shown that the average teacher using an MCE system is able to make her signs correspond to her spoken English somewhere between fifty and eighty percent of the time.[1] So naturally, the MCE proves very difficult for you to understand. It requires a knowledge of English and of the MCE system. Nevertheless, the examiner, like the teacher, expects you to understand her, and to fill in the gaps as best you can.[2]

Suppose that when you use your signed language, the examiner is able to understand only one-third to one-half of what you say.[3] You are a bright, adaptable human being, and you attempt to use the language of the examiner by adjusting your signing to reflect the level of the adult's. You do this, though you are uncertain of what the examiner knows and uncertain of the sign forms the examiner might recognize or choose to use. You hope the examiner will request more information from you when he or she doesn't understand, but you have learned in your short life that adults feel they know more than children, and so tend to avoid acknowledging any sort of weakness. How well would you do on the test?

As you move through school, the hearing adults responsible for imparting knowledge about the world to you continue to be unable to carry on a conversation of any complexity with you. These same adults openly acknowledge that they have great difficulty understanding Deaf children like you, yet they believe that the major obstacle to your educational success resides in you. Hence they perceive you to be a slow learner, and they proceed to change the information they choose to teach you by reducing its language complexity. Teachers present the information to you as if you were in the first or second grade, even though you are twelve years old and in junior high school.

Functioning in such an environment depends on your skill at figuring out what the instructor is actually presenting to you and then figuring out what it really means. Your past experience with adults who do not sign very well suggests that you will have great difficulty deciphering the signs themselves, and even more difficulty discovering the sense of the whole. You develop a great knack for guessing and create a system of strategies that you depend on when trying to obtain information. For example, if you recognize the sign for a person, place or thing and believe that it is the first-named item in the sentence, you assume it is the "doer" of whatever action comes along. This will get you in trouble sometimes. You may misunderstand *Bobby was bitten by Jennifer* to mean *Bobby bit Jennifer*.

If you become frustrated and withdrawn, or constantly ask that information be repeated, you may be perceived as having an intellectual or emotional disorder. If you make the mistake of reacting to the first thing the teacher says, you may find yourself labeled impulsive. If you constantly try to get the teacher's attention and thereby disrupt the class, you might be considered to have a behavior disorder.

Such, more or less, is the educational environment faced by most Deaf children. In the next few chapters, we explore the various manifestations of this environment in some detail and discuss how it came to be so, the consequences for the DEAF–WORLD, and what, from the perspective of the DEAF–WORLD, should be done about it.

DEAF EDUCATION AND THE LAW

In the 1970s two laws were passed by the U.S. Congress that have profoundly affected the education of Deaf children. Intended to make life easier and more productive for people with disabilities, among whom the hearing world includes the Deaf, they are the Rehabilitation Act of 1973, in particular Section 504, and the Education for All Handicapped Children Act (PL 94-142), passed in 1975 and later renamed the Individuals with Disabilities Education Act (IDEA). Together these laws require that local school districts and states provide a free and *appropriate* education to every disabled child, starting when the child is three years old. (The most recent law concerning people with disabilities, the 1990 Americans with Disabilities Act, or ADA, is a civil rights law, and is discussed in chapter 12.)

Under IDEA, the Federal government became responsible for defining "appropriate education" for children with disabilities, and it proceeded to issue guidelines specifying a range of acceptable placement options. At the time the law was passed, many children with disabilities, in particular those with mental retardation, lived in separate residential facilities, where they frequently received poor educational and social training. IDEA was intended in part to ensure that such separate facilities, often referred to as "institutions," would be the last place a state or a public school district would choose to send a child with a disability. To this end, the act specified that every such child was entitled to an education in the "least restrictive environment" (LRE) possible; thus, the range of acceptable placements for the child became a hierarchy in which residential facilities ranked at the bottom. In fact, according to the strictest interpretation of the principle of the LRE by the Office of Special Education and Rehabilitation Services of the federal Department of Education (OSERS), the preferred locale of educational services for the child with a disability is the neighborhood school, and the child should be placed in as close proximity as possible to his or her peers without disabilities, which in the case of the Deaf would be hearing children in a regular classroom.

The problem for the Deaf was, and still is, twofold. First, under the LRE principle as interpreted by OSERS, the residential schools for the Deaf, which are a core element in the very identity of many members of the DEAF–WORLD, and where the Deaf children of hearing parents may encounter peers and adults fluent in ASL for the first time, are referred to as "institutions" and hence positioned at the bottom of the placement hierarchy. Second, most Deaf children require the use of a unique, visual language, which is the language neither of instruction nor of conversation in the preferred setting for the education of most children with disabilities, that is, regular public schools. Thus, the laws that were created to protect those with disabilities carry with them conflicts for the Deaf child and, often, for the Deaf adult who wishes to obtain a quality education. These conflicts are grounded in the issues of language and culture that mark the interface between the DEAF–WORLD and the hearing world.

The Disability Dilemma

The DEAF–WORLD faces a dilemma with regard to the provisions in the laws concerning children with disabilities. On the one hand, disability legislation aims to provide Deaf children and adults with an education, access to information, and protection of their civil rights; they must have these provisions if they are to live fulfilling lives and to be participating citizens in our democracy. Therefore, the DEAF–WORLD supports such legislation. On the other hand, the DEAF–WORLD is a linguistic and cultural minority quite unlike disability groups and with a distinctly different agenda (discussed in chapter 15).

Moreover, to be Deaf is not a disability in Deaf culture, and most members of the DEAF–WORLD see no disability in their way of being. To give up their legal rights would be self-defeating; to demand them under disability law seems like hypocrisy and undermines the Deaf agenda, which aims for acceptance of ASL and Deaf culture.

PLACEMENT: PARENT-INFANT AND PRESCHOOL PROGRAMS

In chapter 2, we described the parents of Deaf children—in particular hearing parents, but Deaf parents as well—struggling with an enormous amount of information regarding the best path to follow in raising their children. Especially in urban areas, the array of options available, starting with parent-infant and preschool programs, is staggering—as many programs, it sometimes seems, as there are professionals who serve Deaf children.

Given the small numbers of Deaf children and their unique communication needs, traditional educational programs for them did not offer early intervention; thus, hospitals, local speech therapists, and some private schools for the Deaf stepped into the breach.[4] Not surprisingly, early intervention programs based in hospitals or speech and hearing clinics (along with most programs based in colleges and universities, which tend to be operated by speech therapists or audiologists who have been trained in hospital-based programs) nearly always see in the young Deaf child only problems posed by disability. In other words, they think that the child is in need of a plan to correct his or her inability to hear. There is very little discussion of the child using vision to learn a language, and there is no mention of the benefits of ASL as a language model. Hearing parents are taught how to encourage and train their Deaf infant to use speech—an approach that tends to put the burden of success or failure on the hearing parents. Since the Deaf infant's ability to acquire speech depends on many things, most of which are not predictable from audiological testing, this approach is embarked on without anyone really knowing whether the child will benefit.

Following the passage of IDEA, with its requirement that school systems make appropriate education available starting at age three, there was a virtual explosion of publicly funded school-based early intervention programs for children with disabilities, including the Deaf. However, the act and its associated funding cover children only starting at age three, and because of the low incidence of hearing loss in the general population, publicly supported parent-infant programs for Deaf children in the first three years of life are few and far between. Services may be offered to parents and their Deaf infants by a counselor or a consulting teacher of the Deaf in connection with an educational program, often in a local elementary school. In rare instances some programs have Deaf professionals who function as parent liaisons. More typically, the Deaf professional is found only in residential programs, which may be an unsuitable placement for very young Deaf children.

For somewhat older children with disabilities, there is an eclectic array of publicly-funded state and regional early-intervention programs, and these are open to Deaf enrollments. (In the years immediately following passage of IDEA, eighty-eight percent of school systems began offering programming for children with disabilities from ages three to six.[5]) Because of the low incidence of Deaf children, however, such programs rarely have professional staff trained to work with them, and the

Deaf child may well be grouped with children who are able to communicate rapidly and easily with the staff in English. In such groups, the Deaf child will at best have very limited access to the spoken language of the teachers and the other children.

Sometimes there is a complicating factor in such early intervention programs that may restrict the Deaf child's development even more. Because the Deaf child cannot speak English, he or she may be categorized with hearing children who also do not communicate in spoken language, including children with learning or emotional disorders. In such cases, the Deaf child lands in a program that greatly underestimates his or her cognitive, social, and academic capabilities. Typically, there is no expertise among the teachers or administrators of such programs on how to serve Deaf children. Responsibility for teaching them usually falls to a speech therapist, who is responsible as well for speech therapy for all the other children who require it and who are hearing.

In most states there are also early-intervention programs based in residential schools for the Deaf, which frequently provide a comprehensive educational program for the Deaf child from infancy through high school. While the law's focus on children age three and older means that the parent-infant portions of these programs may not always be funded properly, typically they are the only parent-infant programs with strong continuing ties to the DEAF–WORLD.

Because of the Total Communication movement in schools and programs for the Deaf, many early intervention programs changed from oral-only to oral with the addition of signing, relying in particular on one of the invented systems of signing that we have called, generically, manually coded English, or MCE systems. As we shall see in chapter 9, MCE systems have proliferated in Deaf education in the last two decades. Although the practice is not sustained by research, programs at all levels have adopted MCE, including programs for the Deaf infant in which parents are trained to use an MCE system as the visual input for the Deaf child. Although these MCE programs may not emphasize speech, they urge parents to speak and sign (using the MCE system) simultaneously.

With the growing recognition of ASL, a new type of parent-infant program emerged in the late 1980s that uses ASL as the basis for enhancing language development in Deaf infants. Typically, a professional who is Deaf provides services to hearing parents and their Deaf infants both in the home and at the school site. When the services are provided in the home, hearing parents have an opportunity to come into contact with Deaf adults, who can be role models for their Deaf children on the parents' and children's own turf. In the resulting non-threatening atmosphere, parents can ask knowledgeable Deaf professionals questions about the future of their child that hearing professionals are unlikely to be able to answer.[6]

All the various types of early intervention programs are further subdivided according to the age of the children enrolled. Indeed, when parents seek to learn about educational programming, they find that the term *early intervention* can cover just the infant-to-three age range, or infant-to-six. Parent-infant programs only provide services until age three. After that, the child must transfer into a different, school-based program. The private hospital-based programs will serve a Deaf child as long as there is third-party payment (usually health insurance). The Deaf child may thus continue with costly speech therapy in a hospital-based program for many years, even while he or she also attends a school-based program.

When Deaf children reach three years of age, they are eligible for the numerous preschool programs federally funded under IDEA and offered in public and private schools—programs of the kind that Roberto attended and that reflect the various elementary education programs available in general. There are programs that function like parent-child tutorials, where parents are taught how to work with their Deaf child in somewhat of an extension of the parent-infant programs. These programs tend to focus on the speech, lipreading, and auditory skills of the Deaf child; they may be solely oral or they may involve the use of signs, but their primary purpose is the development of the child's ability to use spoken language.

In contrast, there are also cognitive-academic preschool programs that tend to focus on knowledge as the fundamental tool for learning. Such schools put less emphasis on hearing and speech and much more on presenting content for the young Deaf child to learn.[7] Teachers in these programs almost always use one of the MCE systems when communicating with their pupils, not ASL.[8] Although a number of preschool programs now have some Deaf professional staff who work with parents and Deaf children, there is still widespread reluctance to use ASL, in part because of the mistaken belief that spoken language is superior for the cognitive and linguistic development of the Deaf child.

Research shows that programs that combine a cognitive-academic approach with the use of signs are significantly better at boosting subsequent academic achievement than those that stress articulation skills.[9] There is very little information on the later academic achievement of the graduates of the few preschool programs that use ASL and Deaf professional staff; the programs are too new. Some of the preliminary findings, however, suggest that both hearing parents and their Deaf children benefit greatly from this programming in the areas of acceptance of the Deaf child, ease in communicating, reduced feelings of stress, increased skills in behavior management, and better academic achievement.[10]

The transition between parent-infant program and preschool program is rarely coordinated. There is little contact between hospital-based and school-based programs, and not infrequently they are in conflict.[11] When, a few years ago, Maryland adopted as a policy that newly identified Deaf children would be referred to the Maryland School for the Deaf, the hospital-based and local speech and hearing clinics protested vigorously (all the more, perhaps, because the Maryland School had a new Deaf superintendent and encouraged the use of ASL). The Alexander Graham Bell Association, promoting the teaching of speech to the Deaf, attempted to discourage parents from participating in the program at the school for the Deaf, and it lobbied the state legislature for a change in policy. This effort failed, and now the School for the Deaf must be notified by hospital-based programs of all newly identified Deaf children. Although proponents of a clinical approach to Deaf children lost this battle, the underlying struggle continues and, as we shall see in part 3, has many other locales and forms.

PLACEMENT: THE DECISION-MAKING PROCESS AND THE INDIVIDUALIZED EDUCATIONAL PLAN

IDEA not only requires that local school districts and states fund the education of children with disabilities from the age of three, it mandates that every such child have an Individualized Educational Plan (IEP), which specifies the services that the school district and the parents agree should be provided to the child. In essence, it is a curriculum guide based on the child's capabilities as determined by formal and informal assessments.

Those assessments of the child are carried out by professionals in the local school district or in a speech and hearing center, typically based in a hospital. Required to be completed annually for each child with a disability by a core team within a school district, the IEP should include the following:[12]

- A description of the current academic and social levels of the child.
- A statement of annual goals and sub-goals for academic achievement and socialization.
- A listing of the specific educational needs of the child and the services required to meet those needs.
- A schedule of when the services will be implemented and, if applicable, terminated.
- A plan that specifies how to evaluate whether the objectives have been met.

At the most basic level, the decisions made as part of the IEP process determine where the child with disabilities will be educated and by whom and how. When it comes to Deaf children, the IEP is commonly fraught with conflicts and contradictions.

One problem that is omnipresent involves the all-important placement and achievement evaluations, a subject we will examine more closely in chapter 11. Here, we only need say that there is almost always a serious problem of communication between the professional doing the evaluating and the Deaf child, although good communication is necessary for any valid evaluation. On the one hand, Deaf children from hearing homes may not be fluent in any language. On the other, the professionals—educators, psychologists or speech therapists—are commonly not fluent in signed language, although their clients may be. Deaf children of Deaf parents are capable by the time they are four years old of complex and sophisticated discussion in ASL. In our experience, the result of the communicative impasse is almost inevitably an assessment that underestimates the abilities of the child. And while the parents have the right to bring in independent professionals to assist them, it is a right that, because of cost and the intimidating and cumbersome nature of the appeals process, is not easy to exercise.

By law, parents have the ultimate responsibility for decisions concerning their Deaf child. However, as we saw in chapter 2, those parents must struggle with an enormous amount of often conflicting input regarding the best course to pursue, and it takes time for them to learn about their rights and responsibilities when developing IEPs. The professionals, on the other hand, know the intricacies of the law and the guidelines, and they may be influenced by other factors as well in deciding what path to recommend—factors such as the economic situation of the town, or the desire to maintain a program they have already established.

Moreover, parents are confronted from the outset by two major groups of professionals with different guiding principles, the speech-and-hearing professionals and the special educators. Typically, the speech-and-hearing professionals, as described in chapter 2, focus on the child's hearing loss and the possibility of mitigating it. This focus distinguishes the category of Deaf children from most other children with disabilities. Special education, on the other hand, tends to approach children with disabilities in a non-categorical way; that is, to see all such children to a considerable degree in the same light. Couple this special-ed reluctance to make provisions for various subgroups with the ideology that the best educational setting—the Least Restrictive Environment—for most children with disabilities is the regular classroom, and you end up with strong pressures for the so-called *full inclusion* of Deaf children in classes with their hearing peers.

In the educational establishment, then, there is no single "voice" for Deaf children, least of all the voice of the DEAF–WORLD, whose members have not been included in the debates on what is the best possible education for Deaf children.[13] Because of the barriers to participation by Deaf professionals, over ninety-five percent of the professionals who make decisions and create programs for Deaf children are hearing.[14]

We will go into some detail below on the pros and cons of the various school placement options, which range from boarding in a residential school to being fully mainstreamed in a regular classroom with or (more typically) without support services. For now, suffice it to say that from the start, many school districts have followed the recommendations and desires of parents, but many have not. Some school district personnel have tended to intimidate and manipulate parents into accepting their approach to educating Deaf children, sometimes because they have had a program in which they were invested, and accommodating parents who wished to do something different was difficult, or expensive, or both. One of the more common contentious issues between parents and school districts has arisen when the parents concluded that their Deaf child would make more educational progress in a residential program for Deaf children, but the district was unwilling to pay for this placement, maintaining that its own program better served the needs of the child. In sum, many school districts have not respected provisions of IDEA that required them to offer parents a range of educational placements for their Deaf children. As a remedy, in 1992, the Office of Special Education and Rehabilitation Services issued guidelines reminding school districts that they must make a range of options available to parents and inform them of the full spectrum of possible placements and their potential benefits for their Deaf children.[15] Even with these new guidelines, however, parents may have to invest enormous time and energy to obtain the services they desire for their Deaf child. If they elect to buck the received wisdom of their local system, their efforts may not, in the end, succeed.

Although parents have the right to decide where and how to educate their Deaf child, when the school district professionals and the parents disagree, there is an intimidating semi-legal procedure that must be followed, involving a pseudo courtroom appearance, with lawyers, defendants, and plaintiffs. The parents, often lacking in resources and isolated, are pretty much on their own. Moreover, the officials who make the final decision are likely to be special education officials from another school district and just as unaware of the needs of a Deaf child as the school district personnel who disagreed with the parents in the first place.

Even if the child has Deaf parents, school districts may disagree with them as to the best program or the services needed by the Deaf child. A famous case that went to the Supreme Court involved a Deaf child of Deaf parents, Amy Rowley, who was functioning at grade level in a regular school classroom without the services of an interpreter. Her parents thought she could do much better academically if she had a signed-language interpreter and they requested one. Because of the cost involved, the school district refused; the parents contested the decision and the lower courts ruled for the parents, stating that Amy needed a signed language interpreter to make classroom instruction fully accessible. On appeal, the

Supreme Court affirmed that children with handicaps have a right to receive the services they need to benefit from their education; however, the Court ruled that Amy herself did not need an interpreter since she was doing all right without one. A majority of the Court ruled that Congress did not intend to give children with disabilities a right to "strict equality."[16]

Placement Options

As you may glean from the intricacies involved in early intervention programs for Deaf children outlined above, determining the educational placements where Deaf students will be most successful is becoming a very complex business. Increasingly, special-education professionals desire inclusion of the Deaf child with an interpreter in a regular classroom in the midst of hearing pupils. Many hearing parents may be reluctant to accept a school where signing is used. Professionals in audiology and related medical fields continue to push for an emphasis on speech; if the child has had cochlear implant surgery (discussed in chapter 14), the hospital team and the parents may insist on special classes for Deaf children where primarily spoken language is used. In some settings, the content of the curriculum may be simplified to make it accessible, and teaching staff may be isolated from the latest developments in pedagogical practice. In others, a Deaf child may have no peers with whom he or she can communicate.

For 150 years, separate facilities, either residential schools or, in large cities, day schools, were the main setting for the education of the Deaf. Since the 1960s, various forms of what is called generically *mainstreaming* have been encouraged, ranging from the self-contained day class within a regular public school (with interaction, if any, with hearing students limited to activities outside the academic program), to *full inclusion* of the Deaf in hearing classrooms. More recently, as we have noted, there has been a strong push for inclusion, with (or without) the provision of signed language interpreters and other support services like resource rooms and itinerant teachers.[17]

In the following pages we will look at these options largely in terms of three factors parents should consider in determining where and how to obtain the highest quality education for their Deaf child. These factors are the language of instruction; the academic quality of the program, including the subjects offered and the level of instruction; and the degree of social interaction.

Separate schools for the Deaf: *Residential schools and day schools*

As we saw in chapters 3 and 5, residential schools for the Deaf—large, centrally located schools providing education from preschool through high school (and, in some cases, adult education)—were at one time the center of the DEAF–WORLD. However, as we also saw, starting in the 1860s, and especially after the Congress of Milan in 1880, oralists took control of the residential schools in the U.S and abroad, virtually eradicating the influence of the DEAF–WORLD. From then on, the teaching staff and administrators were hearing, instruction in almost all schools was oral throughout the elementary years, and the Deaf staff were relegated to nonacademic posts with less influence on academic achievement, posts such as dormitory supervisor, coach, shop instructor, and custodian.

As a result of these changes, the students acquired much of their information and, unless they had been born into the DEAF–WORLD, all of their language, from other Deaf students or the after-school staff. The elementary and middle-school academic personnel especially did not know ASL and therefore could not communicate effectively with their students.[18] Since the students' success was measured by what they knew in English, but most had great difficulty learning English (or much else) through oral instruction, the level of accomplishment was low, both as measured, and in fact. The result was drastically lowered expectations and, in consequence, the drastic lowering of curriculum content. The advent of the special education laws and the change from strictly oral instruction to the combined use of signs from ASL and speech in the 1960s improved matters somewhat, but one of the major drawbacks of the residential schools remains to this day. That is the low expectations they have for many of their students, and the low quality and limited variety of their academic offerings.

Residential schools typically are divided into a lower school, a middle school, and an upper school—designations that may signal the low expectations of the staff. The upper school will include students of high-school age but may well not offer high-school-level instruction. At each

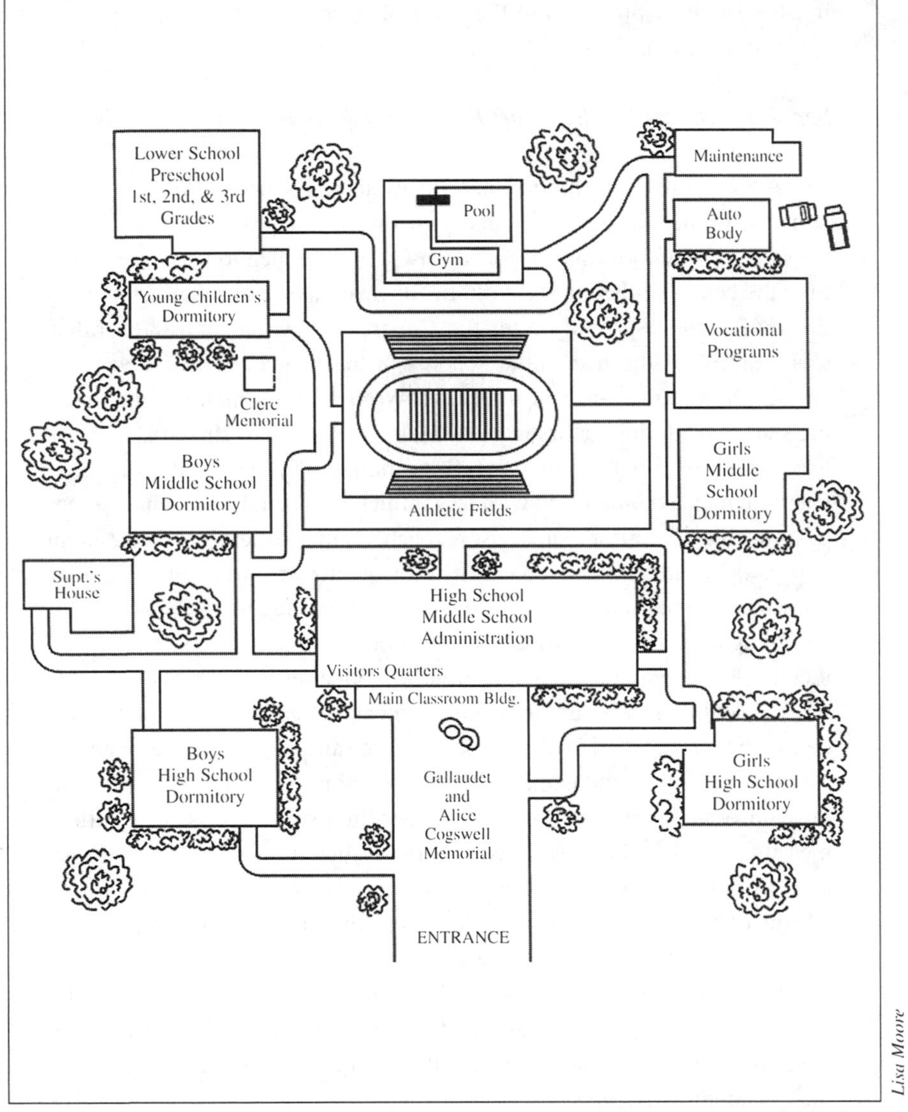

Fig. 8-2. **Diagram of a typical residential school for the Deaf in the U.S.**

grade level, the curriculum that many residential schools offer is much less demanding than that offered to hearing students at the same grade level in most regular public schools, and materials are created or adapted to match the low reading levels of the students. Isolated and insular, the schools find it difficult to incorporate new educational strategies into the curriculum, and they even tend to lose sight of what hearing students of a given age are expected to know.

These are admittedly generalizations; happily, there are residential schools that have changed and that challenge many students appropriately. However, a consequence of the situation generally is that residential school graduates tend not to enroll in college, nor are they prepared to do so. Most students are encouraged to pursue vocational training in high school, with courses in printing, computer data entry, or auto body repair, rather than pre-college courses. In any case, the residential schools can offer only a few of either type of course, given the small size of the school population and consequently the limited number of students who would be taking each subject. Sometimes, to complement these reduced course offerings, the residential schools collaborate with local vocational centers and high schools for hearing students to permit the Deaf students to attend classes.

If, however, most residential schools are below par academically, they do have a great advantage for the average Deaf student: as they always have, they do an excellent job of socialization. There are several reasons for this. For one, since all the children in the school are Deaf, participation in extracurricular functions, such as school government, sports, or dramatic performances, is not dependent on the level of speech one may have, or on the use of an interpreter, as it is in non-residential programs. Moreover, because all their students are Deaf, some hearing teachers in residential schools become proficient in some form of signed communication (though usually not ASL) and are therefore able to converse with students and with Deaf staff to a much greater extent than their counterparts in general education.[19] Children in residential schools can thus participate in every aspect of their schooling beginning very early in their academic careers.

The most important advantage of the residential schools in this regard is the large number of Deaf staff who traditionally work in them (residential schools are the largest single employer of educated Deaf adults). Although some Deaf staff are teachers, most, as we have noted, are employed in non-educational activities as dorm counselors, groundskeepers and cooks—all the many functions besides teaching that make a boarding school work. These people are able to communicate fluently and efficiently with the Deaf students. In addition, like Deaf parents, they tend to have high expectations for Deaf children. (While the paucity of Deaf teachers—typically only seven percent of the teaching staff is Deaf, and they tend to be concentrated in the middle or upper schools—is largely the consequence of history, that the scarcity continues today may also be due in part to the fact that teacher certification requirements in many states make it difficult if not impossible for a Deaf teacher to obtain certification.)

In fact, nowhere other than the residential school, is the Deaf child likely to come into contact with so many Deaf role models, including not only Deaf staff, but older Deaf students and alumni as well. The latter, with whom the residential schools maintain strong ties, support their schools as centers where the Deaf may meet, hold workshops and become involved with students. It is through these contacts that Deaf children, especially Deaf children of hearing parents, may begin to understand that there is a Deaf society, a Deaf culture—a DEAF–WORLD—where they may feel at home. They also have the opportunity to learn a great deal from a Deaf perspective about how to function as a Deaf person in the hearing world.

As a result of all this, most students graduate from the residential schools with healthy self-esteem. Integrated into the DEAF–WORLD by virtue of their attendance at the school, especially if they were residents, they have many friends and are able to take advantage of the DEAF–WORLD's sophisticated networks as they begin their adult lives.

Imagine if strategies to enhance the teaching of content were incorporated into the curriculum and expectations were raised so that the Deaf students in residential schools might become the scholars many of them were before the oralists took over Deaf education after Milan! For many in the DEAF–WORLD, this would be a happy development indeed. Unfortunately, however, the very existence of the residential schools is threatened.

Before the 1960s almost eighty percent of the Deaf children in the U.S. attended residential schools. Today only about thirty percent do. This sharp reversal is mostly a result of the push of the mainstreaming and inclusion movements, coupled with the expansion of interpreter training programs, which have changed the way residential facilities operate. When Deaf students get older, some tend to move to mainstream settings to take advantage of the wider course offerings available in regular high schools. And as enrollments decline, funding becomes a more and more serious problem. Not only does the hearing world consider the mainstream to be the most inclusive and positive educational setting (the Least Restrictive Environment) for all students with disabilities, among whom the Deaf are included, but also the desire of state legislatures to minimize state expenditures on residential schools reinforces the bias in favor of the mainstream placement.

By contrast, the DEAF–WORLD considers the residential school, one of its core institutions, to be the most inclusive and the best placement (the Least Restrictive Environment) for Deaf students. Particularly since the Gallaudet Revolution (see chapter 5), members of this minority have been resisting the mainstreaming movement, aiming to regain control of the schools, to upgrade their academic programs, and to ensure that they survive. We shall explore these developments further in part 3, but two kindred developments should be noted here. First, in the 1990s, we have begun to see a "reverse flow" of Deaf students from the mainstream setting to the residential schools, in some cases when they are "old enough" for boarding school (Americans in general do not like to send young children away to school), and in some cases when, as teenagers, they have become desperate for the company of people with whom they can communicate readily.[20] Second, several states have lately adopted an educational bill of rights for the Deaf child that guarantees a spectrum of placement options, including the residential school (see chapter 15).

Henry, in the story of the Deaf club, attended another kind of separate educational facility for the Deaf, the day school. Indeed, many students, typically fifty to seventy percent of the school population, commute daily even to the residential schools, which effectively also makes them function as day schools.

Since the commuting time for students is limited to an hour each way by law, separate day schools are located in urban areas and tend to serve inner-city populations. Many have large minority populations and their students may also come from immigrant families, where English is a second language. As a result, the day schools must be concerned not only with the problems of the education of Deaf children per se, but with the functioning of the Deaf child within a multicultural framework.

Day schools have the disadvantages of many of the residential schools, without their advantages. That is, generally the teaching staff is hearing, and because of difficulties in communication and low expectations, the curriculum is severely degraded. There is no large number of Deaf non-teaching staff with whom the students may associate after school. If there are Deaf staff members, they tend to be aides in classrooms. Because they leave for home after classes, younger pupils at day schools also seldom come into contact with the older students. ("I would just go home after school," Henry said.) The lack of Deaf role models means that the child attending such schools often does not discover the DEAF–WORLD until much later in life. Henry seemed to come into his own as a Deaf person only when he went away to study and live at the National Technical Institute for the Deaf. For other day school students who are not so fortunate, identity crises can be severe. As in the residential schools, pressure is now being exerted by individuals in the local DEAF–WORLD where the day school is situated, and by local and state associations of the Deaf, to see that more Deaf teachers are hired.

Mainstreaming: *From self-contained classes to full inclusion*

The most popular program for the Deaf child of elementary school age consists of separate, self-contained day classes that are housed in regular schools but are not part of the regular academic program. Interaction with hearing students, if it occurs, will mostly take place outside the normal academic schedule—during lunch, recess, or between classes, etc. Because self-contained classrooms are on the grounds of the local school, their proximity to hearing classrooms means that more options are available to those (relatively few) Deaf students who have the background, skills, and desire to participate in classes with hearing children (see below).

Created in response to the requirement of IDEA that local school districts offer a continuum of options for the education of Deaf children, self-contained programs are typically structured so that there is one class, taught by a teacher of the Deaf, for each elementary grade level. Because there are so few Deaf children, such programs are frequently established through the collaboration of a number of neighboring school districts to increase the size of the pool from which students are drawn. The pool has to be quite large, however, for this type of program to truly succeed.[21] A large pool means significant numbers within each age group so that there are many peers from among whom friends can be chosen, a range of intellectual capabilities, and older children with whom the younger ones can interact. It is crucial that young children have Deaf models from whom they are able to learn in addition to hearing adults.

Even programs that are sufficiently large have disadvantages, however. For example, many Deaf children must spend hours every day on school buses, which, as at the separate day schools for the Deaf and the day programs at the residential schools, effectively prohibits their participation in activities after normal school hours. Distance also makes it difficult for parents to oversee the schooling of their Deaf children; the extra travel means less time for work, family, or just plain smelling the roses. By the time the Deaf child reaches high school, many parents are approaching exhaustion. They have already devoted a great deal of their energy during the elementary school years to trying to ensure that their child will receive a quality education, and they are enormously frustrated when the child's level of academic achievement does not reflect the time they have put into it. On top of that, the power of parents to affect decisions concerning their child is particularly limited in collaborative programs. We have already seen that, while the law puts a certain amount of power in the hands of the parents of children with disabilities, it does not provide a guarantee that parents' wishes will be implemented. In the case of those who are unhappy with their child's progress in a collaborative program, or who wish to influence the program, the problems are compounded, because the parents cannot go directly to the collaborative administrators; instead, they must take the matter to their local school district through the IEP process. This puts parents in the position of having to contend with two administrative entities, and not many are able to commit the enormous amounts of time, energy and resources required. As a result, local school districts usually have their way, setting aside parental wishes because of their superior resources, including access to lawyers and credentialed experts. It is a far cry from sending one's hearing child to a local neighborhood school, where parents who live near each other and the school can band together to become a power bloc, whether in voting for school board members or speaking out against a policy or an administrator. Instead, parents of Deaf children must proceed on their own when they disagree with the quality and type of program presented by local school officials, many of whom are unfamiliar with the needs of Deaf children. The situation amounts to a kind of segregation in reverse.

There are very few self-contained programs at the high school level, where mainstreaming takes the form called *inclusion*, in which Deaf students are included in classes with their hearing peers (see below). The self-contained programs that do exist confront real problems connected with the size of the Deaf student population and the type of high school involved. In programs where there are not many Deaf students, there is almost inevitably a severe lack of social interaction; friends with whom one has anything in common (except being Deaf) are likely to be very hard to come by if the choices are limited to five or six peers. That was just Roberto's experience; he was painfully lonely in high school. The distance between the Deaf student's home and school is also a critical factor. After-school programs that help most high school students develop a sense of their place in the world are often unavailable to the Deaf. Either the transportation problem limits participation or the competition for the few slots on, say, the varsity soccer team, requires Deaf students to have skills that far surpass those of their hearing peers to make up for the disadvantage of being unable to hear the coach's shouted commands.

Many educational programs for the Deaf that consist of self-contained day classes located within regular schools offer the Deaf student various levels of so-called *integration* with hearing peers. Some Deaf children, like Roberto, attend one or two classes with hearing children, usually in non-academic subject areas like gym or art. Deaf children who are placed in the hearing academic program are usually above average in academics compared to the other Deaf children. Many can understand spoken English, albeit with some difficulty, and these students may have intelligible speech. Sometimes those who do not have intelligible speech but who outperform their peers academically are integrated; these students may have a signed-language interpreter accompany them to classes.

Sometimes there are additional services provided to support Deaf and hard-of-hearing students who have been included in regular classrooms. One of these is called the *resource room*. Deaf children who are in regular classes with hearing peers during most of the school day leave the regular classroom for the resource room, where they receive special tutoring, from a teacher of the Deaf, in English and language arts (reading, writing, etc.). These are the subjects found to be most difficult for Deaf students, and it is on these subjects that their success in any class with hearing students largely depends. Almost all resource rooms are managed by hearing professionals.

Another support service for the Deaf child attending classes with hearing students involves itinerant consultants, typically speech-and-hearing clinicians or teachers of the Deaf, who are not based at a particular school but work for a few hours a week in a large number of schools where they assist the regular classroom teacher and provide some tutoring services. The children they serve are usually the only Deaf children in the class, often attending with an interpreter. The itinerant consultant monitors their performance, continually reassessing their ability to keep up with their classmates. For a Deaf child to function with an interpreter requires that the child have great language facility, high intelligence, and a strong background in school-related tasks, as well as a skilled interpreter. Such children are rare; such educational interpreters rarer, as we shall see below. Even Deaf children of Deaf Parents, who have the advantage of access to both the hearing world in school (mediated by the interpreter) and the DEAF–WORLD at home, find it very difficult to perform well in regular classrooms with hearing students. Success has been demonstrated with only a very small number of students, and they have been selected for integration based on their already excellent academic skills. The Deaf child of hearing parents who attends programs like this is encased in a hearing environment day and night in which life is a constant struggle and the child always the outsider.

Least Restrictive Environment and Inclusion

By definition, *least restrictive environment* means the most appropriate educational placement for the child, the setting in which the child's capacities may be developed to the greatest possible extent. We have noted above that the hearing world in general, and special educators who are not familiar with the DEAF–WORLD in particular, tend to see the full integration of the Deaf child into the hearing classroom as providing the least restrictive environment for the education of that child. The DEAF–WORLD clearly sees things differently. Now that we have an understanding of the various program types and educational services offered, it is time to consider this issue.

The paradox of inclusion

In chapter 7, as part of the story of the Metro Silent Club, we learned something of the educational background of several members of the DEAF–WORLD who had been educated in one or another of the programs outlined above. As adult members of the DEAF–WORLD, however, none of them was young enough to have experienced a full-inclusion program, which came into fashion starting in the early 1990s.[22] Advocates of full inclusion for children with disabilities seek to make the educational system keep the promise that mainstreaming in special self-contained classes failed to keep, namely real integration in school—education of children with disabilities alongside children who have none. And for many children with disabilities, special classes are indeed not necessary, though for others, such as some children with multiple severe handicaps, they are. But from the perspective of the DEAF–WORLD, full inclusion is a disaster. Roberto spoke of his loneliness and dependence on his interpreter when integrated into classes of hearing children. What must it be like for a child who is the only Deaf child in all her classes starting in preschool days? Here we consider such a child. We'll call her Dorothy with malice of aforethought for, as we shall see, she finds herself in a Land of Oz.

At four years old, Dorothy is a bright, happy child with well-educated hearing parents who decide that she will obtain the best education if she is included in classes with her hearing peers. Both parents have been learning one of the MCE systems for the past two years and are pretty good at using what they have been taught.

In the classroom, Dorothy is assisted by an interpreter who spends all day with her. The interpreter is a young hearing woman with a high school diploma who attended a two-year interpreter training program and has been interpreting for the past three years using contact sign (PSE, see chapter 3). She functions as interpreter when the whole class is involved, as tutor in small-group activities and one-on-one projects, and as a counselor providing Dorothy with the information she needs to function in school. No one in the school knows ASL and the interpreter is the only person there who even knows some signs; so the other pupils, Dorothy's teacher, and the other staff rely on the interpreter to communicate with Dorothy. No one is able to judge the interpreter's skills.

The teacher, who wants to provide a positive integrative experience for Dorothy, collects children's books about signing and throughout the first year attempts to teach everyone else in the class "how to sign" so they can interact more effectively with Dorothy. The children learn the signs for *apple, boy, cat, dog, elephant*, etc. There is no ASL grammar taught; no sentences are presented. The children rely on spoken English to string the signs together. Of the twenty-five hearing children in the preschool class, twelve learn a good number of individual signs. Dorothy is keeping up academically with the hearing children because of the interpreter's tutoring and the many hours her parents, especially her mother, spend working with her after school.

When Dorothy graduates to first grade, her new teacher decides to empower her (as the teacher views it) by having her "teach the class sign language." Because this is one of the few times Dorothy is really in control, she is excited and looks forward to the sessions. By the second grade she has spent many hours teaching her hearing peers signs, but of the twelve children in her preschool who initially were motivated, only three have stuck with it to the extent that they can actually converse a little with Dorothy. Halfway through the second grade, one of the three students moves away. Despite the best efforts of her parents and teacher, Dorothy is now in a situation where, out of a class of twenty-five, only two can communicate well enough with her to be friends. She did not choose them; they were selected by their ability to use the sign vocabulary they had learned.

In the second grade, Dorothy also begins to have difficulty learning how to read at the same pace as her peers and is put in a remedial reading program. No longer seeing herself as equal to the hearing children in her class, she starts to develop behaviors that signal a loss of self-confidence.

For example, she begins to respond to all questions with requests for confirmation; that is, whenever she answers a question, she gives her teacher a questioning look, essentially asking the teacher to confirm that her answer is correct. If the teacher shows any doubt, Dorothy immediately changes her answer, searching for the response that will be satisfactory. Sometimes this occurs so quickly that the teacher, unaware of Dorothy's strategy, appears to agree to a wrong response when a correct one was given moments before. Interpreter errors and inherent delays compound the problem. Soon Dorothy starts to feel inferior, and her academic work slips some more. But a tutor is obtained, and the interpreter and Dorothy's mother work hard to keep Dorothy at close to grade level.

In the fourth grade, however, Dorothy has a fight with one of the two children who have learned to sign, the one whom she considered her best friend. Although Dorothy has not been really good friends with the other peer who learned to sign, she is forced now to rely on her for companionship. This friend is better than no one.

Dorothy is also slipping farther behind in class, as literacy becomes crucial to advancement. It is during the fourth grade that reading for the sake of reading changes to reading for meaning. Now success in school, for hearing as well as Deaf pupils, begins to be dependent on gaining a great deal of information from print. Dorothy has become pretty good at identifying many words in English, but has great difficulty with the pronoun references in paragraphs and especially across paragraphs. Idioms like *to keep him company,* or *to take charge of the class* also cause serious problems. Much of Dorothy's school day is now spent trying to figure out the idioms and not enough time is spent learning and remembering the information.

By the end of fifth grade, Dorothy is slipping badly both in school and socially. She is now twelve years old, and her social group consists of her two friends from school (she has made up with the friend with whom she quarreled). But this is a time when differences among children begin to be played down and group conformity among peers becomes important. The telephone becomes important, too. Boys are often the subject of discussion. Unable to participate, Dorothy becomes very shy and hesitant in her interactions with her peers and with the hearing adults at school. She feels she cannot trust her interpreter, who is, after all, a grown-up employee of the school, with the confidential exchanges she now wishes to have with her friends. And the interpreter is not available when the hearing children get together after school to do homework. Dorothy is forced to rely on her mother as her primary tutor.

The two friends she has made because of their signing ability have become amateur interpreters for Dorothy in groups outside the classroom; however, this has created a schism between Dorothy and her classmates, because one of the signing friends in particular has begun to feel the power inherent in the interpreting situation. In any encounter with her classmates, attention is focused not on Dorothy but on the amateur interpreter, who enjoys the control she has over the conversation and the praise she receives from adults for helping out and giving the adult professional interpreter time off. Dorothy can't help resenting her dependence on this friend, who is privy to her private life and controls her interactions with her hearing peers. She becomes more socially withdrawn and self-dependent, showing by her behavior that she wants no help from anyone. The adults in her life consider this part of the normal teenage push for independence, but Dorothy, unable to interact freely with peers or with adults—she knows no one who is Deaf—is actually withdrawing angrily into herself. She continues to work hard in school; because she is very bright, she has managed to keep up with the class, but her rank is near the bottom.

Then, finally, when she is fourteen years old, Dorothy learns that there are two Deaf teenagers in her neighborhood and seeks them out. She hasn't encountered them before because they attend a residential school. The conversation flows easily and comfortably when these new acquaintances converse with each other, less easily when they speak with Dorothy, who is not familiar with fluent ASL and is used to seeing signs in English word order. But through happenstance, not educational design, Dorothy, like Henry and Roberto and Laurel, has at last begun her acculturation into the DEAF–WORLD.

What happens to Dorothy as she grows up?

Adolescence is almost always a time of turmoil, stress, and learning about who you are, where you belong, and what you plan to do with your life. As the teenager seeks independence, parents become both confidants and opponents. While conflicts rage over issues of freedom and control, adolescents also look to adult models for direction, feedback, and support. Primarily, however, they depend on their peer group to help get them through this stage in life, forming friendships, stealing kisses, dating.

For Deaf students who are isolated from their Deaf peers and can depend only on hearing students for support, friendship, and collegiality, the problems of adolescence are compounded. Dorothy, for example, has one friend who has acted as her interpreter all through elementary and junior high school. But in high school, for the first time, they will almost certainly be in different classes, either because they have different interests or because they have different academic skills. There will be times, in any case, when Dorothy will not want the hearing friend to interpret for her. There will be times when the hearing friend will not want to be burdened with the responsibility of interpreting. But the link forged by interpreting has become a chain of dependency. The hearing friend will continue to enjoy the power inherent in the role of interpreter. Dorothy will become either more needy and more dependent or will withdraw from hearing friends completely to avoid having to depend on this one.

In an effort to become more independent, Dorothy will probably seek to confide in the classroom interpreter, but will become conflicted as to what the boundaries are when discussing school and personal issues. As the interpreter becomes more enmeshed in Dorothy's problems, another cycle of dependence and resentment is created. Dorothy needs to confide in someone, but does not want to confide in her peer who signs (the problem may have to do with the friend, for example), so she confides in the interpreter. The interpreter, trying to help, goes beyond academics and begins to engage Dorothy in examining her personal problems. Eventually, however, Dorothy will learn that the interpreter cannot really be a confidante, because she is one of the school authorities, with all that that implies.

Dorothy would turn to her Deaf acquaintances, but their attendance at the residential school means that she seldom sees them. Moreover, her parents, who have been counseled that congregating with Deaf people is a negative influence, object strongly to her associating with them at all. Dorothy may ask to be transferred to the residential school; her parents, afraid of "losing her" (their term), may refuse. As time passes, almost inevitably, Dorothy will become more and more withdrawn and secretive and angry—at her parents, at the school, at the hearing world in general. Like Laurel at the Metro Silent Club, she may remain angry long after she has quit school and found her way to the DEAF–WORLD.

So, what is the Least Restrictive Environment for children like Dorothy? For one thing, it seems to change between elementary and high school. Many Deaf students who have been in putatively integrated and even in self-contained settings for their elementary years, and who may have the academic skills to go to a hearing high school, may opt to attend a residential school so that they can have some social interaction with their peers. On the other hand, those Deaf students who have been in attendance in a residential school may well feel competent and secure enough to enter into a regular hearing high school because they have the social development and peer network to make the experience meaningful, as well as the language skills (English and ASL) to function well in the regular classroom, where the academic level is generally higher than in residential or day programs for the Deaf.

The education of the Deaf student in any setting is a problem. The overall dropout rate of Deaf high schoolers has been estimated at twenty-nine percent. One in every five Deaf students who "graduate" does not meet the academic requirements for a diploma and leaves with a certificate instead. Thus only half the Deaf students who enter high school graduate with a diploma. The lowest dropout rates are found in the residential schools, seventeen to twenty-three percent. For Deaf students who are placed in integrated settings in regular high schools, the dropout rate is thirty-seven percent. If a Deaf student is placed in a self-contained program and is not integrated into the school's regular classes, the dropout rate almost doubles to fifty-four percent (recall that many of these programs will not have any Deaf teachers or contact with the DEAF–WORLD). Different kinds of Deaf students go into different kinds of programs, so the dropout rate reflects both the kinds of students and the type of programming. In all types of programs, if a Deaf student has disabilities, such as a putative learning or behavior disorder or blindness, the dropout rate is fifty-seven percent, and if the Deaf student is Hispanic, the rate is thirty-six percent. Thirty-three percent of Deaf females drop out of high school.[23]

In general, the Least Restrictive Environment for Deaf students is probably the one that allows the freest and fullest communication with teacher and peers, which is a prerequisite to academic progress and psychological and social development. For the vast majority of Deaf students, enjoying the communication conditions that their hearing counterparts take for granted requires teachers and peers fluent in a visual/manual language—ASL in most of North America. That requirement, combined with the small numbers of children who are Deaf, favors specialized educational programs with significant numbers of Deaf children. If we further seek not to restrict the Deaf student in participation in extra-curricular activities and in exposure to pertinent role models, the LRE is the residential school.

In concluding in favor of the residential schools, we must acknowledge the pain that hearing parents (but, significantly, not Deaf parents) feel at the prospect of sending their young child to a boarding school. We Americans like to keep our children close to home. The hearing parents must wonder, too, whether an institution can give their children the attention and care they need. It should be reassuring that Deaf parents who have attended such schools and know what they have to offer are grateful to *their* parents for having sent them there, and they do likewise with their own children if Deaf, even though they are in some ways in a better position than hearing parents to provide at home what the Deaf child requires. The sense of shared language and culture at these schools and the presence of healthy, happy and smart Deaf children is a counterpoise to the regimentation and anonymity that can arise in boarding schools. We have repeatedly cited drawbacks in the residential schools, but many of those drawbacks can be corrected and are being corrected in the most progressive schools today. Teachers have better training and higher expectations, and curricula are being enhanced. Meanwhile the residential schools' traditional strengths, such as better communication, more Deaf role models, and opportunities for personal growth, are being reinforced.

Those in favor of integrated education of Deaf children with hearing children might argue that the major drawback of that placement, the language barrier separating Deaf children from peers and teachers, can also be corrected with the will and the funds by supplying interpreters. In fact, as we shall see below, this is virtually impossible to achieve.

Interpreters and inclusion

The movement for full inclusion of all Deaf children in the regular classroom, which has been precipitated by professionals outside the field of education of the Deaf and without input from Deaf professionals, has put a spotlight on interpreters—their training, their function, their skills, and, underlying all of these, the issue of language.

In the past two decades, interpreter education programs have been created throughout the U.S. in which interpreters are educated in the tools of their profession and prepared to interpret in ASL, contact sign or, in a few cases, one of the MCE systems. There are short-term courses not for university credit; there are two-year associate degree programs in community colleges, four-year bachelor's level programs, and a two-year master's level program.[24] Because there is no state-level consensus on what standards a graduate of such programs should actually meet, interpreter skills and knowledge vary widely.

The National Registry of Interpreters for the Deaf (RID) is the national professional organization of interpreters; it has a special interest group for educational interpreters. The RID promotes interpreter evaluations and standards and has a certification program, but it has no power over state and local authorities, and no official role in the licensing of interpreters, although some states require RID certification for court interpreters. A few states have instituted licensing or certification programs of their own. Unfortunately, however, the general lack of standards at the state and local level, where interpreters are hired, means that there are no incentives for interpreters to follow the RID guidelines on minimum qualifications, nor any incentive to obtain RID certification, which is an expensive, selective and time-consuming process.[25] Those few states that do require licensure or certification of interpreters apparently do not make distinctions between adult interpreting of various kinds and educational interpreting.

Two additional factors create problems among states: the language the interpreter is to use and, related to this, the type of interpreting he or she is prepared to do. A majority of programs train students to interpret between English and contact sign. The curricula of many interpreter education programs include some ASL, but the level of mastery varies widely. What we have, then, is a large number of interpreters who use signs in a variety of ways, which have been neither described nor standardized. Programs that teach ASL have developed in recent years, but as we have seen, the use of ASL with Deaf children has traditionally been avoided. Few programs prepare their graduates to work in educational settings.[26] This is true even though by 1984 approximately half the Deaf students in the U.S. participated in some type of mainstreaming in classrooms with hearing students, and over one-third of the graduates of interpreter education programs become educational interpreters.[27]

Since the supply of educational interpreters does not come close to meeting the demand, what happens is that most educational interpreters are simply taken at face value. They are considered educational interpreters because they say they are.[28] Administrators of mainstream programs for the Deaf, responsible by law for seeing to it that interpreters are provided, are almost universally lacking in the necessary expertise to evaluate and assign interpreters. In fact, virtually none of the administrators of local schools have the skills to assess properly the language and accuracy of the educational interpreters and the teachers of the Deaf. Even requiring RID certification is no guarantee that the interpreters hired will have the requisite skills. RID certifies that minimum standards of competence have been met in two distinct domains, interpretation and transliteration. The former certificate, CI, concerns interpreting between English and ASL. The latter, CT, concerns interpreting between English and contact sign. Unless an administrator knows what the different certificates mean and what the particular Deaf student or students in question require, relying on the RID imprimatur can be seriously misleading.[29]

Compounding the problem of inadequate training is the fact that there are very few programs for educational interpreters that offer opportunities to work with children, yet interpreting for young children is very different from interpreting for students of high school level or above.[30] For one thing, children who speak ASL fluently but do not know English will have difficulty understanding and using the contact sign that the interpreter may well be using. Moreover, children have more difficulty than adults in adapting to variation in the signing of the interpreter. And the Deaf children of hearing parents—the vast majority of Deaf students, remember—are unlikely to have the fluency and background in either ASL or English to carry on an in-depth conversation about a topic they may want to discuss.[31]

It is no small challenge to adjust one's level of signed language to a young child, and the skill involved requires a much more comprehensive knowledge of ASL than that required to interpret for a high school student. In high school, the Deaf student might be quite capable of filling in areas where the interpreter either doesn't know ASL vocabulary or structure, or is not sure how to interpret the information. On the other hand, the young child will not be sophisticated enough to know whether the interpreter is performing correctly, and the child may not be able to understand the interpreter because of the vocabulary, structures, or register used, or because of the information presented. These language problems create the potential for enormous tension among interpreters, school officials, and Deaf students.[32]

One more matter of great concern connected with the qualifications of educational interpreters is that many do not have sufficient background in either methodology or subject matter, if indeed they have any at all.[33] Thus, for hearing students, a teacher may be required to have professional training and to continually upgrade that training, and may be evaluated annually by the school district. Yet a Deaf student in that teacher's class may well have to rely on an interpreter who has no training in child development, learning theory, English (either literature or linguistics), never mind pedagogy or, say, mathematics or history. The act of interpreting involves understanding the message presented by the instructor and translating that message into another language. Not surprisingly, the higher the educational background of the interpreter, the better the performance, especially at the high school and college levels.[34] Yet many educational interpreters are employed in high school honors or college classes, but have never attended college themselves.[35] If the interpreter is not knowledgeable about the topic, how can the accuracy of the translation be assured?

Interpreters in the educational setting, at whatever level, many times must function like classroom teachers. They must make the translation understandable, interesting, and accessible. Like teachers, therefore, they should have a college education. Requiring one would be beneficial in two ways: first, a college education provides a substantial background of knowledge that greatly enhances the interpreter's skill; second, it gives interpreters the status of professionals. Because they are in great demand and short supply, educational interpreters frequently are able to command a fairly high hourly or contract wage. To receive this high pay, which is often equivalent to what the classroom teacher receives, it is appropriate that they be required to hold a college degree.[36]

This brings us to what the role of the interpreter is, what it should be, and who is responsible for seeing to it that the proper role is performed. There is a great difference between the conversational or face-to-face setting encountered by most interpreters most of the time, and the one-way communicative setting common to many classrooms and other public forums. In the face-to-face setting, the interacting partners consist of three persons (the two interactors and the interpreter), who must manage the conversation to ensure that the information provided by each interactor is interpreted for the benefit of the other. For example, if one party begins to either talk or sign while the other party is still presenting information, the interpreter is responsible for calling attention to the interruption.[37] In a public forum, on the other hand, the interpreter functions more as a conduit for information being presented.[38] The problem is that in education, especially in elementary school, both types of contexts—conversational and one-way—may be encountered often, sometimes within minutes of each other. Yet the skills involved in interpreting in each case are quite different, and shifting gears between the two modes is not easy for even the most highly skilled interpreter.

On top of this, the educational interpreter is expected to perform other roles that may be in conflict with the roles of interpreters in non-educational settings, and some of which may even be inappropriate.[39] Thus, it has been suggested that the educational interpreter also do the following: remind students about homework or other responsibilities; facilitate social interaction with hearing students; tutor both hearing and Deaf students; act as a classroom aide; be a liaison between the child and the regular classroom teacher; and apprise appropriate individuals (school administrators, parents) of problems children are having.[40]

There are serious conflicts, some quite obvious, inherent in such a list. For one thing, in assigning to the interpreter the responsibility of, say, reminding a student to do homework, the teacher in effect abdicates a responsibility not abdicated with hearing students, and then transfers that responsibility and the authority that goes with it to the interpreter. But this means that the Deaf student now must answer to two authorities in the same classroom, which is not equivalent to the situation for hearing students, and gives rise to further questions. For example, if the interpreter is responsible for reminding students about their homework, does the interpreter become responsible for seeing that the homework is completed? Or, suppose that the interpreter is also the child's tutor. Is it the interpreter's responsibility to see that the Deaf child learns the material, or is the teacher responsible for that? At what point does the interpreter's responsibility end and the teacher's begin?

The educational interpreter is also expected to facilitate social interaction with hearing students. But how can the interpreter who functions with the authority of a teacher simultaneously encourage, support, and facilitate interactions with the hearing students without the authority role getting in the way? The answer is, the interpreter almost certainly cannot. The hearing students, for example, may feel obligated to interact with a Deaf pupil, while not really wanting to be part of the situation. (It is here that Dorothy's friend who likes to be the interpreter can obtain power and authority, by taking over for the educational interpreter.) The hearing students may not like the fact that an adult who is seen as part of the teaching and administrative staff is hanging around with them outside class.

It would be helpful if both Deaf and hearing students in a classroom that involves an interpreter were trained beforehand in what to expect. Many times Deaf and hearing students in the regular classroom are unfamiliar with the purpose, the scope, and the procedures for using an interpreter. A training program for high school students that focused on the appropriate roles not only for the interpreter, but for both the Deaf and hearing students as well, might create an environment much more conducive to learning, not least by reducing the imbalance of power between the Deaf and hearing students who decide to become friends.

The criss-crossing of the lines of authority and responsibility in the educational setting, as the interpreter attempts to play the roles of interpreter, teacher, tutor, counselor, and friend, must inevitably cause conflicts, not least of which are conflicts with the interpreter's code of ethics. An interpreter is supposed to remain discreet with regard to information learned about clients during the interpreting process. A 1994 task force on interpreting stated that the primary role of an interpreter should be interpreting. How does this jibe with the expectations of the administrators of school systems who create the job descriptions for educational interpreters?[41] Even if any single professional could function well in all these roles, it would seem that conflicts of interest and contradictions must render the position untenable.[42]

One reason that interpreter education programs do not teach the skills necessary for educational interpreters is that there is no agreement among educational administrators, interpreter preparation programs, educators of the Deaf and educators in general, on what roles they should perform, if any, beyond interpreting.[43] Such agreement is essential, but it requires in the first place a systematic discussion among all these parties—a discussion that should include members of the DEAF–WORLD.

In a nutshell, the problem is, how can we determine the necessary and sufficient qualifications of a professional who is cross-disciplinary? The answer is not immediately apparent. On the one hand, the needs of an interpreter include fluency in two languages (more on this below) and adherence to a certain code of ethics. On the other, the educational interpreter must function as a teacher. How is this possible? And if it is not, what does this imply for the education of Deaf children included in the hearing mainstream?

There is one more issue of vital importance to the education of Deaf children: Which language or signing system will be used? In the next two chapters we will consider this matter in some detail. Here we will look at it in relation to educational interpreters.

The decision on which language to use in the education of the Deaf is of supreme importance, yet it is seldom addressed in a logical way in the educational systems serving Deaf students. The selection of a means of communication in the classroom is even more problematic when it depends on the skills of the educational interpreter, who may very well have little or no training in the educational needs of the Deaf child; or on the advice of an educator of the Deaf who has been traditionally trained before recent advances in our understanding of signed languages; or the policies of an administrator who, however well-intentioned, probably has little or no background to relate to the circumstances of the Deaf child.[44]

Unfortunately, the situation of the majority of Deaf children, who have hearing parents and no early contact with anyone from the DEAF–WORLD, means that their first exposure to signing of any kind will be at the hands of hearing interpreters and teachers, who will ipso facto function as their signed-language model. (This is true even of children like Dorothy; both Dorothy and her parents learned the MCE system they used from hearing teachers.) It is a situation that receives much attention in specialized programs and classrooms created to serve Deaf children, but almost none when Deaf students are mainstreamed. Yet educational interpreters rarely use the language of the DEAF–WORLD, ASL, and the interpreter's skills are decisive for what language is used in the classroom.

If the young Deaf child is going to depend on the interpreter as the sole language model, then the interpreter's background and training become paramount, and issues pertinent to language acquisition and language learning apply. We will go into this more deeply in the next chapter. Here, let us simply state what that discussion will show: that logic dictates that ASL is the language that should be used with the young Deaf child; that, in fact, there are only two languages the young Deaf child must learn, ASL and English; and that the use of any of the MCE systems, which are not true languages and are incompatible with the visual/manual modality, may serve only to delay acquisition of both languages.[45]

If we examine the language processing the interpreter must perform in a classroom with a young Deaf child, further difficulties come to light. Even if all signed-language interpreters in educational settings with young Deaf children were fluent in ASL (and such are now being trained), and even if all young Deaf children knew ASL, it remains true that ASL and English are very different languages and the challenge of interpreting rapidly and well between those two languages is commensurately great. Moreover, educational interpreters must perform this feat for very long stretches and on topics with which they are frequently unfamiliar.

The time that elapses between the production of a message in the source language and its interpretation into a target language is called *lag time*, or *processing time*. Other things being equal, a short processing time is desirable, so that the messages the Deaf student receives are only a little out of synchrony with events in the classroom, and so that if the Deaf student says something the utterance will arrive only a little late in the flow of classroom speech. However, shorter processing times are associated with more errors in interpretation. There is some threshold below which the lag cannot be reduced if there is to be accurate processing of information into ASL.[46] Processing time and accuracy reflect the interpreter's mastery of ASL and the subject matter. An educational interpreter who is unskilled, and we have just seen many of them are, might present substantially erroneous information to the Deaf student. When the interpreter is working with children, there is no cross check on the interpreter's accuracy. It would be helpful if school programs using ASL interpreters contracted with members of the local DEAF–WORLD to establish procedures for systematically evaluating and controlling the quality of interpreter services. But even in the best of circumstances, the child who receives an education through the mediation of an interpreter is seriously handicapped.

Finally, while the fact that interpreters need to be fluent in two languages is generally accepted, the vital importance of fluency in both expressive and receptive modes when interpreting for young Deaf children is not fully recognized. Interpreter education programs spend most of their training time on production of the signed language; little time is spent on translating the signed form into spoken English. In educational interpreting, this mirrors the expectation that the Deaf child will say very little, since frequently he or she understands little and cannot immediately volunteer a remark with relevance given the time lag involved in mediation by the interpreter. The result is that many interpreters function reasonably well when they have to interpret *from* English but less well interpreting *into* English.[47] In some cases this disparity reflects a lack of mastery of ASL, which the interpreter approximates when signing but finds difficult to decipher when voicing in English. If an interpreter is limited in this way, obviously Deaf students' comments and responses will not be well translated, and they will appear to know less than they may in fact know. This is a common problem with interpreter services for Deaf adults, and it no doubt occurs much more often than it should in the schoolroom as well.

In sum, there is no real evidence that using an interpreter in a hearing classroom is in fact the least restrictive environment for a Deaf child under any circumstances, and there are many reasons to think otherwise. In addition, after twenty-five years of mainstreaming, it is impossible to state unequivocally that both Deaf and hearing children benefit from physical proximity. Deaf children are unable to interact at other than a very superficial level with their hearing peers. Most of those peers will not learn signed language, and the few that do progress at a snail's pace. Even a Deaf child arriving at school without any ASL soon outpaces them. And several studies show that the typical Deaf child, like Dorothy, tends to associate with other Deaf children, even when given the option of associating with hearing peers.[48]

Thus, for the young Deaf child, inclusion does not mean being included or integrated. For all children, being truly integrated means having access to one's peers and to one's teachers. As we have seen, this is manifestly not the case when Deaf children are placed in hearing classrooms. Some researchers have referred to the limited communication between the hearing and Deaf children in these situations as if "the hearing children were talking to their pets."[49]

The problems with educational interpreting—poor training, no standards, conflict of teaching and interpreting roles, lack of academic knowledge, inherent delays—remind us that the Deaf child is led into these dangerous waters by a placement decision. The parents' desire to have their child closer to home in the neighborhood school; the school's desire to utilize the special programming it has created for children with disabilities; the professionals' desire to promote an ethically laudable philosophy of integration—all these are understandable. But what about the desires and needs of the Deaf child? In the abstract, and neglecting such issues as the Deaf child's socialization, heritage and language rights, it may seem that a regular classroom can accommodate that child with the simple provision of an interpreter. Now that we have looked more closely at that placement, it should be clear how handicapping it usually is for Deaf children and why.

Deaf children should receive what we desire for hearing children as well: an education delivered in their best language. Anything less is not equal educational opportunity. Since their best language is different from that of their hearing peers, their education needs to be conducted separately, at least in part. But a separate program by itself does not ensure that the children's best language is used. In the next chapter, we will see how a variety of invented signed systems that we call, generically, *MCE systems*, is used in the education of America's Deaf children, and we will look at the penalty those children pay for the continued reluctance to use their natural language, ASL.

❧

Chapter 9

Language and Literacy

IN chapter 8 we discussed the various settings in which the Deaf child may be placed for the purpose of education, ranging from residential schools for the Deaf to full inclusion, sometimes accompanied by an interpreter, in classes with hearing children. Here we will focus on the methods that are commonly used in the instruction of Deaf children and what accounts for the dismal educational results.

As we saw in chapter 3, during the nineteenth century, ASL was the dominant language of instruction in the schools for the Deaf in the U.S. After the Deaf teachers and their language were expelled from the schools late in the century, the national oral language prevailed. That is, classes were taught orally, and in many schools signing was forbidden.

The rationale for this educational approach, called "oralism," was essentially a cliché, one that continues to be heard today: "This is a hearing world, and Deaf people must learn to cope with it." The oralists believed that to cope, Deaf children must speak. The way to ensure that they did so was to make the abilities to speak intelligibly and to understand speech the focus of their education. Besides, if you could speak and lip-read you could understand and communicate with the hearing teacher, as almost all teachers of the Deaf now were, and so you could learn more. Since reliance on ASL would inhibit the achievement of intelligible speech, it was believed, ASL should not be used.[1]

For nearly a century, then, instruction in the classrooms where the Deaf were educated concentrated on the teaching of "language," which in the U.S. meant the teaching of the oral production of English. For young children, most of the day was spent on this, leaving very little time for the teaching of academic content. That the average Deaf student, upon leaving school, had an academic achievement level equivalent to a hearing student in the third grade was ascribed to his or her failure to learn, not the school's failure to teach. The fact that schools for the Deaf, before signing was banished, had turned out numerous well-educated graduates was suppressed to the point that very few, even in the Deaf community, were aware of it.[2]

Total Communication and the Development of MCE Systems

In the 1960s and 1970s, numerous studies compared the academic achievement of Deaf children of Deaf parents with that of Deaf children of hearing parents. The results were consistent: Deaf children of Deaf parents do significantly better academically than the Deaf children of hearing parents, including in reading and writing English—an achievement that is all the more remarkable when we reflect that Deaf children of Deaf parents often come from poorer homes (generally a disadvantage in academic achievement), and that the schools they attend do not capitalize on their native language. Research also showed that children arriving at school with a knowledge of ASL are better adjusted, better socialized, and have more positive attitudes than their counterparts.[3]

It was largely as a result of these studies that the educational system for the Deaf was transformed from one that used primarily spoken English to one that used Total Communication, which meant, in effect, signs in conjunction with speech.

Initially, however, there was great resistance to the use of signs in the classroom, since the hearing parents of most Deaf children were led to believe that signing would inhibit the learning of speech. Other reasons for the relative advantage of Deaf children of Deaf parents were suggested. For example, they may not have some of the additional disabilities found among the Deaf children of hearing parents, whose hearing loss often results from illness. Another explanation offered was that the Deaf parents' ability to manage their own hearing loss leads them to be more accepting of the hearing loss of their Deaf children. In consequence, the children feel more self-confident and are able to maintain this self-confidence in school, where it is critical to success.

Additional studies were conducted to try and sort out the answers. While the significance of parental acceptance is certainly not negligible, the studies all affirmed the importance of a signed language to the (relative) academic success of the Deaf children of Deaf parents.[4] It was a result that proved embarrassing to advocates of teaching Deaf children to speak English, because those advocates, including educators and speech pathologists, have generally been opposed to signing of any sort. By the 1980s, the pure oralists had been virtually routed and since then, some form of signed communication has been in wide use in classrooms for the Deaf in the U.S.

The form of signing used is not, however, the natural language of the Deaf. One reason is historical: as noted above, educators of the Deaf have long viewed ASL as a problem, not a resource, because it is purported to inhibit the learning of speech.[5] In addition, at the time when the shift to Total Communication began, ASL was still thought to lack the components of a proper language, such as grammar (this was some years before the linguistics research described in chapters 3 and 4 showed that it was in fact a language of great richness). And even allowing that ASL is a language, it has no written form; How then, educators have reasoned, can it be useful for school-related tasks? Besides, it is difficult for hearing teachers to learn, and since the ravages of the Milan Congress of 1880, almost all teachers of the Deaf have been hearing.

Thus, when the studies referred to above proved the benefit of adding signed language to preschool and elementary education programs for Deaf children, and the teaching method called TC was developed and marketed successfully among the educators of the Deaf, ASL had no constituency within the profession of Deaf education. Almost none of the hearing teachers or other hearing staff knew the language. Instead, they knew how to use spoken and written English, and so this became the main avenue along which change was driven. You will recall that TC, as introduced, was a strategy for classroom communication that urged the teacher to mobilize all means at his or her command. However, it devolved into speaking English and simultaneously signing the prominent words in what was spoken—in English word order of course, and without most of the grammar of ASL.

It was but a small leap from this style of classroom communication to the proposal to *systematically* code *all* the elements of the spoken English sentence on the hands. This might initially make communication more difficult (see below), but it held out the tantalizing hope that English might finally be made visible to Deaf children in a way they could understand and master. Thus were invented the several systems for "English on the hands" that we have called MCE (*Manually Coded English*) systems. In general, the inventors of these systems borrowed ASL vocabulary and arranged the signs in English word order, paralleling the spoken message. In addition, where there were no signs that directly corresponded to certain English words, such as the auxiliary verbs *is, are,* and *was*, signs were invented. There were also no ASL signs to pair off with English suffixes that show tense and part of speech, nor any for articles, adverbs of manner, and so forth, because ASL has its own means of expressing those, primarily using space and movement. Thus signs had to be invented for each of these English components. Teachers, professionals and parents were encouraged to produce signs as they spoke. When they arrived at a *was* or an *-ing,* they were to produce the form that had been invented to represent it.

It is this form of signing, a form conceived by professionals in the field to make up for what were thought to be deficiencies in ASL, that has been sold not only as an aid to communication with the Deaf, but as a means to give Deaf children ready access to English by immersing them in a visual representation of that language. Indeed, it was thought that for this vital purpose, the MCE systems would be superior to ASL, because they would present a model of spoken English on the hands.

With the adoption of TC, the simultaneous presentation of signing and spoken English has proliferated among teachers and all other hearing professionals serving the Deaf.[6] Ninety percent of teachers of the Deaf surveyed in a 1990 study reported using simultaneous speech and sign.[7] In over eighty percent of the programs serving Deaf children, from parent-infant to high school, teachers were using (or trying to use) one or another system of MCE, speaking and signing at the same time.[8]

Visual Languages, Codes, and Signing Systems in Use with Deaf People

American Sign Language (ASL): The natural language of the DEAF-WORLD in the U.S. and parts of Canada and Mexico.

Contact sign: A contact language that has arisen from contact between English and ASL. Traditionally known as Pidgin Sign English (PSE). (See chapter 3)

Fingerspelling: The representation of written English words using the manual alphabet.

Simultaneous Communication (sim-com): A communication strategy in which speech and signs are produced at the same time. Also called sign-supported speech.

Total Communication (TC): Initially an educational policy that encouraged teachers to use all means of communication at their disposal, including ASL, English, pantomime, drawing, and fingerspelling. In practice, the Total Communication policy has become simply sim-com.

Manually Coded English (MCE) Systems: Any of several signing systems invented by educators to represent words in English sentences using signs borrowed from ASL combined with signs contrived to serve as translation equivalents for English function words (articles, prepositions, etc.) and prefixes and suffixes. Some function words may be fingerspelled. The systems can be ordered approximately from fewer to more invented signs for the function words and prefixes and suffixes in English. The MCE systems are not languages. The three MCE systems most commonly used in the U.S. are:

1. **Signed English:** An MCE system invented by hearing Gallaudet University professor of education Harry Bornstein in 1973 that uses relatively few invented signs, mostly for articles and common inflections of English verbs.[9]

2. **Signing Exact English (SEE 2):** An intermediate form of MCE, invented by Deaf Gallaudet University professor of education Gerilee Gustason in 1969, and the most widely used MCE system in the U.S. today.[10] The system incorporates many forms borrowed from ASL along with many invented forms, such as adding a fingerspelled -L-Y to adjectives to create adverbs. Some of the forms that were originally ASL signs have been changed extensively. SEE 2 assigns signs to English base words taking into account how those words are pronounced and spelled and what they mean. If any two of those three criteria are the same for two or more English words, then all those words are assigned the same sign. Thus, only one sign would be used for *right* (direction), *right* (correct), and *right* (privilege).

3. **Seeing Essential English (SEE 1):** Invented by a Deaf instructor at the Michigan School for the Deaf, David Anthony, in 1966, SEE 1 is a form of MCE that decomposes English words into their meaningful elements and uses arbitrarily created sign forms to portray them.[11] SEE 1 signs are essentially based on the spelling of English syllables. Thus, the SEE 1 sign for *carpet* contains signs based on ASL CAR and PET (as in, "to *pet* a dog").

The widespread implementation of MCE systems has taken place without any formal evaluation of their effectiveness. As one measure, however, we can look at the academic achievement of Deaf children in an era in which this method has dominated. We have seen that, after nearly a century of oralism, the average Deaf high school graduate had achieved a third-grade education. Alas, after twenty-five years of TC, the results have not improved. (Based on a complicated statistical argument, some scholars contend that there has been a slight improvement in Deaf students' scores, although no improvement relative to their hearing counterparts.) Clearly, Deaf education is still failing at its main task; in the remainder of this chapter we will explore some possible reasons why.[12]

Problems with MCE Systems

The natural acquisition of language by Deaf children is discussed in chapter 3. In this section, we will expand our discussion to explore what happens when the language model to which the Deaf child is exposed is an artificial signing system like the MCE systems. We will then turn to a consideration of what this means for the Deaf child's ability to achieve literacy in English and for academic achievement in general, which depends heavily on literacy skills.

MCE systems as language models

We have noted the striking parallels between the stages in the acquisition of English and of ASL. How can we explain this similarity between two languages that are, on the face of it, so dissimilar? There are in fact significant parallels in the acquisition of all languages, as there are in the rules of word formation and sentence formation. Such universals of language and language learning have led scientists to postulate that the brain contains a language acquisition device, a *bioprogram,* innate in every child, hearing or Deaf, that guides the stages and time course of language acquisition. Children can depend on this bioprogram as a partial guide to the language they are acquiring. They can depend on it even though the language they hear or see (their *language model*) is fragmentary and ungrammatical. The bioprogram allows them to analyze that model to discover the components of signs or words and of sentences and their interrelations, which then enables them to make generalizations that are coherent and valid—"to make sense of the input."[13]

This ability to examine fragmentary input, analyze it, and restructure it towards a language system that is efficient and useful, has been called *nativization*, as we saw in chapter 3. Studies of children's language acquisition have shown that the rules that children abstract from the language samples they encounter differ from adult rules. Over time, further exposure to adult input provides evidence that some of the generalizations made in the course of nativizing are incorrect for the particular language being acquired, whether English, Chinese or ASL. The child then *denativizes*, that is, modifies those generalizations to take account of the specifics of the language being acquired.[14]

The problem for Deaf children in the U.S., however, is that the visual language of the Deaf, ASL, has not generally been accepted as a valid first language for the Deaf child unless that child has Deaf parents, which most do not. And very rarely, as noted above, has ASL been perceived as suitable for use in school. Instead, the several artificial signing systems we call MCE systems were devised to improve "language acquisition" in the Deaf child—with "language" in this case meaning English. This stratagem was destined not to succeed, because the MCE systems are not natural languages that perforce incorporate the principles of the bioprogram. For a language to incorporate those principles, it must be learned as a native language by children who later pass that language to the next generation. Instead, MCE systems entail attempts merely to change the "delivery system" (from voice to hands) of a language that is not accessible to Deaf children (spoken English) and not suited to the visual-manual mode of transmission.[15]

The Deaf child from a hearing home faces great obstacles in school with a teacher whose MCE system may be the child's major source of language modeling, unless the child has access to Deaf adults. For MCE systems are models based on the auditory principles of a spoken language rather than on the visual principles of a manual one—models lacking in the grammar of manual/visual language. Thus there is no way the Deaf child can nativize from an MCE system to develop any true language, signed or otherwise. Here is an example of what we mean. In introducing the grammar of ASL in chapter 4, our theme was the succinctness of ASL, which allows it to have roughly the same pace in communication as English, despite its inherently slower means of producing words using torso, limbs and hands. You may recall that ASL's chief way of achieving this succinctness capitalizes on vision in presenting multiple streams of information at the same time. For example, while the face is marking a clause as the topic of the sentence, and the handshape signals the verb, the movement of the hand indicates the manner in which the verb is being carried out and the location in space reveals which actor is performing the action—all more or less simultaneously. English has none of these devices available because it is not a visual language, but it must still achieve the same ends, marking actors and actions and manner and so on. The spoken language solution exploits the greater speed of speech production to overcome the more limited ability of hearing to analyze patterns—it can make messages longer (compared to visual ones), adding conjunctions, prepositions, suffixes, etc. This is just the wrong solution for a visual/manual language; it undermines the succinctness and slows the pace to an excruciating crawl. Worse than that, it is so alien to the visual/manual mode that the child who is searching for structure in the input makes appropriate but false assumptions; he or she assumes that each successive element in the MCE system must be a major element in the sentence, like an actor or an action for example, and not an element within, or linked to, another word, such as a preposition, article or suffix. In short, the child's bioprogram is bound to proceed doggedly on the assumption that the input is from a language that reflects the visual mode in which it is transmitted; it proceeds with visual principles such as simultaneity. This is all the more true if the child has already constructed a grammar of ASL based on those principles. Because the structure of the MCE system goes counter to its mode, and hence to the child's bioprogram, we will refer to it as *contrarian*. It is, in addition, impoverished with respect to ASL. It does not provide a model from which the child can denativize toward ASL, that is, master the grammar of ASL, including verb agreement, inflections and so forth. Hence the input can serve to help the child build neither a grammar of English nor one of ASL.

Let us look more concretely at the inherent mismatch between mode (visual/manual) and language (spoken/heard) in MCE systems. For example, in an MCE system, the English verb form *working* may consist of two signs: a sign derived from the ASL sign for *work* and a gesture invented to mean *-ing*. When using the MCE system, the ING receives the same stress as WORK. What the Deaf child sees, then, is not the integrated ASL sign WORKING (verb plus inflections) but two separate units (uninflected), WORK + ING, which have nothing to do with each other.* No English speaker would speak in this way, stressing all of the grammatical elements, including those that are unstressed in English; and no one would sign this way in ASL. There is a perfectly good ASL translation for *working*, but in ASL, ongoing action is conveyed by repeating the movement of the verb.

What about the young Deaf child, who has to determine the regularities in the language input to which he or she is exposed? If the MCE system is the child's only language model, what nativization decisions can he or she be expected to make? If there are conflicting regularities between the spoken and visual forms, what denativization decisions might be made by a child who knows ASL? We may get some idea from the following example, an anecdote which we hope will illustrate the problems encountered by children trying to process a contrarian signing system. Remember that the Deaf child will rely totally on the visual input in an attempt to make linguistic sense of what is happening.

In the course of a research project on the acquisition of ASL in Deaf children of Deaf parents, one of us (Bob) filmed an extended conversation with a four-year-old boy who inserted an MCE sign for *-ing* at the end of each of his ASL utterances. Asked why he did that, the boy explained proudly that his teacher had taught it to him in school. The teacher later explained that she was engaged in teaching the English present progressive to her class of Deaf preschoolers. She asked each child to come forward to sign and perform an action sentence, then write the English sentence on the blackboard. Dutifully, each child came to the front of the classroom and performed and signed sentences like the following, in accord with the MCE system used by the teacher.

M-A-R-Y IS JUMP ING
J-O-H-N-N-Y IS KICK ING
S-E-A-N IS TOUCH ING
B-E-T-H IS LAUGH ING

* Neither of these units is an ASL sign, since verbs in ASL would never be signed without inflection and verb agreement.

(This is just the drill that, at the Metro Silent Club, Roberto said he had found so boring and "wacko.") In her effort to teach the *is* verb-*ing* English form, the teacher had, in effect, provided evidence that ING is a signal that the sentence has ended. Since ING has its own independent sign and stress in MCE systems, and is separable from the basic verb, it was appropriate to assign it a function separate from that verb, which is precisely what our bright young friend had done. He concluded that ING is how you mark the end of sentences. Not only was he not learning English (*-ing* does not mark the end of English sentences, whether spoken or written); the signed input to which he was exposed was corrupting the ASL denativization process (ASL contains no ING at all, nor any separable element that signals the end of sentences).

As this example illustrates, Deaf children presented with MCE are able to analyze the visual input, and in attempting to nativize or denativize, are led to make hypotheses about the structure of the input language. The rules they infer may be, and usually are, different from the rules of English, however. For example, the MCE system SEE 2 would assign the same handshapes to *park* (a car) and *park* (the place), following the two-out-of-three rule (see box, p. 272). The handshapes chosen to express both meanings of *park* include an ASL handshape that appears in the verb PARK and also in other signs whose meaning involves vehicles, such as SAIL and SUBMARINE. Consequently, in SEE 2, *park* (the place), *sail*, and *submarine* all are expressed with signs that contain the same handshapes. Since they have handshapes in common, the child infers that the three words have a similarity in meaning. However, the groupings specified by ASL classifiers are not found in English structure. There is no pronoun in English peculiar to vehicles (for example). In fact, there is no utility—indeed, it is counterproductive if you are trying to learn English—to note as a structural regularity that *a park, to sail,* and *a submarine* are related.

The child is led even further in the wrong direction by the general strategy of analyzing sets of signs into their permutations of handshapes, movements, and locations. It seems the child infers that the handshapes, movements, and locations in each sign represent separable meanings and that the meaning of that sign can often be constructed from the meanings of its component handshapes or movements. While that may frequently be true in ASL, the signs presented in an MCE system will not allow the child to predict from their handshapes, movements and locations what the meanings of the English words they represent are. In general, then, we can say that the child forms some hypotheses about the input that are appropriate to a visual/manual language, but later learns that these hypotheses are not supported by further input. The goal of presenting MCE, however, is not to help the child form wrong hypotheses about signed language; rather, it is to lead the child to correct hypotheses about a spoken language, English. And as we have also just seen, MCE systems do not do that either.

To summarize: Deaf children, like all children, are equipped with the innate propensity to develop a language. They have the cognitive and perceptual mechanisms to assist them in doing so. They thereby make sense of the linguistic input in their environment, provided that input exhibits the regularities of form and function basic to one of the natural, visual languages of the Deaf. In other words, given the opportunity, they will construct a grammar of ASL (or another signed language in other lands). We have seen, however, that MCE systems do not employ the natural structures visual children depend on to learn a language.

With an MCE system as input, Deaf children are not able to construct a signed language that contains the rules and generative properties of English. That is, they do not denativize toward English; nor are they able to construct a fully developed ASL (denativize toward ASL). This suggests that the structure of MCE systems and their instructional use may actually limit the development of language in Deaf children. Deaf children with hearing parents, especially, are unable to advance linguistically—to master grammar, vocabulary, discourse styles, registers and art forms—because they have no real first-language model through which to acquire sophisticated skills in either English or ASL. Deaf children of Deaf parents are constrained as well when confronted in school with the contrarian and impoverished language model that hearing teachers use almost to the exclusion of all others. These Deaf children, fluent in their first language, ASL, are unable through the medium of an MCE system to gain fluency in English as a second language.

Conversational language, school language, and MCE systems

Jim Cummins, a Canadian expert on bilingualism, has identified two types of communicative knowledge that the school child must master. First, there are the skills required for social, conversational communication, which Cummins calls *basic interpersonal communicative skills* (BICS). Then there is the type of communication skills that school requires, *cognitive academic language proficiency* (CALP). The two types of skills involve quite different language styles, or *registers* (see chapter 3).[16]

We get our knowledge of BICS through the natural process of language acquisition. The structural components of this conversational register are generally acquired in a highly contextualized setting.[17] By this we mean that the speaker knows the intended audience and whether they can supply the context for his or her remarks—context like the character of the people involved, the nature of the locations and so forth. At home, with Mom and Dad as conversational partners, rules for how one interacts conversationally are taught explicitly, if cursorily, at first (e.g., "No!"). Later, as we mature, the rules may be taught more precisely. For example, at the dinner table, a child may be told, "Say 'Excuse me' before interrupting your mother." These rules follow the cultural patterns of the family, language is used as their carrier, and the rules are stored for future use. When the child (or adult) is engaged in a conversation, the structure of the language required in the interaction is dictated by the setting, the topic, and the familiarity of the conversational partners.

CALP is another matter. It requires both natural language acquisition and explicit learning. In academic language proficiency, the setting, the topics, and the conversational partners will be different from what the child has experienced at home. In addition, to be successful, the child must learn to read, to master a language skill that requires explicit instruction.[18] Most children (except for most Deaf children of hearing parents) enter school with highly developed BICS in their native language. In school they build on these skills to figure out what academic language—the register used by the teacher—is all about, and to learn the language skills necessary to academic success. For children who are native English speakers, this means acquiring two language registers, one natural and acquired mostly at home, and one unnatural and learned in school.[19] Bilingual hearing children whose native language is not English will usually have mastered BICS in their native language at home; at school they must learn both BICS and CALP in English (for more on bilingual hearing children and school, see chapter 10). For Deaf children in the MCE setting, however, the situation is more complicated—and much more problematic.

Like bilingual hearing children, at school Deaf children must learn both BICS and CALP in English. However, they are expected to do this through a medium of instruction that is itself not a natural language, but an artificial MCE system, which they must also learn. To put it mildly, this is not an easy task. As we have seen, MCE systems follow the linguistic logic of neither visual nor spoken language. To conceive of BICS in such a system is virtually a contradiction in terms. It is hard to imagine how one could have a substantive conversation using an MCE system because, as noted above, such systems run counter to the principles of the visual mode. Students are likely to use ASL or contact sign; even teachers highly trained in MCE have difficulty using it in classroom conversation.[20] Although Deaf students may not have BICS in English, they may have them in ASL. However, that repertoire is not called into play. Lacking basic communicative skills in English, which the MCE system has been unable to supply, and with their ASL skills excluded from instruction, the Deaf students have no basis on which to build the academic register of English, and thus literacy.[21]

Deaf Children and English Literacy

Literacy is a misunderstood term in general education. In the education of the Deaf, it is not only misunderstood but misstated and misapplied. We will look further into the real meaning of literacy in chapter 10; for now let us note that one fundamental error is the belief that literacy and the ability to read and write are synonymous. They are not. Reading and writing are components of literacy, but not the only components. They are, however, the central components of literacy in school, and they are the components on which the MCE systems were based and to which they are intended to give the Deaf child access.

What it means to read well

The activity we call "reading" may entail any of three types of literacy: functional, cultural, and critical literacy. Someone who is functionally literate can read a simple newspaper and possibly fill out a job application, but is not able to read most books. Someone who is culturally literate is able to read and understand more elevated journalism and most books. Someone who is critically literate can write an article for the newspaper analyzing a topic in some depth.

People who are functionally literate are able to obtain a very limited message from text that is presented in simplified and commonly used terms. Usually attained by the third or fourth grade, functional literacy implies the ability to accomplish practical, everyday tasks that involve responding to print. A person who is only functionally literate is unable to perform jobs that require some reading facility and hence finds his or her vocational options limited.

People who are culturally literate are able to bring to the text knowledge derived from their culture, encompassing values, customs, and information, including information about the socio-historical context of writing. Cultural knowledge is important because it sets the context in which literate behavior is to occur, defining the rules for the interaction between writer and reader and the purpose of the message. Literate behavior must occur on a common foundation of shared experiences.

People who are critically literate understand that literacy has both a social and a political purpose.[22] Such readers seek to understand the cultural, social and political vantage point from which the text is written and the reasons for it having been written. Thus, they take a critical posture with respect to the information in the text, and are able to see the characteristics of the text as a set of choices in form and content. Likewise, critically literate readers are able to prepare a text that achieves a social or political goal.

Widespread cultural and critical literacy is the primary goal of education in complex societies such as ours. Our schools aim to endow students with the reading skills that lead ultimately to the development of culturally and critically literate adults. Good readers at the elementary level are those who master these skills quickly so that they are able to apply them to texts of increasing complexity in a variety of areas, expanding both knowledge and skills.

Learning to read

Research shows that to be good readers, students must bring a substantial body of background knowledge to the task. That a good part of this knowledge involves the rules of the language in which the text is presented perhaps goes without saying. In addition, however, for reading beyond the most basic level, it is essential to have considerable knowledge of life and the world. Such knowledge helps students create accurate expectancies and hypotheses about the meanings of texts—to abstract meaning from passages of text, not just individual words. It also allows them to remember what they have read, a process that is aided by integrating new information into what one already knows. The kind of background knowledge that is necessary to good reading is more than mere experience, however. It is experience that has been categorized and stored by means of a language. If some of that knowledge is to come from a teacher, or from texts, as it does in school, then a language common to student and teacher, one that also gives access to texts, is needed.[23]

Research on the reading abilities of Deaf children reveals that they have difficulty learning how to read in English because of their lack of knowledge of English language structure, and because they have trouble integrating information from the past and using it in devising predictive and generalizable strategies for understanding print. Deaf children are said to lack these basic abilities because of a lack of exposure to information within their environment, that is, a lack of background knowledge. This lack in turn appears to stem from a number of sources: growing up with little access to language at home and in school; ineffective instruction in school; and excessive time devoted to oral skills and English grammar and vocabulary rather than content acquisition.[24]

Let us, then, take a closer look at *background knowledge*—at what we mean by it, the ways in which language is crucial to its acquisition and development, and how it provides the essential context for the comprehension of texts.

As children we often participate in discussions with parents and others. For example, we chat at the dinner table, when people visit, or when people meet in the neighborhood. It is at these times that we learn our social roles. In addition, through these interactions we learn social rules. We learn who is responsible for what in our home, neighborhood, and community. We learn about rules for social behavior.

This is background knowledge, and the learning process involved is *contextualized learning*, because it occurs in a context where there are a lot of clues to the meaning of the event. For example, suppose there is a rule that requires Junior to tap Mom on the shoulder gently when seeking her attention. He is not supposed to pull on her clothes or stomp on the floor. If he yanks on her dress, she might say "Please, just tap me if you want me." The topic is introduced by the actions of the child within the setting, and the rule is repeated within that setting.

Not all learning at home is so contextualized. For example, suppose later Mom tells Dad what happened. Dad tells Junior not to forget the rule. This reminder is *decontextualized,* that is, it is removed from the original setting and unrelated to the current one. The scenario has been recreated through language. To understand the father's reminder, the child must have stored in memory the original setting, the incident, and the result. And that memory must be retrievable with language in a setting that is physically and socially removed from the incident. Learning how to talk about things in decontextualized or unnatural settings is a precursor to what schooling is all about, and it is a vital part of background knowledge.

The background knowledge that we bring to school, and to the texts that we will read there, also includes such things as tales that have been passed down through generations and adapted to convey the cultural values and mores of our society. They tell us to watch out for strangers; that if we work hard, life will reward us; that beauty is only skin deep, etc. They are part of our cultural heritage, and we remember them. So are the Fourth of July, Paul Revere's Ride, and *Mary Had a Little Lamb.*

Background knowledge also involves everyday things. Before we arrive at school we know that eggs come from chickens and bacon from pigs. We know, too, that print is an important method of conveying information. Signs tell us to stop and go; brand names announce stores and products.

All this knowledge, which we take with us to school, is mediated through language and plays a vital role in our ability to comprehend the peculiarly decontextualized form of language that is printed text. How does this work? Consider a simple activity like going to a store. What kind of knowledge do we have about this activity? Specifically, we know what to wear. Where to go. What we want to buy. This knowledge may be available as a matter of routine, or it may require explicit reflection. The ability to draw on such information, whether it is daily information or a matter of reflection, is critical to becoming literate. Relative to our ability to access stored information, such things as accessing sound waves, movements of the lips, or printed words play only a small part in leading us to understand a sentence. The meaning of each word and its grammatical class are likewise not the basis of comprehension. In interpreting a sentence, in arriving at its sense, we rely unconsciously, and thus much more than we realize, on our knowledge of life. This knowledge is not specific to any particular language. Rather, it is knowledge that comes from general acculturation. It helps us place new information in perspective, providing data from which we are able to make judgments about the meaning of a text. Incongruent interpretations of sentences are automatically ruled out while practical knowledge about the world and society guide the reader or listener at every moment.

What would it be like to try and read a text where one lacked the necessary background knowledge? Most of us have had that experience at one time or another. Perhaps it was legalistic language, instructions for a tax return, or the impenetrable instructions for assembling some unfamiliar device. Here's an example from philosophy:

> We now reiterate the procedure, that is, we extend the absolute notion of a possible world to that of a world (M', V') possible relative to a given world (M,V,). (M', V') is such a world if M' is any structure, with the same domain as W, for the non-modal sentences, in which all such sentences 'A' for which V assigns to '□A' the value *true* are true, and V' is any admissible truth-value assignment . . .[25]

This passage presents information in words that we all know but it is clearly "context reduced." We know the words, but we probably have no clue about the meaning of the passage, because we lack the background knowledge to make sense of them when they are arranged in this way (unless we are familiar with formal logic).

In addition to background knowledge about the physical and social world and about culture, we bring to the activity of reading background knowledge about reading itself—what is called literacy knowledge. We scan a sentence, parse it, begin to sketch out its structure in our mind, place the clauses in the right relations, identify actors and actions and so on. What would it be like to lack this kind of background knowledge, which helps us find structure where there is only a series of words and some punctuation? Perhaps the following passage will help us simulate that:

> Thispassagecomesfromabooktitledfregethephilosop
> Hyoflanguagewrittenbymichaeldummettfroma
> Llsoulscollegeoxfordenglandthebookisverydi
> Fficulttounderstand

In this case, the background knowledge required to comprehend the passage is not knowledge of content, but knowledge of *form*—of the mechanics of the reading process, a type of "meta-reading knowledge." When printed this way, this text does not demarcate the words or contain punctuation. So we, as the readers, must invent a strategy for discovering words and sentences in the stream of letters. Only after inventing and applying that strategy can we execute the subsequent stages of reading, such as finding the word in our vocabulary, updating hypotheses about the structure of the sentences, their place in the story, and so on. Because the process is cumbersome, the unfamiliar search-and-find strategy may confound us, and the entire process may overload our short-term memory for a while. Nevertheless, in the end, we probably will succeed in figuring out what the passage says. We know that there are words in this passage, so we look for them. Once we find them, we reconstruct the sentence. Our expectation of how things are supposed to look gets in the way at first, but in fact there is no inherent need for word separators (the Romans, for example, didn't use them). Ultimately, our background knowledge of words and syntax, and the very fact that we are discussing reading, gets us through.

For Deaf children, learning to read presents obstacles analogous to these two samples. Like all children, they need literacy knowledge to find the words and sentence structures and to devise predictive and generalizable strategies for making text intelligible. They need knowledge of the world and cultural knowledge so they can recontextualize, as far as possible, decontextualized writing, and thereby derive meaning from it. Unlike other children, however, Deaf children, particularly the Deaf children of hearing parents, commonly reach school age without acquiring any cohesive language at all. Unable to store their experiences in memory because they lack language, they cannot help but arrive in the classroom extremely deficient in the background knowledge so essential to reading. What other children have learned incidentally and sometimes formally at home, they must be explicitly taught. And of course, they lack as well fluency in the language that is in print, English.[26]

Deaf children often lack substantial background knowledge also because many of the sources of that knowledge that are available to hearing children are not available to them. Deaf children of hearing parents are very likely to be excluded from discussions about everyday life, and about local, national and world events. When hearing parents attempt to read to their Deaf children, the focus tends to be on language, and the child is able to extract little if any background knowledge from the passages. Since there are probably no other people about who speak ASL with one another (as there are, say, at the Deaf club or the Deaf family table), the child is unlikely to pick up incidental information that is addressed to someone else. Deaf children of hearing parents could learn a lot from older Deaf friends—if they had any. School should be an important source of background knowledge for them, but all too often class time is devoted to the form of what is said rather than its content. Because teacher and students do not have one full language between them, there is little substantive exchange. Finally, texts are an important source of background knowledge, frequently on the job and in everyday life, but especially in school. Background knowledge gleaned from texts grows exponentially, for the more one gathers knowledge from texts, the greater the range and depth of texts that come within one's reach. Deaf children's background knowledge from texts does not multiply across the years, however, for texts are, at the outset, impenetrable for the Deaf student, and they largely remain so.

Deaf children's problems with reading

First-language (ASL) acquisition, second-language (English) learning, and learning how to read, are all bound together for Deaf children. Some Deaf children arrive at school without a first language because they have been deprived of accessible language models. Those who have not been so deprived are likely to find that their native language is not acceptable or understood in school. Without a language they can use in school, both groups will find learning English and English literacy a great challenge. Lacking literacy knowledge in English, such children make characteristic reading errors. For example, several studies investigating the Deaf child's knowledge of English syntax have reported that Deaf students make the most mistakes with so-called *function words*, that is words that work primarily to convey the grammatical structure of the text—words like *of, but,* and *by*.[27] Yet a knowledge of English syntax is critical if one is to learn to read at a level beyond the stringing together of content words.[28]

Deaf children also have trouble with English vocabulary, in particular with the organization of words into categorical hierarchies. That is, the Deaf child is said to be unable to choose a more general word that includes a more specific word in its meaning; for example, *fruit* as a general category to which *apple* belongs. Some research suggests that the child's difficulty may be due to an inability to integrate, combine, and compare different levels of English vocabulary in memory for future use.[29] It seems that in learning English, many Deaf students attend excessively to individual words and their restricted dictionary meanings, thus limiting the possibility of finding a wider reference in the meaning of the sentence.

That Deaf children of hearing parents seldom have contact with signed-language users almost certainly relates directly to their inability to understand and integrate information about language (either signed or spoken). Since in their early years at home and at school, they do not have significant command of any language, they cannot be involved in discussions about language.

It has also been suggested that these characteristic reading errors result from "impoverished educational experiences,"[30] possibly the overreliance on the low-level reading materials commonly found in classrooms for the Deaf child.[31] Another contributing factor may be educational practices that insist too heavily on teaching vocabulary in isolation and on verbatim recall, which would lead students to focus on specific meanings in specific contexts, as opposed to the variations of meaning across sentences and text passages.[32]

It may be that the very MCE systems that have been designed to make English accessible to Deaf students and thereby to enhance their reading skills are actually part of the problem. When Deaf students in a classroom where an MCE system is the medium of instruction are asked to "read aloud," they are often told to "sign every word." That is, they must follow the English precisely. In order to do this, they must use the MCE system they have been taught, with its manufactured signs for *-ing* and *the* and so on, and they may be corrected whenever they miss a word or a word ending. This is bad enough during reading class. But it also happens in other contexts, when teachers may admonish students for not using the ING or the S (signifying the plural) sign when responding to a question in social studies or science class, or describing something, instead of reacting to the content of what they say.

Reading for the Deaf student thus becomes a process of attending to details—the very details that good readers learn to gloss over early in their reading development, because most of the time they are irrelevant to the purpose of reading. Normally, people read to gain information from a text. With this goal, good readers may sometimes skip words that are not familiar to them if these words are not essential to understanding the passage.[33] Indeed, focusing on unknown words for the purpose of discovering their meaning as individual words may detract from one's ability to derive meaning from the passage as a whole.[34] For the Deaf child, then, school reading tends to focus on reading for the sake of reading, not deriving content. In fact, teachers of the Deaf generally continue with this approach well into high school.

There is clearly much that could be done in the home and the school to help Deaf children achieve higher levels of literacy. But we suspect that poor pedagogical practices are not the sole reason for the reading problems of Deaf children and that they may have an inherent disadvantage compared to their hearing peers in processing the alphabetic writing system of their second language.[35] Let us characterize an important component of the task of reading for hearing children at its most rudimentary level: recovering spoken words that have been transcribed into printed words. To accomplish this task, hearing readers know unconsciously the principles by which sequences of English sounds are represented by sequences of letters. They also know the inventory of elements (vowels and consonants), rules for their combinations in words and, most important, hearing readers know the spoken words themselves (for the most part). Thus, once hearing readers have recovered from print the original utterance, they can recover the meaning if they know the spoken words (they may also learn a direct connection between the printed word and its meaning). Deaf readers who have not acquired English by ear tackle this same task with a significant disadvantage. As we discussed in chapter 4, the best Deaf readers have mastered the system of elements that comprise English words, and they call on that representation when reading. We speculated that Deaf readers who have mastered that system have done so using indirect evidence such as fingerspelling, analyzing patterns in print, lipreading, etc. With such sources of information, one may arrive at a fragmentary (and perhaps in places erroneous) system of representation for printed words. But once the Deaf reader has recovered with that representation what at least some of the utterance must have been, there is still a serious problem: he or she may well not know that spoken English word.

We also said in chapter 4 that Deaf readers apparently use other strategies that involve associating signs from ASL with printed words, and even associating meanings directly with the shapes of the words. Both of these strategies do not use the alphabetic principle which underlies the patterning of the text. Perhaps this limited discussion of the problem is sufficient to suggest the important challenge for the psycholinguistics of reading presented by Deaf readers and our uncertainty concerning how much of the shortfall in reading achievement is due to the failure to build a solid foundation in ASL. It is probable that a large share must be attributed to that, however, since native speakers of ASL achieve much higher reading scores on the average than their Deaf peers who are not native speakers. It is important to keep in mind that no generalization about Deaf readers, such as average scores, captures the wide range that is actually encountered. There are some crackerjack Deaf readers who have achieved outstanding cultural and critical literacy.

LANGUAGE AND LEARNING IN SCHOOL

In the previous sections of this chapter, we focused on the language of the classroom and literacy. But the language used in school not only affects the child's achievement in language development, it also influences the child's ability to learn other content the school is supposed to teach. For all children, success depends on the quality of the instruction; the time spent actually learning the subject matter, called "time on task"; the size of the classroom; and the use of out-of-school time.[36] The two most important variables for Deaf students appear to be the quality of the instruction and time on task.

Given the discussion we have presented so far, it will be no surprise that the quality of instruction the teacher can deliver depends on the language used in the classroom. Simply put, without a valid, consistent, and viable language, teachers cannot be understood by students. Since most teachers of Deaf children report that they are quite weak in ASL, it seems likely that they may not have the language skills to instruct their Deaf pupils in ways that challenge them intellectually. If children are unable to use the language they know, and if they interact with teachers who are unable to present information appropriately, then learning will be slow and often thwarted.

Just how bad is the language situation among teachers of the Deaf? One survey of teachers found only thirty-eight percent capable, in their own judgment, of producing "signs" as well as English. Only one-fourth said they could *understand* "signs" as well as English. (Note that producing and/or understanding "signs" are lax criteria of signed language fluency; probably only a very small fraction of these teachers were using ASL.) For most teachers, learning a signed language is akin to learning a second spoken language. One of the most effective ways to increase proficiency in any second language is to interact with the community of users. Yet only one in five hearing teachers in the residential schools reports any outside social interaction with Deaf adults. That number drops to one in ten in non-residential programs for Deaf children (the most common type of program).[37] Nine out of ten teachers of Deaf children owe all their knowledge of the DEAF-WORLD and ASL to hearing faculty and textbooks. Roughly one-fourth state that they learned whatever ASL they know from their students.

There is no other field where the instructors or professionals learn the language of instruction from the students they teach.

Even these figures may not truly show the seriousness of the communication problem. Since so few hearing teachers are able to understand older Deaf students and Deaf adults well enough to carry on a substantial conversation, Deaf people often adjust their signing to accommodate the hearing person. For example, they may use simpler syntactic structures. They may introduce anglicisms. They sometimes slow their rate and stress individual signs. They may address simpler topics and, when possible, speak of things in the immediate environment. This may give the hearing person too favorable an impression of his or her ability to communicate in signed language.

We have already discussed the severe limits on the ability of Deaf children, particularly the Deaf children of hearing parents, to gain information via MCE systems. The inadequacy of these language models, coupled with the reduced exposure to content that results from the simplifying of materials, creates some overwhelming obstacles to learning content.[38]

Deaf children of Deaf parents do better because, though they are also exposed to MCE systems and to the same teaching styles, they have a language base from which they are able to make some sense out of the signed input they receive. Since they come equipped with substantial linguistic knowledge and language decoding skills in ASL, they can rapidly test various hypotheses about how the signs they see might be reordered and grammaticized in order to become interpretable in ASL. Knowing the meaning of the sentence translated into ASL, they are in a better position to puzzle out the regularities in the sequences of real and invented grammatical signs of the MCE system. Their problem is that the information in English is presented at such a low level that their potential is seldom realized; they have the advantage of a full language, but the school doesn't use it. Some of these Deaf children succeed in spite of the system of education to which they are subjected.

Turning next to time on task: One study found that hearing teachers of Deaf students sign between forty and fifty percent of classroom time. If the class lasted an hour, for example, there was at best thirty minutes of information presented visually. However, Deaf students only paid attention, on average, for half of a class period.[39] During the remainder, they signed among themselves or were distracted by other events in the classroom. All in all, there were only about fifteen minutes of accessible instruction in each hour.

Interestingly, teachers who are Deaf apparently often have a teaching style that significantly enhances the attention Deaf students pay to classroom instruction, so they may deliver more time on task.[40] Deaf teachers who are skilled speakers of ASL are able to interact with their students most effectively and present substantial academic information; they have been found to be better at keeping attention focused on a topic and seeing to it that the topic is mastered.[41] Thus the teacher's language competence may underlie both formulas for success—the quality of instruction and the time spent on the task.

It has been observed that, even apart from the language they use, the in-class behavior patterns of Deaf teachers of the Deaf are very different from those of hearing teachers.[42] Deaf teachers, for example, use DEAF–WORLD attention-getting behaviors, like tapping pupils on the shoulder or flicking the lights on and off, at appropriate times. This suggests that teachers of the Deaf who are not fluent in ASL might use similar behavior to better hold their students' attention and thus increase the academic content Deaf students receive, though the limited ability of most hearing teachers to communicate with their Deaf students will still probably prevent the students—except those quite competent in ASL and English—from divining what is supposedly being taught.

Class size is not among the factors that make a difference in learning in Deaf children because, as a consequence of the fact that there are so few Deaf children, virtually all classes for Deaf children are extremely small, with a student-teacher ratio in most states of eight to one or less. It is interesting that these small classes have not resulted in relatively high academic achievement, as would be predicted with hearing children. We may speculate that the reason involves the teacher's lack of competence in signed language. Teachers of the Deaf often compensate for poor instructional delivery by requiring students to do more work in their seats and by providing them with more individualized attention—which sounds like an advantage until one realizes that it means there will be very little dialogue among the students, who will also be unable to profit from exchanges between teacher and students.

Since out-of-school activities contribute to academic achievement in hearing children, their lack in most non-residential Deaf education programs in the U.S. today may be contributing to the poor achievement of most Deaf students. As we saw in chapter 8, after-school activities in elementary programs for the Deaf housed in regular schools generally do not exist (although parents may enroll their children in the Scouts and the like). Usually Deaf students are bused home and spend most of the afternoon and early evening watching TV. In one study of eighty-one Deaf students in day and residential schools, seventy were commuters or non-boarders; the activity listed as accounting for the majority of time spent at home for sixty-four of the subjects was watching TV.[43]

Language issues in the elementary programs for Deaf children are magnified in high school. Many Deaf students enter high school with conversational ASL skills far beyond those of their hearing teachers. This is one of the reasons that Deaf teachers in the residential schools are most often assigned to high school classes. High school students faced with the limited signing abilities of most hearing teachers are likely to be bored, to say the least. Most Deaf teachers are able to interact more effectively with older Deaf students, in significant part because of their language skills.

But if Deaf high school students are on average much better at using signed language than their hearing teachers, their English language abilities tend to be much below high school level, as we have seen. Yet the normal high school curriculum places far greater demands on English reading skills, and the severe "dumbing down" of content we have noted at the elementary level has catastrophic consequences in high school, as the students attempt to master more complex ideas.[44] It is also during the high school years that a great deal of class time is usually spent in "collaborative" learning. This has a special meaning when it comes to Deaf students, because those who are capable of understanding the teacher often serve as interpreters for the others. It is not uncommon to see individual Deaf students re-explaining the content the teacher has just attempted to provide in a lecture. Is it surprising that the average Deaf high schooler gains only one grade-level of academic achievement in four or more years of high school?[45]

The issue of language is clearly central to the education of the Deaf child. What we have learned in this chapter raises the question: What language will allow the Deaf child to achieve the maximum success in school and out of school? The evidence indicates that in the first half of the nineteenth century, when the natural signed language of the Deaf was used in school, many Deaf children achieved academic success comparable to that of their hearing peers.[46] We know that one hundred years of oralism was disastrous for Deaf education. Twenty-five years of MCE systems in TC programs has not produced the rise in achievement that was expected, and in this chapter we have explored some of the reasons why.

Since our efforts to understand the failure of Deaf education keep leading us back to language, many educators of the Deaf and Deaf leaders have concluded that the greatest hope for reform of Deaf education lies in ensuring that teacher and student have a shared fluent natural language at their command for conducting learning. For most Deaf children, that language can only be the natural language of their DEAF–WORLD; in the U.S., ASL. In the next chapter we will explore the implications of this for Deaf children, for the professionals who serve them, and for the future of the DEAF–WORLD itself.

❦

Chapter 10

Bilingual and Bicultural Education for Deaf Children

IN the preceding chapter, we explored the relationship between language and the education of the Deaf, in particular the role of language in the failure of education to assure that the average Deaf student achieves at the level of his or her hearing peers. Here we shall contend that if ASL were looked upon as a useful tool within the educational setting, it could provide the foundation for building knowledge about both conversational and school language. This knowledge is critical to the development of literacy skills.

Basically, ASL is the native language of the Deaf child in the U.S. (see chapters 2, 3). To those who say, "Not for the Deaf child of hearing parents, it isn't," we reply: ASL is the best language model that is within the biological reach of the Deaf child in this country. It is the language he or she will be able to learn naturally, easily, appropriately, and fully. Because ASL is a natural language, it is rule-governed, predictable and generative; hence it can be used for full communication and as a means for acquiring new knowledge, including the knowledge of other languages, specifically English. Even if fluent in ASL, many Deaf children will still remain at a disadvantage when it comes to English, whose written form involves the representation of sounds they may never have heard. However, it is our view that approaching the learning of English as a second language through ASL offers the best chance for the Deaf child to succeed at the task.[1]

For over a quarter century, the federal government has steadfastly pursued the reform of American education to accommodate children whose primary language is not English. It has used a carrot and a stick. The carrot is the 1965 Bilingual Education Act, which provides funding for a wide variety of programs promoting the use of minority languages in schools. The stick is composed of civil rights statutes, which, the Supreme Court has ruled, impose an affirmative duty on schools to give children who speak a minority language an equal educational opportunity by lowering the English-language barrier to their education.[2]

The Bilingual Education Act specifies "that there are large and growing numbers of children of limited English proficiency; that many such children have a cultural heritage which differs from that of English proficient persons; and that the Federal Government has an . . . obligation to assist in providing equal educational opportunity to limited English proficient children." The law goes on to say that "a primary means by which a child learns is through the use of the child's native language and cultural heritage" and concludes that "therefore large numbers of children of limited English proficiency have educational needs which can be met by the use of bilingual educational methods and techniques. . . ."[3]

According to the regulations implementing the law, the test for whether a child is covered by the act is whether he or she normally speaks English. For the purposes of the act, it does not matter what language the child's parents speak. What matters for the success of the child's education, and therefore for bilingual education programs, is the language the child speaks. According to the regulations, if the child normally speaks a language other than English, then the child's native language is not English, and if the child has limited English proficiency, then he or she can benefit from the programs funded by the act.[4]

Bilingual/bicultural instruction includes several components. Academic subject matter is taught, transitionally at least, using the pupil's primary language. English is taught as a second language. Students are instructed in the history, culture and language arts of their minority-language group. In addition, equal attention is given to learning about American culture and history. The goal is to teach the student English so that he or she can ultimately be educated exclusively in English, while assuring that the student does not fall behind in other studies. This objective is met by (1) fostering a healthy self-image in the learner, (2) developing the student's cognitive powers, (3) creating a bridge to the learner's existing linguistic and cultural knowledge, and (4) developing the student's reading and expressive skills in English.

While it was Congress that directly provided the carrot to motivate the schools to serve their bilingual children, it was the Supreme Court that provided the stick by ruling in *Lau v. Nichols* (1974) that the Civil Rights Act of 1964 requires local school authorities receiving federal financial assistance to provide special instruction to language minority students. The Court wrote: "We know that those children who do not understand English are certain to find their classroom experience wholly incomprehensible and in no way meaningful [if the language of instruction is exclusively English]."[5]

Congress weighed in again in 1974 with passage of the Equal Educational Opportunity Act, which explicitly requires local authorities to take "appropriate action to overcome language barriers that impede equal participation in the instructional program."[6] And in 1978 the Court ruled in *Rios vs. Read* that the Civil Rights Act and the Equal Educational Opportunity Act and other laws "mandate teaching [minority-language] . . . children subject matter in their native tongue (when required) by competent teachers . . . and [strongly suggest] the requirement of a bicultural [component] as a psychological support to the subject matter instruction."[7] The Court explicitly found that a school district was not in compliance if it merely provided students with intensive training in English while they fell behind in their other subjects, and it ordered officials of the defendant school system to add three features to its bilingual education program: to educate teachers about the special cultural problems of minority language children; to train all instructors in the teaching of English as a second language; and to actively seek and employ instructors of the same minority group as the students.

The Bilingual Education Act is really based on a simple idea. Americans want their children to be educated and in command of English. For children to achieve this goal, if their most fluent language is not English, they should be instructed using their most fluent language until they have achieved a sufficient command of English. This accords with the weight of the evidence. There is a substantial scientific literature comparing monolingual and bilingual education for children whose primary language is not English. A comprehensive review of that literature finds a consistent advantage favoring bilingual education on tests of reading, listening, language skills, mathematics, social studies, total achievement, and attitudes toward school and self.[8] It surprises no one to learn that students are more successfully educated in a language they understand well, that if you want to teach geography, say, to Hispanic-American children whose primary language is Spanish, you will be able to teach that subject more effectively in Spanish (presuming you are fluent in it). What is more surprising, at least at first, is that English fluency gains by this detour through the child's best language, even though the detour takes time away from practicing English. A paradox? Not really. For students to make progress in learning English as a second language, the input must be understandable. And the greatest aid to understanding messages, as we explained in chapter 9, is background knowledge. Thus time spent providing background knowledge in the students' primary language is time also invested in their acquisition of a second language. Moreover, literacy development in the students' primary language builds skills that transfer, in part, to learning literacy in their second language, skills such as interpreting formal language registers.

A major study of bilingual education in the United States found that the majority of Hispanic children who were taught to read Spanish before learning to read English learned later to read English quite well. The children who had difficulty learning to read English were not those who spoke Spanish at home but those who had poor language and prereading skills, whether the home language was English or Spanish. And if those children did not get assistance in their native Spanish, they did not do well in later years. The best readers of English, on the other hand, were the children with the best skills in Spanish.[9]

A Canadian study of children from Russian and other language minorities who were learning French came to a similar but broader conclusion: Those children who could read and write in their minority language outperformed nonliterate children on all measures of French achievement, not just reading French. There was evidence, furthermore, that the results were not due simply to the children's spoken fluency in their minority language; what mattered for success was their literacy in their native language.[10] A later study involving two thousand Hispanic-American students in bilingual education in five states compared English-only, transitional, and maintenance bilingual programs.[11] Transitional programs aim to make an early transition from using Spanish exclusively to using English exclusively (all by the fourth grade in this study). In maintenance programs, on the contrary, the goal is to build Spanish fluency and literacy while developing English-language competence. In this carefully constructed study, children in the maintenance programs had the highest rates of academic achievement in English reading and language, and in mathematics.

This finding concurs with extensive research on bilingual education in Canada. A review of that literature found that the greater the incorporation of minority students' language and culture in the school curriculum, the greater their success in that curriculum.[12] While incorporating the students' language gives them access to information and builds second-language literacy, incorporating their culture helps to create a positive attitude toward their own identity and toward the school, and these enhance academic achievement as well.[13]

In his 1986 book summarizing research on bilingualism, psychologist Kenji Hakuta concludes that bilinguals also have an advantage over monolinguals in cognitive flexibility.[14] A Canadian expert on bilingualism, Wallace Lambert, reached the same conclusion about a decade earlier: Bilinguals are more sensitive to semantic relations among words than monolinguals; they are better at analyzing sentence structure and discovering rules generally; they are more able to reorganize perceptual situations; they are more creative in solving problems.[15] A 1991 review of this research in the last three decades finds most studies showing clear superiority for bilinguals in cognitive tasks.[16]

The implications for most Deaf students, who must learn English as a second language, are clear. Bilingual education using ASL as the language of the classroom will teach subject matter better and it will impart background knowledge and skills that will facilitate learning English. As such Deaf students become bilingual, they will be more capable of a variety of cognitive tasks.

This reasoning based on theory and findings is persuasive, but, you may ask, is there research in the U.S. that supports these claims for bilingual education of ASL speakers in particular? No, there is not, nor is there any for bilingual programs using Norwegian, Xiamen, and scores of other minority languages here. Surely the merits of bilingual education for children who speak minority languages need not be proven anew for each language.

There are multiple ancillary benefits that should accrue from extending bilingual/bicultural programs to ASL-using children. Such programs could spawn new ideas and methods for teaching this minority, including new strategies for teaching them English. Bilingual education for Deaf students, by improving English literacy, should lead to improved academic achievement scores, as it has for other language minorities (see below). When the child finds his or her own language and culture used in the school, self-esteem and emotional adjustment improve, leading to decreased need for counseling services. If both teacher and student were fluent in ASL, there would be no need for the very small classes required to assure individualized attention. Bilingual/bicultural education for Deaf children may decrease dropout rates, as well as underemployment on school leaving. Such programs naturally increase the bilingual fluency of classroom teachers. They clearly open careers to adult minority-language users. Increased bilingual fluency of teachers and cultural awareness between teachers and students may enhance communication between teacher and pupil, ultimately leading to enhanced mutual respect between hearing and Deaf people.[17]

Bilingual education has its ardent opponents.[18] Their chief criticism is that the steps taken to support non-English speaking students' native language tend to support separatism and to absorb time and energy and resources that should be focused on the essential task of learning English. The schools do not keep their promise, they say, to move surely and early into English as the language of instruction. Countless Americans, they remind us, arrived on North American shores ignorant of English, acquired it, and made their way into American society and culture without bilingual education.

Defenders of bilingual education have rebuttals. Separatism is fostered by oppression, they say, and the rejection of the minority's language is symbolic of that oppression. The way to achieve political integration and economic well-being for a minority is to respect their language rights in education as elsewhere. In a school where the child's language and culture are not acknowledged while those of his or her peers are, the minority child often becomes submissive and unmotivated.

Whatever the merits of these arguments (and we believe that the evidence and arguments in favor of bilingual and bicultural education are compelling), it is undeniable that in the U.S. in the mid-1990s considerable hostility to language minorities has developed, along with a political backlash against so-called special rights, including the right to a bilingual/bicultural education. There is a movement to declare English the nation's official language. Two major lobbying groups have raised millions of dollars to press for a constitutional amendment that would prohibit government's use of languages other than English in many situations. Surveys indicate that about three Americans in four support this initiative.[19] Given this situation, it is especially important, therefore, to recognize that the arguments against bilingual education lose force when applied to children whose primary language is a signed language. America's Deaf children will not learn English merely by "making their way" in our society; spoken English is not accessible to them. The inability of any spoken language to replace signed language is a unique characteristic of signed-language minorities. Moreover, when educators of Deaf children in the U.S. take measures to enhance mastery of ASL, they are not taking time and focus away from learning English. On the one hand, if the history of the education of the Deaf over the past 125 years proves anything, it is that employing spoken languages or artificial signing systems does not lead to English mastery or to academic success in general. On the other, the evidence for the relative academic success of native ASL speakers, along with the accomplishments of the education system for the Deaf before the oralists took over, and the success of the modern bilingual Swedish system (see chapter 6), all strongly support the claim that bilingual/bicultural education has a much better chance of improving both English mastery and school achievement. Even the charge that bilingual education may betray the goal of a transition into English does not apply to signed-language minorities. In the end, English can never totally replace ASL either as the language of instruction or in the work-a-day world, because the Deaf cannot hear conversational (spoken) English. All in all, then, the main objections to bilingual education do not apply to children who speak ASL. Conversely, the main reasons favoring bilingual/bicultural education—fluent communication, positive self-image, and a basis for English mastery—remain valid for Deaf students.

Little wonder, then, that the 1988 Congressional Commission on the Education of the Deaf strongly recommended that awards should be made under the Bilingual Education Act to schools that seek to improve the quality of education of children with limited English proficiency whose native (primary) language is ASL, as they are to schools for children with other primary languages.[20] The National Association of the Deaf formed a lobbying group known as COED-15 (for the name of the commission and the number of its recommendation on bilingual education), which, as of this writing, has been meeting with officials in the Department of Education to press for implementation. They are making slow headway, however, despite professions of good will on all sides. No doubt the underlying reason is that officials find it difficult to see children in the DEAF-WORLD as members of a linguistic minority, all the more so as another division in the same federal department funds education programs for children with disabilities and includes schools for the Deaf.

The gains to be had from bilingual/bicultural education of Deaf children will not accrue automatically merely by changing the orientation of the education system. There must also be a phase of development in which new materials and methods are conceived, tried out, and modified. For example, a rational approach to teaching English as a second language to ASL speakers begins with a contrastive analysis of English and ASL grammar. That analysis guides a progression through English grammar, with lessons conducted in ASL. Materials such as teacher and student workbooks, videotapes, and examinations must be developed. Courses must be designed and materials created to teach ASL, its grammar, art forms, registers, so that ASL speakers can study their language throughout their academic careers, just as English speakers do. Teachers must be trained in new ways and new subjects, not the least of which is ASL. However, fresh approaches also open up to teaching most subject matter. For example, American history can be taught in conjunction with American Deaf history; areas of mathematics can be presented with an emphasis on visual representations, rather than notation, from the start. In addition to developing new materials and methods, means must be found for greatly increasing the numbers of teachers and administrators drawn from the Deaf minority. Such professionals are teachers, they are a resource for their hearing colleagues, and they provide powerful role models. Their very presence helps the Deaf pupil form a deep personal relationship to the school.

A key element in ensuring the success of a bilingual program has to do with the training of the instructional staff. It is extremely important that teachers be skilled in using ASL and have a great resource of knowledge about ASL structure. Without the latter, instruction will tend to be based on English knowledge, and teachers may be at a loss as to what principles in ASL are directly comparable to similar or contrasting principles in English. Where the success of bilingual programs for hearing children belonging to language minorities has been called into question, the level of teacher competence in the languages involved has been a recurrent concern.[21]

Literacy, language and bilingualism

In the preceding chapter, we discussed literacy in general and the inability of the prevailing system of education of the Deaf to fulfill what is arguably its most important mission: to give the average Deaf student the ability to read and write English (one aspect of literacy) at a level commensurate with the demands of today's world. Here we return to the subject from the perspective of bilingual/bicultural education. In particular, we look at what it would mean if the signed language of the Deaf were to be welcomed among the professionals serving the Deaf as the Deaf person's first language. What if they saw ASL not only as an aid to learning English, but as a resource to be cultivated and enhanced in its own right?

As noted in chapter 9, there are two registers of English at work in schools. One is the language of schooling, the other is the conversational language of the home. In America both of these registers are usually registers of English. Children from minority families where English is not the first language generally have difficulty in using English in school. However, they all have acquired a first language. This gives them knowledge of what a language is and how it operates. They can build on such knowledge even if their school program ignores or denigrates their native language.

In bilingual/bicultural programs, the minority students' native language is not denigrated. Rather, it is used to teach the language of schooling with a three-part strategy. First, it enriches the children's command of their native language to include the school language register and literacy. Second, it helps them to bring to awareness and to talk about the structure of their language and its registers and art forms. (The language used for description of language is called *metalanguage,* and the ability to discuss and compare languages is a *metalinguistic* ability.) Third, using that expanded repertoire in their first language, it teaches first-language literacy and various cognitive tasks that school involves. With these abilities—first-language fluency and literacy, metalinguistic skills, and cognitive skills—students are better equipped to develop the corresponding set of abilities in English. Acquiring school language skills at the outset in the first language provides the bilingual child with an understanding of the purpose of school, with exposure to high-level content in the first language, and with a model from which metalinguistic tasks may be learned.

The native language of Deaf children, ASL in the U.S., has not been capitalized on in this way because of historical opposition to ASL on the part of many of the professionals who serve the Deaf. In fact, as we saw earlier, that opposition has resulted instead in the creation and widespread use of MCE systems as the vehicle for instruction—systems that involve not only "borrowing" ASL signs and using them in English word order, but the invention of signs to provide a visual match for English grammatical structure. As we also saw, this widespread approach to the development of both language and literacy has delivered neither. Taking a natural visual language and creating an artificial system that purports to represent natural spoken English visually cannot reasonably be expected to enhance—and has not enhanced—English language fluency and literacy in Deaf children. Clearly, using only spoken language with Deaf children, the practice for many decades in the U.S. and still the predominant practice in many nations, has not produced the results we desire either. This leaves us with the perspective that Deaf children will have to acquire American Sign Language naturally, master ASL literacy, including the registers and art forms of ASL (see below), and study English. This will allow them to build English literacy on a foundation of ASL literacy and metalinguistic awareness of the two languages' similarities and differences.[22]

As we saw in chapter 9, finding meaning on the printed page does not rely for the most part on the text in front of the reader, or what scientists call "bottom-up" information. While this obviously plays a role, the reader's expectations of what words, sentences and paragraphs are likely to be encountered, and his or her ability to make interpretations and predictions concerning the message of the text, are provided not by the page alone, as it were, but by the reader working with the page. The reader's general background knowledge, cultural literacy, and metalinguistic knowledge all contribute to comprehension. If theories of reading that emphasize this kind of "top-down" knowledge have captured an important principle, as it seems, this bodes ill for novice Deaf readers using present instructional methods. From the bottom up, print is a representation of a spoken language they do not know. From the top down, the failure to use ASL to teach them (and allow them to teach themselves) about the world, and the failure to use it to develop their understanding of metalinguistic processes, deprive them of essential resources when reading. If many of the bilingual approaches to literacy that are used with hearing children were used with Deaf children, then the Deaf child could rely on the learning of a natural language, ASL, and separately learn about ASL as a language (the metalinguistic skills). This metalinguistic knowledge could then be used to transfer some of the principles from ASL to learning about English. For example, developing an understanding of how particular structures in ASL operate, such as which classifiers are appropriate as references for which objects, or that one classifier can refer to more than one type of object, can enable the Deaf child to see that the same operations are available in English (i.e., in super- and subordinate categories of words). Similarly, knowing how to identify nouns and verbs, synonyms and antonyms, and so on in ASL would make it possible to develop strategies for identifying the same categories in English. By the same token, the child's background knowledge, which is available for recall and reference through the first language, could also be brought to bear.

Literacy in ASL

In considering the possible role of ASL in the bilingual/bicultural education of the Deaf, it is vital that we recognize the significance and complexity of the cultural component. ASL, like all languages, is a cultural resource. As we saw in part 1, the language and the culture of the Deaf are inseparable. Much of cultural knowledge is learned and numerous cultural activities are engaged in with the mediation of language. The stories told in Deaf clubs, in residential schools, by Deaf parents to their Deaf and hearing children, are all part of the literature of Deaf culture, learned, remembered and passed on from generation to generation. We consider this a part of ASL literacy, for we subscribe to the view that expands the notion of literacy beyond reading print and refocuses it on the language registers that must be mastered. These include the formal storytelling register, with its coherent, complex, decontextualized language, which exists as assuredly in ASL as it does in English.[23]

Schools and programs for Deaf children have ignored the rich narratives and folk tales of the DEAF–WORLD because, as Deaf education foolishly equated language with English, so it has equated literacy with English print literacy. But signed languages as well as spoken languages have various texts that literate speakers can perform, interpret, and pass on to the next generation. Storytelling, be it face to face or in print, allows cultures to pass on their values, teachings, philosophy, and cultural rules. Stories are one of the major resources for learning, because through the language of stories, children extract much of the cultural information which applies to events in their lives as they mature.

ASL literacy is similar in some ways to the literacy of many cultures where print is not available to carry messages from one generation to the next. Stories are developed which have particular structures, specific themes, and an established set of goals. The common structures make it easy for the members of the culture to recognize a story for the cultural artifact that it is, to identify with the elements of the story, and to remember it.[24] The ability to understand and recognize the structure and theme of these stories is part of ASL literacy knowledge.

The denial of ASL as a valid language, then, has led to more than its denial as an instructional tool. It has led to a denial of the riches of Deaf culture and the failure of the educational system to use the cultural resources of the DEAF–WORLD in the education of Deaf children. This denial influences all levels of education. Many if not most Deaf children begin to learn ASL in the course of their education, even though it is not used in class. But because it is not cultivated, not only do Deaf children have a long-term problem accessing information, they are also not given credit for what they may already know with respect to ASL or to general knowledge about the world. Education professionals do not know what Deaf children know. Indeed, almost all education research with Deaf children has been based on examining what they do *not* know. And while research in other fields, such as psychology and linguistics, has given us some tools to evaluate what the Deaf child does know, this information has not been incorporated in any coherent way into the educational system.

How do we create an environment in school and at home that takes advantage of the strengths of the first language of Deaf children (ASL in the U.S.) to eventually lead them into literate behaviors in their second language (English)? Achieving English literacy is vital to the success of the Deaf child as he or she grows up in our hearing society. However, to be fully successful, Deaf children will need skills to be able to function in the DEAF–WORLD as well. If we apply research judiciously from the field of bilingual education to the problem of literacy in Deaf children, we can identify skills and approaches that will prove useful to Deaf people as they attempt to cope with the two worlds in which they live, and we can identify methods of teaching that will help them to achieve English literacy along the way.

The principles of bilingual/bicultural education that are most transferable to the education of the Deaf are (1) respect for the language of the child, (2) incorporating heritage information in teaching, (3) using the language of the child to increase understanding of content information, (4) increasing the complexity and metalinguistic knowledge of the language of the child, (5) developing transfer strategies from one language to another to gain information, and (6) developing a strong metalinguistic awareness of English and how it is used in different settings and situations, such as the ways in which conversational English is different from textbook English, for example, and how creatively written stories are a combination of both registers. To be good students, Deaf children need the skills to develop strategies for contrasting and comparing usage and styles in both English and ASL: for example, recent research demonstrates that ASL narratives have a structure different from English stories.[25]

As noted above, however, bilingual/bicultural education for the Deaf child cannot be exactly the same as bilingual/bicultural education for hearing children, primarily because transitional bilingualism, where students move from using their native language to using English all the time, and which is the major goal of bilingual education programs in the U.S., is neither a feasible nor an appropriate goal for Deaf children. The major goal for Deaf children should be maintenance, indeed, cultivation of ASL and ASL literacy, throughout the Deaf child's educational career, with English, as a second language, to be used at specified instructional times. To achieve this, it is critical that throughout their education, Deaf children have access to literate models in both ASL and English, not just in English alone.

ASL in early childhood and the Deaf child of hearing parents

We have seen in previous chapters that ASL is the natural language of Deaf Americans, that when they encounter it they learn it readily and automatically. We have also noted, however, that as with other natural languages, there seems to be a critical period during which the foundations of one's first language may be most readily and firmly laid (see chapter 4). Deaf parents with a Deaf child can model an accessible language for that child from birth onward, as can hearing parents with a hearing child. Hearing parents with a Deaf child must make special provision to introduce the language of the DEAF–WORLD into their home. Yet the parents of Deaf children are often not encouraged to come to know Deaf people, their language, and the DEAF–WORLD. Deaf adults, often parents themselves, could teach hearing parents strategies for communicating with their Deaf child and for solving the everyday problems they confront. They could inform the parents about the culture their child typically will enter, and they could help the parents model language for the child.

With the widespread recognition of ASL as a full-fledged natural language, educators have begun to debate the merits of introducing the language into parent-infant programs. Would language acquired early in this way, they ask, be likely to pay dividends in school and later in life? And can parents learn to use ASL, even an ASL heavily influenced by their native English, in the time they usually have to devote to the task? Parents who are expected to come to a hospital or school program weekly and learn ASL in a group setting will have a difficult and prolonged learning curve. Such programs cannot be a substitute for parents building bridges to the DEAF–WORLD, and yet that is commonly how the programs operate. To make matters worse, this learning process occurs at the same time parents are deluged with information about Deaf education, child development, and so on.

The rare programs in which Deaf professionals have a major role provide a different model of learning for hearing parents and their Deaf children.[26] One way to reduce the learning time for both parents and Deaf children is to work with parents of young Deaf children in their home, the practice in Sweden, you may recall. This approach avoids several pitfalls that can slow language learning. Deaf professionals who meet with parents in their home regularly are able to discuss with them what it means to be a Deaf person in today's world. They are able to interact with the parents either individually or in small groups for the purpose of learning ASL. They can interact in ASL with the Deaf child, modeling in timely fashion the language the child is to acquire.

Deaf professionals who are part of the hospital or school team may visit the parents regularly for the express purpose of teaching ASL. These professionals are trained not only to teach the language, but also to support the parents in their quest for information. Another possibility is for parents who have the means to house a Deaf student from a local university or college in exchange for baby-sitting or nanny duties. This permits the Deaf child to have the necessary language model, and it also allows parents to exercise their newfound abilities in ASL on topics of keenly felt relevance to their roles as parents. There is evidence that early intervention in families with Deaf children that leads them to use a signed language gives the children in those families an advantage over their counterparts from families that did not receive early intervention.[27]

As noted, published guides for parents of Deaf children and hearing professionals often counsel parents against using ASL. (Most Deaf parents ignore this advice; hearing parents usually do not.) Several reasons may be offered. For one, ASL is said to be too difficult for hearing parents to learn. No research has been conducted to test this hypothesis, but professionals often assume it to be true, even though great numbers of American college students nowadays learn ASL as their peers do French or Chinese. Parents are also steered away from learning ASL when their

Deaf children are young because of the orientation towards speech on the part of the professionals who guide most of the parent-infant programs and preschool programs for the Deaf (see chapter 8) and who continue to counter suggestions that ASL be used in such programs with the assertion that parents and professionals must speak with Deaf children so they will learn English. However, it is Deaf children of Deaf parents who, as we have seen repeatedly, achieve the highest English scores, and their parents primarily use ASL with them, not spoken English.

Many parents with Deaf children must wonder what their children will say one day, as adults, about their upbringing. Here, one Deaf adult, Jack Levesque, eloquently responds to that unspoken question.

My Mother's Last Words

At the age of eighty, my mother asked me, "Did we do the right thing by sending you to the Clarke School for the Deaf? Was an oral education right for you?" At eighty-one, she said, "I should have learned signed language. But we were told it was not the right thing to do by the staff at the Clarke School. I can now see the difference in communication, and I see that it was a mistake not to learn signed language."

On July 10, 1992, at 10:20 a.m., my mother, Ruth Miller Levesque, passed away. I was at her side when she died. I had about three last hours to spend with this courageous woman before she slipped into a coma and passed away. It was obvious that we had very little time left, so we tried to say all the things we had in our hearts. I talked and lipread her. Toward the end, she wanted to tell me something. I didn't understand and asked her to repeat it. Twice more, I asked her to repeat. Then finally I gave her a piece of paper. She was only able to write the letter *O*, or maybe *C*, before her eyes closed and the deep sleep of coma overtook her.

In the weeks and months before my mother's death, we spent many hours going over issues and preparing for her death. It was done verbally—not comfortably, but adequately. My mother had made sure I got the finest oral education around. She was proud of my speaking ability and impressed by my less-than-perfect lipreading. But we never had a real conversation. Oh, I knew she loved me. I knew she was proud of me. But I'll never know her last words to me.

Her death was, in a way, a blessing. She had been in pain for two years due to cancer. I am comforted to think of her at peace and free of that pain. But the frustration of our final moments together will haunt me. If she had learned signed language, she would have been able to tell me clearly whatever it was that was so important to her. That moment was a painful one. It made me think of all the other things she might have told me over the years, but didn't.

I can't change anything. I can't go back and make her hands fly easily. But I can make a plea to other parents of Deaf children: *Learn signed language.*

Communication between parent and child, or between any two people, is just too vital to be embroiled in communication methodology. The simple truth is: If you want fluent communication and a meaningful exchange of ideas, emotions, thoughts and love with your Deaf child, *sign* it.

Parents, don't let idealism and rhetoric get in the way of realism.

The point was made painfully clear to me that sad morning a few weeks ago. I shall always wonder what my mother wanted to tell me.

It's too late for me. Is it too late for you?

(Adapted from Levesque, 1992.)

In recent years, in accord with the Total Communication movement in education and the incontrovertible evidence for the superior performance of the Deaf children of Deaf parents, some professionals have recommended that the hearing parents of Deaf children learn one of the invented sign systems that seek to present English in a visual-manual form, believing that such MCE systems are easier to learn than ASL and have the added advantage of presenting English to the child in a form that the child can perceive. There is no evidence for the belief that it is easier to learn a manual form of English than to learn ASL. On the contrary, as discussed in chapter 9, there are reasons to think otherwise. Moreover, there is no body of research establishing that Deaf children who use these invented systems learn English faster or better. Such evidence is unlikely to be forthcoming since, from the Deaf child's point of view, what is most visible when the MCE system is used is not English, which is spoken, and what is most English—speech—is not visible.

Numerous studies of Deaf children of Deaf parents acquiring ASL have demonstrated that Deaf parents often present ASL to their young children even when the parents have mastered English and have had a college education.[28] In addition, these Deaf parents frequently make a conscious effort to teach English to their Deaf child. The Deaf parents assist their young Deaf offspring in learning how to make metalinguistic judgments about English and reading—skills vital throughout a child's educational career. Many Deaf parents actually discuss with their children how English works. They fingerspell some English words, explain the classes of nouns and verbs, and demonstrate the processes involved in translation from one language to another.[29] During the course of one study investigating how children acquire ASL, one Deaf parent, who was fifth-generation Deaf and the best educated of all the parents in the study, vehemently denied that she used ASL with her children. In subsequent viewings of videotapes of her interactions with her children, however, she was amazed at the amount of ASL she used and at its complexity. Not only had she exposed her children to the language, she had discussed the differences between English and ASL with them extensively. For example, she explained in one sequence that fingerspelling was used to represent the letters of English in print, but when she signed she did not fingerspell a great deal. Her children had the advantage of arriving at school knowing there were two different languages and with some inkling of how they both worked. Such information gives children like these a huge advantage over their peers with hearing parents, who are almost always just beginning to acquire a system of signs—signs which are presented in the format of the spoken language at that.

It is true that Deaf children of Deaf parents also have other advantages, such as access to a substantial amount of background or incidental information, acquired especially from peers and from observing their parents when they are conversing with each other or with other Deaf people. It is also true, for hearing parents, that learning ASL means learning a second language, and one that is difficult for many English speakers because it is so different from English, not only in mode of expression, but in form and structure. (Likewise, Chinese, which is very different from English in form and structure, is more difficult for English speakers to learn than, say, French.) Hearing parents (and siblings) of Deaf children who undertake to learn it may never become thoroughly fluent (though the siblings may well do so if they start when they are young). But a parent's lack of fluency does not mean that the effort does not make a difference.

Deaf children of hearing parents do better in academic programs using Total Communication than in "programs oriented towards speech, socialization and parent adjustment,"[30] and the former programs present at least some signed language, albeit in a much impoverished form.

Several studies have further shown that when parents and young Deaf children are able to exchange information, that interaction provides a kind of scaffolding on which more social interaction can be constructed.[31] Parents who are able to communicate with their Deaf children are less overprotective and develop a more realistic set of expectations for their children.[32] Less overprotection and more challenging expectations, in turn, promote interaction and increased learning. Thus, the young Deaf child who learns to sign is more likely to be socially mature.[33] Studies of parents who communicated orally with their Deaf children and who rejected any form of signed language found them often so focused on the quest to normalize their Deaf child that they were unaware of the accomplishments their child was demonstrating.[34]

A particular advantage that parents who use ASL or contact sign bring to their Deaf child involves the vital task of learning how to read. It is very important in a child's reading development to give the child, whether hearing or Deaf, early exposure to and knowledge of books. The more any child's parents read to him or her, whether the child is Deaf or hearing, the better reader that child will become.[35] Knowing what books are for, realizing that print carries messages and has meaning, is essential to entering the reading process. In an alphabet book for a child who is just beginning to learn to read, there are letters on the pages. Adjacent to each letter is a drawing of an object with its written name ("*A* is for Apple," and so forth). The child who names the picture while inspecting its written name has taken a first step toward learning the complex skill called "reading" and toward succeeding in school. Parents who speak ASL can read to their child, translating as they go. They can also help the child access environmental print, such as brand-name advertising and traffic signs, thus teaching that there is a purpose to print.

One other advantage accrues to the Deaf child of hearing parents if ASL is introduced into the home and used in preschool programs. The child and family come into close contact early on with members of the DEAF–WORLD. We noted above that culture is carried by language, and

Deaf culture is no different. Introducing Deaf culture to Deaf children can be an enormous benefit, furthering their understanding of the world and assisting them in developing a fund of information from which they can approach the learning of literate strategies and academic information.

The Deaf child's Deaf culture does not oppose, but rather potentially reinforces the child's mastery of the culture of the parents. Again, the basic principle of compare-and-contrast as a strategy for learning can be used to help Deaf children understand what it means to be Deaf and what it means to be hearing. Professionals, Deaf or hearing, who promote access to such cultural knowledge, have no intention of creating a divide between hearing parents and their Deaf children. If anything, increased knowledge on the part of both Deaf children and their parents will lead to better and more positive interaction, since each group will have a better understanding of why things are done in particular ways. The bitterness that often characterizes the relationship between Deaf young adults and their hearing parents, like the estrangement between Laurel and her mother, may be avoided.

Aspects of Deaf culture (and of other cultures with which the Deaf child may identify) should be introduced to a Deaf child as early as possible, together with the comparable aspects of mainstream majority-language culture. For example, discussions around how to introduce people can easily be used in cross-cultural comparisons to demonstrate that each group of people uses different strategies. Some cultural differences are traps for the unaware Deaf child. For example, in the DEAF–WORLD, maintaining eye contact shows that you are paying polite attention to the speaker. However, in some contexts in U.S. hearing culture, extensive eye contact is viewed as threatening. Cross-cultural comparisons and analyses enable the Deaf child to realize that different ways of doing things need not make close cross-cultural relationships impossible, while the hearing parents may obtain a better understanding of why their child functions better in some settings than others, and they may be able to better accept the child's belonging to both the DEAF–WORLD and the hearing world.

The bilingual/bicultural approach to raising and educating Deaf children provides them with a storehouse of tools, both linguistic and cultural, to allow them to cope successfully with both the DEAF–WORLD and the hearing world. Using those tools to whatever extent they deem necessary, they can decide how to manage the two worlds at a much younger age than is now the case, and then can acquire the sense of autonomy and independence, as well as the skills, that will make it possible for them to choose their own future path.

In the last three chapters we have presented a selected set of topics about the education of the Deaf and have tried to clarify the complex issues that are faced by Deaf children, their parents, and professionals in the field. The myriad options that confront parents almost from the moment when hearing loss is diagnosed, the variety of placements, the confusion over making predictions based on hearing level, the inability of the professionals to bring parents together with members of the DEAF–WORLD (professional and non-professional), and the attitudes that prevent Deaf professionals from joining in policy decisions—counseling parents and becoming teachers and administrators—all serve to maintain the failure of education for the average Deaf child.

It is a failure that can no longer be tolerated. We are living in an increasingly technological world. Nearly three-fourths of all jobs now require technical training beyond a high school diploma. Projections for the year 2000 show that the average new job will require 13.5 years of education. This means that the people who fill these jobs will have to have some college training. Such education will be required for an *average job*, just to bring home a paycheck. In the past, there were many jobs available to the average Deaf high school graduate, often connected to the printing and garment businesses. Deaf people like Roberto and Henry were able to sustain a middle-class lifestyle with that kind of employment. Today those jobs are disappearing. In this new era of information technology, the price Deaf students are paying for the rejection of the language and culture of the DEAF–WORLD in Deaf education gets higher every day. Either Deaf education must be reconceptualized and restructured to match the education of other language minorities, or the field of special education must prove adaptive enough to accommodate the needs of this distinct cultural group.

One central educational issue affecting a Deaf person's school years and adult years concerns evaluation. A great deal rides on evaluation in the school years, including placement, tracking, and teacher expectations. It is equally important at the end of school, when most Deaf people are evaluated for career choices. It is deeply disturbing then, to find that evaluation is as sorely beset by language barriers as education itself, presenting further obstacles to the successful and fair treatment of Deaf people. Evaluation applied to the members of a minority is often just the systematic account of how people in the majority perceive them. Because the profession of Deaf education has proceeded essentially with a disability model, rather than the model of a linguistic and cultural minority, evaluation procedures and findings have tended to paint a picture of Deaf people as disabled. From the vantage point of Deaf culture, many hearing people, unfamiliar with signed language and Deaf mores and values, can be viewed as communicatively disabled and culturally ignorant. This reminds us that evaluation of the members of a minority is never power-neutral; minorities such as African-Americans, Native Americans, and Americans with disabilities are likewise underestimated and misjudged in education and employment. Once evaluation quantifies and, as it appears, establishes the nature of Deaf people's disabilities, the hearing technologies of mitigating those disabilities—among them special education—have their raison d'être. Thus, we now turn to the evaluation of Deaf people and its consequences for hearing intervention with Deaf children and adults.

❦

Chapter 11

Evaluating Deaf People

COUNTLESS hours and a great deal of money are spent quantifying how the individual Deaf child differs from other children. The Deaf child is first tested by an audiologist when the parents suspect a problem, although there is now a push to give audiometric tests to all newborns in the U.S. before they are released from the hospital. The Deaf child will be tested again for hearing, for intelligence, for adjustment, and for much more, and the testing will be repeated in preschool, elementary school, and high school, where vocational testing will be added. After high school, the young Deaf adult may be tested in college or on the job.

Despite all the testing, it is surprising how little the test results count for. One reason for this is that the practitioner knows the data are not a valid basis for action. A 1994 book on auditory rehabilitation, for example, states that measures of someone's hearing loss are not an adequate guide to that person's impairment or rehabilitation needs.[1] Then, too, because of limited resources, there are often no educational strategies that link up to various test outcomes. One might ask, then, why all this individuation? All the individual testing, and the strong emphasis on individual differences, tend to minimize what the Deaf child has in common with others, the bonds of language and culture that unite the Deaf child to the DEAF–WORLD. Instead, the testing maximizes the view of the child as, technologically speaking, "disabled."

Today's widespread practice of testing children and adults began in the last century, when a French minister of education asked an eminent psychologist, Alfred Binet, to develop a test that would identify students who were unlikely to succeed with regular schooling and would need special schooling if they were to take their place in the newly industrialized society. Binet needed a criterion of success in school that his test would predict when perfected. Nowadays, experts in testing (psychometricians) who want to predict academic success, take grades in school as their criterion measure. They develop tests that can be shown to predict grades reasonably accurately for a small group of students. The test is then said to have *criterion validity* and an individual's score on such a test is taken as a guide, or *predictor*, of the grades the student will likely achieve. Rather than using grades as a criterion measure, Binet chose teacher ratings of student success. Next he developed an experimental test, with questions testing memory, perception, abstraction, vocabulary and so on. He added and deleted questions in repeated administrations of his experimental test in an effort to make students' scores on the test correlate as closely as possible with their teacher ratings. When he was done, he could predict a student's ratings reasonably well given that student's score on his test, and so he felt justified in presenting his test as a predictor of academic success. Binet called his test an intelligence test. It was obvious to him, however, that it did not measure native mental ability.[2] After all, a child's success measured by teacher ratings obviously does not depend only on native mental ability; it also depends on whether the child's best language is the language of instruction, whether family values and resources promote serious study, whether the child comes from the majority culture or a minority culture, and so on.

IQ testing and the new science of psychometrics came to the United States in 1916 and quickly became a tool in the hands of the eugenics movement that sought to ensure the "purity of the race." Eugenicists argued that crime, poverty, disability and deviance were the product (not the cause) of inferior IQ—an expression of "bad blood." American authorities on Ellis Island used IQ testing to label large numbers of immigrants arriving from southern and eastern Europe as idiots and to deny them entry.[3] To this day, there are social scientists who contend that Black Americans obtain lower average IQ scores as the result of an innate biological limitation, and that success and failure in the American economy is substantially a matter of genes.[4] The more widely accepted view, however, is that IQ tests are biased in their language and content in obvious and not-so-obvious ways, to the detriment of members of various cultural minorities. For example, when the Binet test was adapted at Stanford University in 1916 for use in the United States (and thus came to be called the *Stanford-Binet Intelligence Scale*), it contained a drawing of a white male child used to identify the parts of the body. That drawing has since evolved into a multicultural child of ambiguous gender in an effort to remove racial and gender bias. Similarly, there are vocabulary questions (such as "Define *mundane*") that are biased in favor of children whose parents have more education, and questions on the relations among things ("How are boots, sandals and sneakers alike yet different from gloves?") that are biased in favor of children who possess those things.

There has been a lot of attention to evaluating Deaf children and adults in the twentieth century, but insufficient attention to such larger issues as the language and cultural bias surrounding their evaluation. If Deaf people are to evaluated effectively and the results of those evaluations are to be interpreted wisely, we must first ask, Who is evaluating whom for what declared and undeclared purposes? Evaluation by test is a form of description, and descriptions of stigmatized groups can rarely be taken at face value. Tests allow the authorities to engage in a ritual of power, to "effect distributions about the norm," and thus to justify their role in regulating the persons tested.[5] Technology, we are told, can isolate deviance and more technology can correct that deviance. The child or adult's deficits on the tests are presented as the reason that we must have specialized treatment establishments. So there is a marriage between the technology of testing and the technology of correction in which each partner depends on the other. For example, the existence of an establishment devoted to auditory prosthesis and rehabilitation fuels Deaf children's need for hearing tests. As sociologist Robert Scott has explained, "The needs of the blind are those [needs] blind people must have if they are to fit into and be served by programs that have arisen for other reasons."[6]

PSYCHOLOGICAL TESTING OF THE DEAF

There is a body of literature on the personality traits of people who have grown up Deaf that is known as the *psychology of the deaf.* It has been published for the most part by hearing professionals in several disciplines and presents the results of administering a wide variety of tests to Deaf children and adults. Deaf people are predominantly characterized in that literature as socially isolated, intellectually weak, behaviorally impulsive, and emotionally immature. This description of Deaf people as a collection of individuals with various deficits contrasts starkly with the DEAF–WORLD's description of itself as a society of interrelated people with a bonding culture, history, language and social structure. Thus, the hearing research literature about the Deaf attempts to make individual and medical what is communal and cultural. It is as revealing to note what that literature does not measure as it is to note what it claims to measure. Culturally relevant information is not gathered. Fluency in ASL is not measured, nor is its relation to academic and vocational achievement. Bilingualism in the DEAF–WORLD is not assessed, nor are patterns of intermarriage, profiles of Deaf leadership, the dimensions of the Deaf cultural renaissance, or even the number of ASL speakers. Because of its failure to recognize Deaf language and culture, the body of research proves to be so severely flawed in numerous ways that it simply isn't possible to make any accurate generalizations about Deaf people based on that literature.

Tests are cultural artifacts: different cultures test in different ways and even the same culture tests differently at different times. The authorities present test results as the basis of opinions of what individuals and groups can do, but in fact the authorities' opinions of what those individuals and groups can do form the tests: evaluation presupposes representation. As long as Deaf children are viewed as defective members of the majority culture, it is natural to attempt to use tests designed for majority children to quantify and characterize "Deaf defects." If Deaf children were viewed as members of a language minority, various tests that are used with majority children would be developed in ASL for ASL-speaking children, as they were, say, developed in Spanish for Spanish-speaking children with the advent of bilingual education. However, since Deaf children are not viewed as a language group but as individuals with a disability, there has been very little effort expended on language-appropriate testing of Deaf children. (Two examples of positive developments, a personality test in ASL and an ASL fluency battery, are discussed below.)

Thus, what the Deaf child can do does not determine the test outcome; rather, the test outcome determines what the Deaf child can do. Once children are labeled inferior in some regard, they are often treated in ways that tend to conform to that label, thus making it more true over time. For example, children mistakenly labeled "learning disabled" may be placed in less educative environments and thus learn less. Evaluation is part of a regulatory system. Our views and practices in describing, educating and rehabilitating Deaf children are interlocked, as are the numerous professions that shape and even regulate the lives of Deaf children and adults. For example, test results are used to describe the putative needs and abilities of the Deaf child in his or her Individualized Educational Plan, and that IEP determines where the child can go to school and the curriculum the child follows once there. If that schooling is not appropriate, the child may later become a client of a vocational rehabilitation program, and tests will be used once again to determine whether the client can have access to adult education, job training and selected job openings. The decision to construe and shape the child's fate in terms of psychometrics, rather than in terms of cultural history, is the most important determinant of the future it claims to predict.

Deaf people, their families and friends, and hearing professional people who work with the Deaf, should be aware of the main pitfalls in evaluating Deaf children and adults. This should help them to avoid some of those pitfalls and to make them wary of claims about Deaf limitations. Much of the published research is untrustworthy in the first place, because of faulty test administration. For example, it is essential that the testee receive clear and comprehensible instructions, but examiners are commonly unable to provide them in a natural language accessible to the testee, such as ASL. They simply rely on the child's ability to read the instructions, or they resort to ad hoc pantomime, or to some other contrivance, such as speaking and signing. It is not humanly possible to speak and sign while using the grammar of ASL, so the hearing test administrator has the illusion of making sense, but the ASL-speaking child is likely to be at a disadvantage when instructed with such impoverished language.

Clear and consistent administration of personality tests is a particular problem. The Deaf child's reticence when presented an ink blot or a picture from the Thematic Apperception Test (TAT) may have much more to do with lack of communication with the examiner than with personality dynamics.

Selecting the language of the test itself is the second pitfall confronting those who would validly evaluate Deaf people. To illustrate: A study of the questions that proved more difficult for Deaf than for hearing students taking the Stanford Achievement Test found six basic groups of such questions. However, these difficult groups were not based on the *content* of the questions but on their *form*. The following groups of questions (in English) were harder for the Deaf students: those containing conditionals (if, when); comparatives (greater than, the most); negatives (not, without); inferentials (should, could, because, since); pronouns (it, something); and long passages.[7] The test is supposed to measure academic achievement, but it seems largely to be measuring English reading skill.[8] For the same reason, it comes as no surprise to learn that eighty-five percent of Deaf students taking another test, this one a test of aptitude for college study, the Scholastic Aptitude Test, have lower scores than the average hearing applicant.[9] Of course, this is not an accurate measure of the aptitude of Deaf high school students, as their high scores on nonverbal IQ tests remind us.[10] In fact, the Scholastic Aptitude Test does not predict the scholastic achievement of Deaf students, who on average outperform its sorry predictions; nonetheless, the test is widely used with Deaf students.[11] The outcomes of many personality tests, with their numerous questions in English about behavior and feelings, are even more dependent on the English-language skills of the subject. One authority estimates that the testee must have a tenth-grade knowledge of English to take most personality tests meaningfully.[12] For example, here is one of many questions from the most widely used personality test, the Minnesota Multiphasic Personality Inventory (MMPI), that combines complex English with cultural bias: "In a group of people I would not be embarrassed to be called upon to start a discussion or give an opinion about something I know well." Presuming you have understood the question, you realize that for Deaf students to answer it, they need to know whether the group of people is hearing, mixed or Deaf. But the average Deaf student leaves school with only a third-grade command of English, and only one Deaf student in ten reads at eighth-grade level or better.[13] Is it reasonable then to expect the typical Deaf student to even understand the sentence in the first place? If not, then how can we accept Deaf people's answers on this test as valid indicators of their personalities? We must reject the results of most personality testing done with Deaf people, and with them most of the unfavorable attributions in the psychology of the deaf.

Test content is the third source of evaluation bias against Deaf children and adults. A host of items on the MMPI patently presuppose hearing ("I would like to be a singer"; "At times I hear so well it bothers me") while others are more subtly biased ("I enjoy reading love stories"). Perhaps a fourth of the items are inappropriate.[14] Should it count as paranoid if a Deaf person confirms that "People often stare at me in restaurants," when indeed they do generally eye his signing? Nearly all the other tests whose results constitute the literature of the psychology of the deaf have likewise not been revised in content for Deaf populations or standardized with them.

The psychological literature concerning Deaf people is further invalidated by examiner bias. This bias frequently includes the belief that Deaf people cannot be fully normal in cognition and behavior; as one investigator put it, "common sense considerations would suggest that the Deaf would have an increased risk of developing schizophrenia."[15] To aggravate the problem of bias, a child or adult who is acting up and who also does not respond to English commands represents a double threat to the examiner, parent, or teacher.[16] When the assessment of the Deaf person is subjective, as it is with rating scales, checklists, and interviews, a biased examiner can unwittingly influence the scores and therefore invalidate the results. Nevertheless, just such subjective scoring methods are used by the TAT (Thematic Apperception Test), the Rorschach, the Vineland Social Maturity Scale, the Bender-Gestalt, and many more tests whose findings make up the literature on the psychology of the deaf. Thus examiner bias frequently compounds the invalidity introduced by the language of the examiner and of the test, and by test content.

Studies using behavioral rating scales are especially vulnerable to bias, since the rater knows the status of the child he or she is rating. That information can be withheld when clinicians score a projective test like the TAT. The weight of the evidence impugns the accuracy and impartiality of teacher ratings, and we should not be surprised. Teachers of Deaf children carry, in the words of a senior investigator, a "tremendous emotional load . . . Often their frustration, impatience, and anger can create additional classroom problems."[17] Likewise, parents of Deaf children "feel powerless and become increasingly angry and shrill," writes a psychiatrist.[18] Parents who think highly of their Deaf children tend to be those who can communicate with them. However, as we have seen, most cannot do so. All things considered, is it reasonable to have confidence in the unproven validity of teacher and parent ratings of emotional disturbance, and to publish their judgments as facts about Deaf children?

The validity of teachers' and parents' ratings is undermined not only by bias but also by lack of consistency, of what is called in testing, *reliability*. Psychologists consider two judges reliable in evaluating a child if most of the time they make independent judgments that agree. A commonly used measure of agreement is the correlation coefficient, abbreviated *r*. It has the value 1.0 when the two sets of scores agree perfectly, and 0.0 when the two sets have no relation to each other at all. Reliability coefficients of .8 or higher are generally considered acceptable. When it comes to rating their own Deaf child's emotional disturbance, mother and father agree $r = 0.63$, mother and teacher $r = 0.45$, and father and teacher $r = 0.16$.[19] Moreover, parental ratings correlate poorly with any other measure of their Deaf child's adjustment.[20] Likewise, teachers of Deaf children do not agree with each other most of the time in rating emotional and behavioral problems of their pupils.[21] When raters do not agree with each other, both cannot be validly rating the child. Whom shall we trust to be making valid ratings of the child's emotional disturbance? The mother? The father? The first or second teacher? Or the test? Perhaps none of the raters is rating validly, which explains why none of them agrees reliably with any of the others.

Finally, research on the psychology of the deaf is seriously marred by its failure to characterize and distinguish its subject populations, reporting average performances of extremely heterogeneous groups and obscuring important differences in performance due to sex, age, race, and social class; cause, extent and nature of hearing loss; mode of communication used at school, at home, and with peers; type of schooling received; command of oral and written English; ethnic group membership; presence of physical or mental handicaps; and the influence of family mental health.

Because of all these flaws in the research evaluating Deaf people, many scholars and practitioners agree that it would be most prudent simply to write off the entire literature. Professionals who work closely with Deaf people, moreover, are aware that the sum and substance of that literature just does not correspond to their own observations and experiences with Deaf people.

Evaluation Instruments

There are legitimate reasons for measuring the academic achievement, social and emotional adjustment, language, and cognition of Deaf children and adults. While some of the pitfalls can be avoided (for example, the pupils' best language can be used when administering the test), other pitfalls are unavoidable (such as the culturally biased content of some tests). The best one can do, it seems, is to be aware of these limitations until better tests are developed and standardized with Deaf populations. The culturally knowledgeable examiner should place more weight than might otherwise be the case on personal judgment and on the coherence of informal and formal evaluation. The Individuals with Disabilities Education Act requires that evaluation materials not be culturally discriminatory, that their language be appropriate to the child's language, and that they have demonstrated validity for the purposes used. Likewise, Section 504 of the Rehabilitation Act of 1973 requires establishing the validity and reliability of any test used in making decisions about Deaf people. Since, as we have just seen, most achievement and personality tests are not able to meet these standards without modification, practitioners must proceed with great caution. In view of the severe problems in testing Deaf students, it is worrisome to read survey results showing that, in order to make decisions about where Deaf children will be placed educationally, eighty-eight percent of Deaf high school students have been given some sort of achievement test, sixty-eight percent some type of vocational test, and forty percent some type of social-emotional test.[22] Likewise, in developing the Individualized Educational Plans required for Deaf children by IDEA, the results of standardized tests often are highly influential, and that is cause for great concern.

The following sections examine the strengths and weaknesses of the tests most widely used to measure Deaf academic achievement, intelligence, social and emotional adjustment, and language mastery. Since there is poor agreement among scores on commercially available vocational tests, which also lack evidence of reliability and validity, that category of test will not be discussed.[23] Our aim is to help our readers interpret test results circumspectly, and to select and administer tests, if called upon to do so, more validly. Additionally, we will look at the ways in which Deaf people evaluate one another within the framework of Deaf culture.

Measuring academic achievement

Although a variety of achievement tests that are widely available have been used to characterize the academic achievement of Deaf children, the practice is irresponsible, since all but one have not been adapted in administration, language, content, and standardization for use with Deaf children. The exception, and thus the one to be considered here, is the Stanford Achievement Test, adapted for the hearing-impaired (SAT-HI) by Gallaudet University's Center for Assessment and Demographic Studies.[24] Most Deaf children who have taken any test for academic placement have taken this one.[25] The SAT is an achievement test designed for hearing elementary and secondary school children that comes in eight different grade levels of difficulty. In addition, there are numerous subtests, most of which are not appropriate for use with Deaf children because they require listening or rely too heavily on a reading knowledge of English to measure achievement in some subject matter.[26] However, the subtests of English vocabulary and reading comprehension are widely used with Deaf children, since the object of these subtests is to measure reading skill itself. Also used are the subtests on mathematics concepts and computation, since these are thought to make minimal demands on reading ability. The same questions are used for Deaf and hearing versions of each subtest, but Deaf students must also take a preliminary screening test. That is because the tests developed for first- through ninth-grade hearing students are too difficult for Deaf students in the same grades, so a Deaf student cannot be assigned a test merely by his or her grade level. There are sixteen screening tests (eight for math and eight for reading), and the Deaf student's teacher selects the one for reading and the one for math that seem appropriate—tests that will avoid a situation where the test-taker merely guesses on the one hand, or performs perfectly (called *topping out*) on the other. The score the Deaf student receives on the screening test determines the grade-level test of the SAT that he or she will be assigned to complete.

An individual Deaf student's scores can be compared to those achieved by hearing and Deaf students and even to those of particular subgroups of students, for example, those in comparable educational programs. Such comparisons are possible because, in its design stages, the test was administered to a sample of some 6,500 students, most recently in 1990.[27] This procedure is called *standardizing*, or *norming* the test: with a large sample of scores in hand, the score obtained by any individual student can be expressed relative to the norm for the student's age level. For example, that student's reading achievement score might exceed the scores of eighty-five percent of the students in the same age group tested in the norming sample; the student would be said to have ranked in the eighty-fifth percentile. The test's reliability was evaluated in two ways (by computing a measure of agreement among the item scores, and by retesting a sample of Deaf students with an alternative form of the test) and was found acceptable.

Although the SAT-HI has proven reliable, very little evidence has been published to show that the test, as adapted for Deaf students, is valid—that it truly measures what it claims to measure, such as reading comprehension, for example. Some scholars have argued that Deaf students have much greater ability to read English in real life situations than is reflected in their SAT-HI test scores.[28] Other scholars have shown that when Deaf and hearing students are matched on their Stanford scores, the Deaf students have much more difficulty on other tests of vocabulary and syntax than their hearing counterparts.[29] Both kinds of results challenge the validity of the SAT-HI. So do reports from several studies indicating that many items on the test are biased. For example, some items depend too much on reading ability, as described earlier.[30] The validity of the Deaf students' mathematics scores are open to question since scores on the subtests for arithmetic applications and concepts are much lower than those on the computational subtest, and it is just the first two subtests that require more reading. This confounding of English-language mastery with mathematics mastery is about to become much more severe with the publication of the ninth edition of the SAT: the computational subtest has been replaced by one with word problems that aims to assess more abstract mathematical reasoning, in keeping with the evolution of our increasingly technological society.

On the one hand, it seems invalid to penalize Deaf students' mathematical reasoning scores because English is not their primary language. On the other hand, if English word problems are a valid measure of later success in American society, it may indeed be true that Deaf students will be penalized in that arena as they are on the test that aims to predict later performance. A positive effect of the change in the math subtests may be to focus the attention of teachers of the Deaf on the importance of mathematical problem solving. One study has shown that the SAT-HI has *content validity* for Deaf students in this sense, that it is related to the content taught in school. Teachers of the Deaf were asked to rate how well the content of test items correlated with content they had covered in class, and most topics had, indeed, been covered. Moreover, students scored highest, on the average, on those test questions that were covered in most depth.[31]

Because the SAT-HI is to a large extent a measure of knowledge of English, as we stated earlier, we would expect Deaf children from homes where English is spoken and who became Deaf after acquiring English to score higher on the test, and that appears to be the case. Conversely, Deaf children from homes where spoken languages other than English are used, those with the least hearing (and thus more likely to be ASL speakers), and those said to have cognitive or behavioral handicaps, score appreciably lower on the test than their peers. We say "appears to be the case" because Deaf pupils differ in numerous ways and it can be a mistake to interpret a correlation between one of their characteristics and their achievement scores as evidence that that characteristic causes the achievement scores. For example, Black and Hispanic students generally score lower on the SAT-HI, but this does not mean that their ethnic status itself is the cause of their lower scores. We know that children from homes with lower socio-economic status have a disadvantage on such tests, and that is no surprise, since such children usually have fewer books in the home, travel less, have fewer opportunities for out-of-school learning, and so on. Now, it is reasonable to presume that the Deaf children from ethnic minority homes come, on the average, from homes with lower socio-economic status. Thus the origin of their disadvantage, one that many white children may share, may be more directly connected to their parents' low economic standing.[32] Deaf children with Deaf parents achieve higher scores on the English language parts of the test than Deaf children with hearing parents.[33] As we have seen, there are many differences in the family life experienced by the two groups of Deaf children that might account for this difference in test scores, but since Deaf children of Deaf parents almost always learn a full natural language "on schedule," this is very likely a particularly important source of their English advantage.

Measuring intelligence

There are, of course, many tests of intelligence available, including the American adaptation of Binet's original test, mentioned earlier. Most of these tests, however, are radically unsuitable for use with Deaf children and adults because their score depends very largely on English mastery. A possible exception is the Wechsler Adult Intelligence Scale (WAIS), designed for persons sixteen years of age and older, and its counterpart for children, the WISC. Both tests have a verbal section and a performance section; only the performance scale is appropriate for Deaf people, and it is the most widely used test of Deaf students' IQ. The performance subtests are: picture completion, picture arrangement, block design, object assembly, and coding. The WISC has been standardized on a national sample of over one thousand Deaf children.[34] When a sample of Deaf children was given the WISC-R, their average IQ scores were comparable to those obtained by hearing peers on the WISC performance scales.

The reliability of scores on these tests has not been established and their validity is open to question as well. While some studies have shown that scores on the WISC correlate with other nonverbal measures of IQ and with some measures of academic achievement, other studies find low correlations with scores on the Scholastic Aptitude Test[35] and the Stanford Achievement Test.[36] Since at best the tests are administered by an examiner using contact sign, it is questionable whether ASL-speaking children, who, as we saw in chapter 10, have difficulty with the contact variety, have the same opportunity as English-speaking children to establish their prowess on the subtests. Interestingly, when the WISC is administered with pantomime to hearing people, their scores are reduced by about five IQ points on average.[37]

In one study, Deaf children were administered both the performance and verbal subtests of the WAIS; instructions were given in contact sign. The subjects' performance-scale IQ turned out to be twenty-four IQ points higher on the average than their verbal-scale IQ, confirming yet again that accurate assessment of Deaf aptitude and achievement cannot be predicated on English mastery. Scores on the picture completion subtest correlate modestly with measures of English reading ability. Not surprisingly, the best predictor of reading ability was the Deaf child's score on the vocabulary subtest of the WAIS; vocabulary knowledge is an aid in reading.[38]

A recurrent and intriguing finding concerning the IQ of Deaf children is that the performance IQ scores of Deaf children of Deaf parents are not only higher than those of Deaf children with hearing parents, but they are also higher on the average than those obtained by hearing children of hearing parents. That is, they are higher than the general population norms.[39] The outstanding performance of Deaf children of Deaf parents was all the more surprising to researchers when they confirmed that many of those children had a disadvantage: they came from homes with lower socio-economic status, on the average, than the two other groups of children. One investigator tested sixty-two Deaf children of Deaf parents and found they had an average IQ of 114. He suggested that hereditary hearing loss is associated with higher IQ because natural selection has demanded this for survival![40] Incidentally, eighteen of these sixty-two children were judged in a related study "clear-cut cases of brain damage" by three clinicians who also administered a perceptual test called the Bender-Gestalt.[41] We mention this to underscore the unreliability of such testing with Deaf children.

The research described in chapter 4 on spatial cognition provides a possible explanation for the finding of a performance IQ-advantage among Deaf children of Deaf parents. That body of research shows that speakers of ASL, especially native speakers, have an advantage in a variety of non-linguistic tasks involving spatial thinking, including generating and transforming images, face identification, and rapid integration of visually presented information. It is possible that these tasks, and some of those on the performance IQ subtests, tap common underlying intellectual abilities. In that case, native ASL speakers would be expected to outperform others on the performance IQ scale, and they would be found particularly among the Deaf children of Deaf parents.

Measuring social and emotional adjustment

Questionnaires are also not a good means of assessing a Deaf person's personality because of their reliance on English and their culturally inappropriate content. Despite these obvious limitations, however, and despite a lack of norms on Deaf people, questionnaires have been widely used in research and practice. These include the MMPI, with its 566 true/false questions, cited earlier. An ASL version of the MMPI has been developed as a research tool; but its utility is limited by the lack of Deaf norms and lack of evidence for its validity.[42] The Social-Emotional Assessment Inventory, consisting of 59 questions normed on about two thousand Deaf children, circumvents the language problem confronted by questionnaires by querying teachers about the children's positive school behaviors and problem behaviors. However, behavioral rating scales encounter the problems of low inter-rater agreement and rater bias discussed earlier.

Projective tests such as the TAT and the Rorschach present other problems. The TAT consists of nineteen black-and-white pictures; the instructions are normally read in English to the testee, who is to invent a story lasting up to five minutes in response to each picture. The story is recorded by the examiner or a stenographer. Clearly, the examiner must be fluent in ASL and knowledgeable about Deaf culture to administer the test and to record and interpret its results. The validity and reliability of this test have not been established. The Rorschach consists of ten inkblots. Again, instructions, recording, interpretation, norms, reliability and validity are all problematic. Since the members of the DEAF–WORLD are visual people, and also have a distinctive culture, it is quite plausible that they react to ambiguous patterns such as ink blots in ways quite different from hearing people.

If questionnaires, behavioral observation, and projective tests are all ruled out as appropriate ways to assess the social and emotional status of Deaf children and adults, what means are there? As radical as it may sound, there appear to be none. Even when clinicians are fluent in ASL and knowledgeable about Deaf culture, which is rare indeed, they are ill-advised to use projective tests, since all the problems of test bias, lack of norms, and uncertain reliability and validity remain.[43] Probably the best move for such culturally knowledgeable people is to use their common sense rather than have illusions about scientific support. Most examiners and researchers are not, alas, even in a position to exercise culturally informed judgment and must forgo not only personality testing but also decision-making based on assessment.

Measuring language mastery

A variety of tests have been used to assess Deaf children's mastery of English. With rare exception, the tests have not been normed on Deaf children and their reliability and validity have not been established. Some of the more widely used English tests are mentioned briefly here. With the Peabody Picture Vocabulary test, the examiner speaks and concurrently signs 175 words, and the Deaf child chooses the one of four illustrations that best matches the meaning of each spoken word. Because the signing is not standardized, it is not valid to compare results among Deaf children. Deaf children's scores on the test do correlate modestly with their scores in English reading achievement, however.[44] The Illinois Test of Psycholinguistic Abilities (ITPA) is an aptitude test designed to assess abilities in English including auditory reception, auditory association and auditory sequential memory. These parts of the test are clearly inappropriate for Deaf people. There are also subtests of visual reception, memory, and association, but these have not been normed on Deaf people. Reliability of the subtests is highly variable and validity has not been established.

The Test of Syntactic Abilities (TSA) is a paper-and-pencil test of nine major syntactic structures in English. There are twenty diagnostic multiple-choice subtests that sample such abilities as recognizing and comprehending questions.[45] Deaf children's scores on the TSA are good predictors of their scores on tests of English reading ability.[46] This is to be expected, since the TSA requires the Deaf child to read the multiple-choice test items. However, that poses a problem since a Deaf child's knowledge of some parts of English syntax might exceed that child's ability to read the relevant questions on the test. Thus, the test is unsuitable for Deaf children below the age of ten. The recognition part of the test requires the child to judge the grammaticality of English sentences. The validity of such a measure as an index of language development has not been established.

The Rhode Island Test of Language Structure presents twenty different English sentence types (e.g., sentences with negatives, relative clauses, adverbial clauses, etc.) spoken aloud and simultaneously signed in English word order.[47] The child responds by pointing to one of three pictures that depict different interpretations of the sentence. For example, for the sentence *The girl hit the boy*, one of the pictures illustrates a boy hitting a girl. The test has been standardized on large samples of hearing and of Deaf children. There is evidence for its reliability. It is hard to know what criterion of language mastery one might use to establish the criterion validity of the test, however. The authors point out that hearing children do better on the test than Deaf children; that hearing children gain higher scores as they mature; that both groups have more trouble with complex sentences than with simple ones; and that Deaf children have particular difficulty with the English passive. Since all of these findings are to be expected, the authors believe they provide support for the validity of the test. To minimize any effects of the child's not knowing the vocabulary in the test sentences (since the test seeks to evaluate syntactic knowledge), the authors relied on teacher ratings of which words were familiar to the children.

Tests have only recently been developed to assess Deaf children's fluency in ASL. As we have seen, because most Deaf children have hearing parents, they frequently enter school with a command neither of English, which is not accessible, nor of ASL, which is not presented. Increasingly, such Deaf children may remain without a full language for many years, especially if they are educated in a mainstream setting with few other Deaf children who know ASL. It seems likely that the children's mastery of the one language they can master would be an important contributor to their academic success, yet this has not been studied directly. In a rational educational setting where teachers communicated with students in their primary language, tests of ASL fluency would take on a further role: they would determine in which classrooms the Deaf child would be educated and whether remedial ASL instruction should be part of that child's curriculum.

A comprehensive test battery for evaluating mastery of ASL grammar has been developed by a group of investigators at the University of Rochester.[48] Both production and comprehension are evaluated with twelve subtests in all. The production tasks each present a series of short videotaped events which the subjects are asked to describe in ASL; the events are designed to elicit single-sign or simple-sentence responses which use the various structures encountered in ASL. The comprehension tasks each present a series of short videotaped ASL signs or sign sentences, which also involve the various ASL structures; the subjects are asked to manipulate an object or to choose one of two pictures in correspondence with the meaning of the ASL form.

For example, in the Verbs of Motion Production Test, each item shows an object, such as a car or a person, moving along a path (e.g., in a straight line or in a circle), with a manner of motion (e.g., bouncing or rolling). The subject is asked, in ASL, to say what happened. The appropriate response should include a verb with the correct classifier, path of motion, and manner of motion. In the Verbs of Motion Comprehension Test, each item shows an ASL verb of motion, and the subject is asked to choose the appropriate object and make it perform the action. The response should involve making the correct object travel along the proper path with the proper manner of motion.[49] As another example, in ASL, verbs agree in spatial location with their subjects and objects (that is, they move from the location of the subject to the location of the object, as we have seen). The Verb Agreement Production Test includes a series of events involving several videotaped participants. Each participant sometimes carries out an action and, at other times, is the object of an action. Testees are asked to describe each event in ASL, and their responses are scored correct if their verb agreement is correct. The tests of the other linguistic structures are constructed similarly, in accord with analyses of native ASL usage. Scoring on each of the tests is performed by native signers. Correct responses have been determined by linguistic analyses and verified with native signers. Therefore, the test-taker can be assigned a score of percent correct. In addition, the specific errors the test-taker makes are analyzed to reveal patterns of incomplete understanding or misunderstanding of ASL grammar.

When hearing people evaluate Deaf people, their purpose is commonly to predict success in a phase of hearing culture such as the school or the workplace. Their criteria for the evaluation tend accordingly to be linked to hearing culture—for example, reading achievement, or ratings of performance by hearing people. Finally, their means of evaluation in such settings is, as we have seen, partly formal: a test is developed to stand in for the criterion performance, such as success in school. Although the test commonly demands quite different behavior than the criterion-performance, people who do well on the test, are evaluated favorably and allowed to learn or do the criterion-performance. Thus it is that students who do well, for example, on the Scholastic Aptitude Test, are evaluated favorably for higher education and admitted to universities.

In describing Deaf culture in chapter 5, we told how Deaf people distinguish themselves among their peers. Clearly, when Deaf people evaluate Deaf people in the DEAF–WORLD, their purposes, criteria, and means are often quite different than when hearing people evaluate Deaf people. The purposes of DEAF–WORLD evaluations tend to be bound up with Deaf culture: the goal is to select a storyteller or a group leader, for example, or a representative such as Miss Deaf America. Similarly, the criteria, such as ASL fluency, Deaf pride, and knowledge of Deaf culture, are embedded in the culture. Finally, the means of evaluation tends to be a sample of the criterion-performance itself. (In fact, a sample of the criterion-performance is often its best predictor.)

Hearing professionals usually do not evaluate Deaf people on Deaf terms, such as ASL fluency, knowledge of Deaf culture, achievements in the DEAF–WORLD and so on. Evaluating language skills provides a good example. Deaf children's relative mastery of ASL in all its complexity, including storytelling, registers, poetry, politeness rules, and so on, has traditionally not been evaluated, because educators have been unaware of that complexity and richness. Worse yet, ASL and other signed languages around the world continue to be viewed as makeshift language prostheses for people who can't hear. We should see in this attitude not only simple ignorance and the common denigration of minority languages but also, and more fundamentally, the exclusive perspective on members of the DEAF–WORLD as people with a disability. That understanding of Deaf people, or rather that misunderstanding, guides most of what hearing people do, generally with the best of intentions, to and for Deaf children and adults. The hearing initiatives that we have examined thus far, such as schooling of Deaf children, and those we will examine in the next chapter, such as rehabilitation of Deaf adults, are indeed predicated on understanding Deaf people in terms of disability. Therefore, we must ask what underlies that construction of the social problem of Deaf people, and what forces have led our society to choose that construction rather than the one held by Deaf people themselves.

❧

Chapter 12

The Hearing Agenda I: To Mitigate a Disability

TO understand the lives of people in the DEAF–WORLD, it is essential to examine the hearing agenda for members of that culture. It is not the case that hearing professionals and the larger hearing society have an agenda specifically for culturally Deaf people. On the contrary, their agenda is designed for members of the hearing world with hearing losses (and it is embedded, as we shall argue, in broader agendas for people with disabilities and for mainstream society). The agenda for hearing people with hearing losses would be a largely irrelevant matter for the DEAF–WORLD were it not for the fact that this agenda treats the members of the DEAF–WORLD as if they were essentially like hearing people who cannot hear. And those who set the agenda have the power to enforce it. Almost all Deaf children (except those with Deaf parents) enter the DEAF–WORLD in the U.S. through the hearing-controlled system that is based, as we have seen, in hospitals and schools. Although they are not members of the DEAF–WORLD, hearing people commonly have the decisive say in the affairs of Deaf people: where they will attend school and how they will be educated; where they will work; what information they will receive; even, in many cases, where and how they will live. This state of affairs, so contrary to contemporary ethics concerning minority groups, in which the majority regulates the lives of the members of a minority, arises for fundamentally two reasons. The first is that the existence of the

DEAF–WORLD was not generally recognized until recently. The second is the unique family situation of its members. Unlike any other language minority, the members of this one generally come from homes where their language, culture and identity have not been shared or valued by their parents. Most parents of Deaf children, because they are hearing people, subscribe to a hearing agenda for Deaf people. In so doing, the parents turn, as does society in general, to professional specialists, who are empowered by law and tradition (but not by Deaf people) to set the agenda for members of the DEAF–WORLD. Nearly all of these professional people, like most parents, are hearing people, and they, too, pursue a hearing agenda.

The hearing agenda for all people with limited hearing, including the culturally Deaf members of the DEAF–WORLD, is based on the premise that all such people have a disability. Therefore, the agenda for Deaf people is fundamentally the same as for all other people with disabilities. What is our social agenda for people with disabilities? To answer that question, we need to reflect for a moment on the concept of disability, how it arose, and the purposes it serves in our society. How shall we conceptualize disability? As we will explain shortly, the Disability Rights Movement is strongly challenging the widely-accepted medical understanding of disability. Nevertheless, that classical definition will serve as a starting point for our discussion. The box gives the official definitions of terms according by the World Health Organization.[1]

Disability Terminology Defined

Impairment: Any loss or abnormality of psychological, physiological, or anatomical structure or function.

Disability: Any restriction or lack (resulting from an impairment) of ability to perform an activity in the manner or within the range considered normal for a human being.

Handicap: A disadvantage for a given individual, resulting from an impairment or disability, that limits or prevents the fulfillment of a role that is normal, depending on age, sex, social and cultural factors, for that individual.

(World Health Organization, 1980.)

"Bodies are the battlefield," wrote the French philosopher Michel Foucault. In several of his works, he argued that political and economic forces in the history of the Western world have fought for control of the human body and its functions. By the eighteenth century, the Western tradition of esteeming "the poor" was replaced by a political analysis of idleness that continues to the present. To make productive citizens out of idle burdens on the state, it was necessary to distinguish those who could not work (the sick and disabled) from those who would not work (vagabonds). In early 1995, the Speaker of the U.S. House of Representatives confirmed this policy-objective of distinguishing the infirm from the indolent: "We want able-bodied people who are taking a free ride in the welfare wagon to get out and pull with the rest of us." Likewise, the British government has stated that the products of special education "should be productive if possible and not a burden on the state."[2] A 1993 Japanese law similarly aims to make people with disabilities independent and thus employable.[3]

To reduce the numbers of those who could not work and must be given a free ride, the state had great responsibility for ensuring the health of the population and could even penetrate the tight-knit family unit and prescribe what should happen to the child's body: hygiene, inoculation, treatments for disease, compulsory education.[4] (Modern schools continue this tradition with many practices that have little to do with education and much to do with the state's interest in regulating the child's body: lunch programs, audiometric screening, athletics, hygiene, etc.) These practices are generally quite desirable and they thus formed a continuing basis for the state's claim on the control of bodies. That claim can also be abused, however, as we discuss in chapter 14.

During this era of the rise of modern medicine and the growing intervention of the state in the health of the family, the first national schools for the Deaf were founded and, in order to ensure that those who could work had work to do, a central purpose of those schools was to teach the Deaf pupils a trade, removing them from their families where they were poor dependents and converting them into productive members of society. The Deaf schools in Europe contained shops to teach trades such as printing, carpentry, masonry, gardening, tailoring, etc. When schools for the Deaf were founded in the United States, they followed this model.

With the arrival of the Industrial Revolution, much larger numbers of people were marginalized; machinery, buildings and transportation were designed for the normative worker. To distinguish the able-bodied who could work in these settings from those with disabilities who could not, and to regulate the health of children and adults, it was necessary to measure, evaluate, create hierarchies, and examine distributions about the norm. For example, "mental defectives" were considered able to work at simple repetitive tasks, provided their impairment was not too severe. Moderate hearing loss (or unilateral loss) was not an obstacle to most employment, but severe bilateral loss was. Hence the brazen power of the king and nobles in feudal society was replaced by a "technology of power" exercised more subtly by the state. The technology that has been developed to aid in regulating and rehabilitating includes such disciplines as medicine, population studies and applied genetics, psychological measurement, physical anthropology and rehabilitation. In order to classify people as mentally handicapped, mentally ill, blind, deaf, lame, etc., and hence unable to work in varying degrees, the state requires techniques of measurement and specialists organized into agencies to do the measuring. The more elaborate are the special services and benefits offered to people with disabilities, the greater the need for complex measurements.[5]

This *social theory of disability* maintains, then, that the category of people with disabilities arises out of the work ethic of our society: people who are legitimately not working are those prevented from employment by disability; they have needs which the rest of society should meet. All other people, such as thieves, vagabonds, and the lazy, are not working for reasons that are illegitimate; they have no claim on our social solidarity, they should work and be self-sufficient.[6] Fully a fifth of the U.S. population between the ages of eighteen and sixty-four is considered disabled for work, so it is easy to see that the construct of "legitimately-not-working-because-of-disability" plays a large role in our society.[7]

Talking about disability as a construct motivated by economics takes many people by surprise. The off-the-cuff view, after all, is that disabilities are characteristics of the people who have them, much like height, say. A little reflection reveals however, that social issues such as disability are constructed in particular cultures, at particular times, in response to the efforts of interested parties. In the U.S. at the present time, we mark out some forms of human variation as functional limitations arising from an impairment, and other forms we construe as normal variations. Thus the following are accepted as normal, human variation: wide differences among people in skin color (but not albinism), height (within limits), obesity (but not gross obesity), baldness, near-sightedness, halitosis, rates of learning (but not mental retardation), mood (but not mania or depression), consumption of alcohol (but not alcoholism), cigarette smoking (but not crack smoking), and so on.

Pediatricians, special educators, welfare workers, and many other specialists have an important stake in what is construed as a disability and are active in lobbying local, state and national government on behalf of their professions. They are frequently opposed by organizations of people with disabilities—the very people they claim to serve—who object to the construction of disability as a tragic individual flaw requiring professional intervention. Self-advocates among people with disabilities reject the medical model of disabled people as "sick people who spend their lives trying to get well."[8] The Disability Rights movement seeks to shift the construct of disability from its focus on the body to the "interface between people with impairments and socially disabling conditions."[9] In other words, disabilities arise when a society fails to accommodate its physical and social environment to the range of human variation that it contains. People who get about in wheelchairs, for example, point out that they have no disability in homes that have access ramps, low counter tops, and the like. The United Nations *Standard Rules on the Equalization of Opportunities for Persons with Disabilities,* adopted by the General Assembly in 1993, states that the purpose of the term *handicap* "is to emphasize the focus on the shortcomings in the environment and in many organized activities in society."

Thus the hearing agenda that impacts the DEAF–WORLD begins by construing its members as people with disabilities, and it then construes people with disabilities as individuals struggling valiantly with tragic bodily flaws that legitimate their sufferers' failure to work. Consequently, the goals of hearing professional people in their intervention in the lives of the DEAF–WORLD have been of fundamentally two kinds: to mitigate and to eradicate. In order to mitigate the effects of limited hearing and reduce the barriers to work and other forms of participation in hearing society, the hearing professions, often with the help of government, provide social services, such as vocational rehabilitation, and they provide technology, such as hearing aids. Measures aimed in part at eradicating the Deaf, taken up in part 3, include efforts to regulate the reproduction of Deaf people and cochlear implant surgery on children.

The Social Services Sector

Access to work

The 1973 Rehabilitation Act (Public Law 93-112) sought to remove some of the barriers to fuller participation in the work force of people with disabilities. It provides for affirmative action programs to get more people with disabilities working for the federal government (Section 501) and for contractors supplying the federal government (Sec. 503). It set up a federal Architectural and Transportation Barrier Compliance Board to make sure that federally funded buildings were accessible to people with disabilities (Sec. 502). It also prohibits discrimination against people with disabilities in programs receiving federal assistance (Sec. 504). For example, many universities receive federal funds; the courts have ruled that this act requires those that do to provide interpreters for students who need them. However, employers are excused from a "reasonable accommodation" to workers with disabilities if it would cause an "undue hardship" on the program's operation.[10] Only an estimated one in twenty American colleges provides interpreters and related services.[11]

Following passage of this act, Deaf people seeking employment frequently turned to the federal government or to large corporations that had federal contracts. Once an agency or company had a few Deaf employees, this attracted others, who learned of the employment possibilities from their friends and who sought a work environment in which there was easy communication with some co-workers. In recent years, the federal government has employed about six thousand Deaf people, mostly in the postal service and the Department of Defense. The 1973 act concerned only the federal government as an employer and employers who had contracts with the government or received grants from it, however. Some seven million private employers and eighty million workers were thus unaffected by the act.[12]

The 1990 Americans with Disabilities Act (Public Law 101-336) extended legal protection to virtually all work sites; Title 1 of the ADA, prohibiting discrimination in recruitment, hiring, discharge, compensation, etc., now applies to all employers with fifteen or more employees. Title II requires state and local government to make all their services accessible to individuals with disabilities. For example, schools, welfare agencies, and hospitals must all be accessible. They must provide TTYs and other auxiliary aids (e.g., visual fire alarms) and services, such as interpreters, that allow Deaf people to communicate with the agency and the agency with them. Title III gives people with disabilities the right to equal access to public accommodations, such as hotels, theaters, restaurants, and doctors' offices.

Title IV of the ADA has had a particularly dramatic impact on the lives of people in the DEAF–WORLD. It requires telephone companies to provide both local and long distance telecommunications relay services. These are services manned by specially trained operators that allow Deaf and hearing clients to exchange information over the telephone. For the first time in history, a Deaf person can call anyone a hearing person can, and any hearing person, even though lacking a TTY, can call any Deaf person. Employers can no longer refuse to hire Deaf applicants, as they have so often in the past, on the grounds that the Deaf applicant cannot use the telephone.

The American DEAF–WORLD has traditionally had a strong work ethic, reinforced no doubt by the emphasis on trades instruction in the network of residential schools where much American Deaf culture was forged. Until the 1960s, the National Association of the Deaf magazine was called *The Silent Worker*, and the NAD franked all its letters with the slogan *Deaf workers make good workers.* The slogan reflects not only Deaf culture's commitment to work, but also an appeal to employers who traditionally have discriminated against Deaf workers—just the kind of discrimination that Public Laws 93-112 and 101-336 were written to combat. The combination of a Deaf work ethic and discrimination against Deaf workers led for many decades to a widely employed but underemployed Deaf work force. A 1971 census of the DEAF–WORLD found Deaf people working in every industry and most occupations, but earning twenty-five percent less than the national average.[13] The majority, like Roberto at the Metro Silent Club, were in the manufacturing sector, working as machine operators, assemblers, printers, and so on. That is just the sector that has been dwindling in recent decades. Information processing and service industries are on the rise (retail, education, health care and the like) but these commonly require education beyond a high school degree. To succeed in these industries, Deaf workers need a good command of English, mathematics, and computers; the average new employee will have two years of postsecondary education. However, nearly one Deaf student in three drops out of high school before getting a degree, as we said earlier; almost half of Deaf students in mainstream high schools drop out before graduation. Of those who do complete high school, between a third and a half go on to postsecondary studies, but only one in five of those achieve a degree.[14] An estimated fourth of the Deaf students are neither employed nor in school one year out of high school. A fifth are in food preparation jobs and another fifth in janitorial and stock handling posts.[15] In short, there is a great and growing gap between the knowledge demanded for employment in our post-industrial society and the knowledge that Deaf education is able to impart to Deaf students. To make matters worse, companies are becoming smaller; it is projected that the majority of openings in the year 2000 will be in companies with less than one hundred employees. These small companies will find accommodation to Deaf workers more of an "undue burden." (Perhaps this was the reason Henry was laid off from his job as a graphic designer.)

Vocational rehabilitation

Hearing initiatives aimed at ensuring that Deaf people can find their place in the work force begin with Deaf education, which we examined earlier. That part of the hearing agenda for Deaf people has generally not been successful. In its 1988 report to the Congress, the Commission on the Education of the Deaf stated that 100,000 Deaf people of all ages are seriously underemployed or unemployed; it put the blame on their poor command of English and lack of psychological, social and vocational development.[16] Into the breach between the Deaf person's abilities at the time of leaving school and the demands of the workplace steps the vocational rehabilitation (VR) counselor. The goal of VR is to enable people with disabilities to become productive members of the work force. The first rehabilitation act aimed at approaching that goal was passed after World War I, with disabled veterans particularly in mind. In the ensuing decades, and especially after World War II, the role of government in assisting people with disabilities in joining the work force expanded greatly. The 1973 Rehabilitation Act created a federal agency (the Rehabilitation Services Administration) in the Department of Education, and established grants for state VR agencies, which were to "return disabled persons, where possible, to substantial gainful activity." Eight thousand Deaf youths every year go from school to work or from school to postsecondary programs, most with the aid of their state VR agency. Indeed, the Deaf student's IEP contains a plan for the transition from school to work and a referral to a VR agency. These agencies assist in the transition from school to work with career counseling, training, job placement, and some on-the-job support. They also pay for some of the costs of college and trade school, and they retrain displaced workers.[17]

In practice, the VR counselor, working with the client, develops an Individualized Written Rehabilitation Plan (IWRP). It takes into account the client's background—schooling, family, and work history—and his or her educational achievement, work skills, and language skills. The counselor is charged with arranging various kinds of assessments; most standardized tests are ruled out, however, because they were developed for hearing people (see chapter 11).[18] The VR counselor can interview the client's former teachers and employers, ask the client's own opinion of his strengths and weaknesses, and possibly obtain a sample of his work. Finally, the VR counselor makes recommendations, which may include a direct job placement, purchase of equipment such as a TTY or a hearing aid, training in independent living skills, or continuation of education in a postsecondary program.

Some states require their VR counselors who work with Deaf clients to obtain specialized training, earning the title RCD, *rehabilitation counselors for the Deaf.* Although it is evident that the counselor who can communicate with the Deaf client fluently and is knowledgeable about the DEAF–WORLD has a great advantage in providing effective and efficient services, such specialization runs counter to the integrationist philosophy that has dominated the disability professions of late, including special education, and thus it is controversial.

There are about ten thousand Deaf students enrolled in postsecondary programs, especially at Gallaudet University and the National Technical

Institute for the Deaf. Other large Deaf postsecondary programs are at California State University, Northridge; St. Paul Technical College in Minnesota; and Seattle Community College in Washington.[19] There are an estimated 150 specialized post-secondary programs for Deaf students in the U.S.[20] However, increasing numbers of Deaf students are electing to attend public and private colleges and universities that have little or no specialized provision for Deaf students. According to Department of Education regulations that implement Section 504 (of the 1973 Rehabilitation Act), educational institutions may not refuse to admit Deaf students or neglect them in their recruitment efforts. In practice, few universities engage in planned recruitment of Deaf students, and most simply gamble that their Deaf students will not hold them to the letter of the law when it comes to accessibility. The regulations further require the schools to adapt academic requirements as appropriate; for example, if a Deaf student does not have standard English skills, tests must be modified. Perhaps most significant, the school must provide interpreters (and other auxiliary aids, such as closed caption TV) at its own expense, even if the student is able to pay for them. Private schools that do not receive federal aid were beyond the reach of Section 504; however, Title III of the ADA, which ensures fair access to public accommodations, applies to such schools, which now must provide interpreters, TTYs and other auxiliary aids.

Compliance with these laws presents some serious challenges to universities. The first concerns money. Providing qualified interpreters for individual Deaf students, each of whom follows a different academic program, is exorbitantly expensive, and most schools are not able to absorb the costs in tuition increases. To add to the burden, there are many other accommodations for Deaf students that are also required, and state VR agencies dispute whether, under ADA, the state has a legal obligation to assume any of the costs. The second challenge in compliance is more subtle. If it is wrong for a university to refuse to adapt the SAT test, for example, so that a Deaf student is not disadvantaged by a lack of English skills, is it right for a university to admit a student who doesn't have the English skills required for academic success?

With the completion of their postsecondary education, Deaf graduates have been joining a small but growing Deaf professional middle class in the United States. A 1987 study of almost two thousand Deaf professional people found that one-third of Deaf students who did complete postsecondary studies got professional and technical jobs or management and sales jobs, on graduation. (Laurel, from the Metro Silent Club, would be among the other two-thirds. Having graduated from Gallaudet, she is employed in a routine job in the Post Office.) Three-fourths of these Deaf professionals, like Jake, worked in occupations serving Deaf people (such as vocational rehabilitation counselor).[21] Most graduated from colleges with Deaf programs and most used personal contacts to get their job.

The typical Deaf VR client does not belong to this elite, however, and the counselor's goal is to ease his or her transition from school to work. The IWRP tends to focus on developing literacy, and on expanding independent living and social skills. Independent living skills include shopping, handling money correctly, appreciating the value of work, developing good work habits like punctuality, and keeping one's home neat and clean.[22] It may have occurred to you to wonder why so many members of the DEAF–WORLD should require an agency to assist them, at the end of their schooling, in acquiring literacy and the skills of independent living, including an adjustment to the world of work. The clear implication is that either their neediness is much exaggerated by those agencies, or their schools and families have fallen gravely short in imparting to them even the most elementary kinds of knowledge (or both). Three national centers active in vocational rehabilitation of Deaf workers are the Southwest Center for Hearing Impaired (San Antonio, Texas); the University of Arkansas Rehabilitation Research and Training Center on Deafness and Hearing Impairment; and the Northern Illinois University Research and Training Center on Traditionally Underserved Persons Who Are Deaf. The professional organization of VR counselors of the Deaf is the American Deafness and Rehabilitation Association (ADARA); it has about one thousand members and publishes a journal. ADARA recently expanded its scope and added to its name, "Professionals Networking for Excellence in Service Delivery with Individuals who are Deaf and Hard of Hearing."

Direct payments to Deaf people

Despite the efforts of the vocational rehabilitation agencies, many Deaf school-leavers and adults remain unemployed. As we have seen, people with disabilities have been historically cast as a category of people who legitimately do not work. Such people require financial assistance to survive, since they do not have an income from work. The Social Security Act provides for cash payments to people with disabilities under several titles. Title II provides Old Age, Survivors and Disability Insurance (OASDI; also known as SSDI); this is an insurance fund that receives payments from social security taxes on the earnings of all employed people. Many people with disabilities have not worked a sufficient number of years, however, to qualify for drawing disability payments from the trust. Therefore, Title XVI of the act provides for cash payments to people with disabilities based solely on their financial need, assessed by a means test. This is called Supplemental Security Income, or SSI. Some people receive both OASDI and SSI payments, when the income from OASDI does not exceed the means-test requirements of their state for SSI.

Although the members of the DEAF–WORLD traditionally have been heavily employed, they have also been viewed as possessing a qualifying disability, allowing them to be legitimately unemployed. Because, moreover, Deaf people traditionally have been underemployed, their wages commonly have been not much greater than the income offered them under social security, particularly if social security income is supplemented by off-the-record employment in odd jobs. Thus, members of the DEAF–WORLD have been provided with a strong disincentive to seek and maintain gainful employment. There is a widespread (but undocumented) belief in the DEAF–WORLD that OASDI and SSI have lured large numbers of Deaf workers away from the work force and that these programs discourage young Deaf men and women from entering it.[23] One study has shown that VR clients receiving OASDI and SSI income are less likely to secure employment than non-beneficiaries.[24]

We asked the Social Security Administration to search their records and tell us how many Deaf people were receiving cash payments. Of course, the administration could not answer that question, because they comprehend Deaf people only in terms of disability, in terms of hearing impairment, but our concern was with culturally Deaf people. What they *could* count for us was the number of recipients under the age of sixty-five who registered for benefits with hearing losses considered severe enough to affect work. In 1993, there were 40,578 such people receiving disability benefits from the Social Security Trust Fund (OASDI); and there were 52,703 such people receiving cash payments based on financial need (SSI).

Members of the DEAF–WORLD pay a high price for going "on the dole": their standard of living remains low; they forgo the psychological benefits that derive from working (pride in accomplishment, for example); and they literally buy into the system which construes the salient difference between Deaf and hearing people to be an impairment possessed by Deaf people. Since members of the DEAF–WORLD do not believe they have a disability, they have been presented with a soul-wrenching choice. Should they take money from the society that discriminates against them, but in so doing implicitly subscribe to the construction of Deaf people as people with a disability? Or should they refuse the cash, which is not offered to members of other language minorities? A parallel dilemma has been created for the members of the DEAF–WORLD in the area of education, as mentioned in chapter 8. Education, including residential school, is offered Deaf children under the disability umbrella. Should the DEAF–WORLD work to reform that special education, thereby implicitly subscribing to a view of Deaf children as having a disability, or must Deaf education leave special education in order to be true to its principles? People unfriendly to the DEAF–WORLD have charged angrily on these issues: "You're trying to have it both ways!" Clearly, the DEAF–WORLD would prefer to have it the right way: effective education, no discrimination in the workplace, and no need for disability payments. The framers of the ADA realized that the stigma of disability can itself lead to unequal opportunities in our society. Consequently, the protection of the law extends not only to people who have physical and mental impairments, but also to those who do not but are widely regarded as having them.[25] As society's understanding of the DEAF–WORLD grows and Deaf people are increasingly given control of their own destiny, there will be fewer such double-binds for the DEAF–WORLD to resolve.

Mental health services

In the period just after the Second World War, the U.S. Office of Vocational Rehabilitation began to use mental health methods in addition to physical rehabilitation to assist its clients, many of them veterans, to become, once again, productive members of the work force. It was not until 1955, however, that the first psychiatric treatment program in the U.S. was established in the interests of Deaf people. This project, at the New York State Psychiatric Institute, was soon followed by others, at St. Elizabeth's Hospital in Washington, DC, the Michael Reese Hospital in Chicago, and the University of California San Francisco Center on Deafness. Laudable as these initiatives were, they were frequently limited by the inability of staff to communicate with Deaf patients, by the staff's frequent lack of knowledge of the DEAF-WORLD, by the lack of psychological tests designed for Deaf people, and by negative stereotypes concerning Deaf people. For example, the Illinois center found depressive illness common among its Deaf patients, but the New York center found it rare. The former group interpreted all the depressive signs as evidence that Deaf people generally internalize thoughts of failure (blame it on themselves); the New York group interpreted the lack of depressive findings as evidence that Deaf people generally externalize failure (attribute it to agents outside themselves). Other studies of the incidence of mental illness among Deaf people find schizophrenia a common diagnosis in the United States but rare in Denmark, where Deaf adults are more likely to be found suffering from paranoia, a rare diagnosis for Deaf Americans. Such diagnostic mayhem not only leads to irresponsible characterizations of Deaf people; it prevents effective planning of the services Deaf people need, and it deprives Deaf children and adults of proper care. Heaven help the Deaf man or woman who really is mentally ill, for earthly help is not likely to be forthcoming.

In order to see how hearing experts portray the mental health of the members of the DEAF-WORLD, one of us (Harlan) reviewed the scientific literature on the "psychology of the deaf" from the last few decades, comprising some 350 journal articles and books. It is rife with statements such as the following from the *Journal of the American Academy of Child Psychiatry*: "Suspiciousness . . . as well as impulsive and aggressive behaviors have been reported as typical of deaf adults. . . . Recent reports tend to confirm these judgments."[26] A widely cited summary of the literature on the "psychology of the deaf" finds "rigidity, emotional immaturity, social ineptness."[27] As part of this review of the scientific literature, each time such characteristics of Deaf people were given, they were placed on a list. Then, terms that meant the same thing were eliminated and the remaining descriptions were sorted somewhat arbitrarily into four groups and alphabetized. Table 12-1 presents this distillation of the literature. In general Deaf people are characterized as socially isolated, intellectually weak, behaviorally impulsive, and emotionally immature. The list of traits attributed to Deaf people is inconsistent: they are both *aggressive* and *submissive; naive/shrewd, detached/passionate, explosive/shy, stubborn/submissive, suspicious/trusting.* The list is, however, consistently negative: nearly all the traits ascribed, even many in pairs of opposites, are unfavorable. Clearly we must suspect that the "psychology of the deaf" consists of hearing stereotypes about Deaf people.

SOCIAL	COGNITIVE	BEHAVIORAL	EMOTIONAL
Admiration—depends on	Conceptual thinking—poor	Aggressive	Anxiety—lack of
Asocial	Concrete	Androgynous	Depressive
Clannish	Doubting	Conscientious	Emotionally disturbed
Competitive	Egocentric	Hedonistic	Emotionally immature
Credulous	Failure—externalized	Immature	Empathy—lack of
Disobedient	Failure—internalized	Impulsive	Explosive
Conscience—weak	Insight—poor	Initiative—lack of	Frustrated easily
Dependent	Introspection—none	Interests—few	Irritable
Immature	Language—none	Motor development—slow	Moody
Irresponsible	Language poor	Personality—undeveloped	Neurotic
Isolated	Mechanically inept	Possessive	Paranoid
Morally undeveloped	Naive	Rigid	Passionate
Role-rigid	Reasoning-restricted	Shuffling gait	Psychotic reactions
Shy	Self-awareness—poor	Stubborn	Serious
Submissive	Shrewd	Suspicious	Tempermental
Suggestible	Thinking—unclear	Unconfident	Unfeeling
Unsocialized	Unaware		
	Unintelligent		

Table 12-1. **Some Traits Attributed to Deaf People in the Professional Literature**

A careful reading of the studies from which the trait attributions were taken reveals many serious flaws, like those discussed in chapter 11. Test administration is frequently unclear and unreliable; test language is commonly incomprehensible to the testee; test scoring is undependable, subjective, and easily influenced by the prejudices of the examiner; test reliability, the agreement between raters and the consistency of each rater, is suspect or very low; test validity, the proof that the test really measures what it claims to measure, is usually lacking and frequently doubtful; test content is unrelated to Deaf experience and schooling; test norms are nonexistent or inappropriate; finally, subject populations are inadequately characterized.

The psychological literature portrays Deaf children and adults as commonly emotionally disturbed. Some psychiatrists believe that this emotional disturbance leads to frequent mental illness. But a majority of experts seems to contend that it does not, that Deaf people do not differ from hearing people in the types and frequencies of their mental disorders.[28] Somehow, the severely disturbed children become healthy adults. This is a happier view, and probably the one we should hold to in the absence of any good evidence one way or the other, but the fact remains that there is no reliable information on the incidence of mental illness in Deaf people. A 1977 estimate had it that 43,000 Deaf people needed mental health services, but less than two percent received them.[29] Estimates of the number of Deaf Americans who need substance abuse counseling have ranged from 100,000 to one million.[30] A survey of VR counselors reported seventeen percent of their Deaf clients had mental health problems, but a follow-up study two years later found nearly twice that percent. These mental health problems included difficulties with interpersonal relations, stress management, problem-solving, and the like—"diagnoses" that leave wide latitude for the counselor's judgment, and biases.[31]

Deaf patients in psychiatric hospitals have longer lengths of stay and yet receive less treatment than other patients. It seems probable that these regrettable outcomes, like the wildly fluctuating incidence estimates, are the result of staff knowing too little of Deaf language and culture. One investigator presented four mental health case studies to eighty mental health professionals; they were to "write up" these four case studies, make diagnoses, and recommend treatment. Half the time, the four case studies were presented as Deaf patients, and half the time these same case studies were presented as hearing patients. It turned out that higher doses of medication and more supervision were recommended for cases when they were presented as Deaf than when they were not.[32] The study also found that the most positive attitudes toward Deaf people came from professionals who had treated Deaf people before, from younger professionals, and from those who were most educated.

The culturally incompetent therapist confronts many pitfalls with members of the DEAF–WORLD. In the first place, what counts as socially appropriate behavior (and hence a sign of mental health) can be quite different in Deaf culture than in the therapist's hearing culture, as we have seen. Eye-contact, facial expression, interpersonal distance, greeting and parting, politeness, decision-making, privacy and confidentiality, all function differently in the DEAF–WORLD than in American society in general.[33] Depression, for example, could go undiagnosed because the therapist mistakes the patient's terseness for a communication problem. On the other hand, if the client expresses frustration with communication barriers, the unaware therapist may misinterpret the display of emotion. Symptoms of physical illness may be misread by a therapist unable to collect a case history.[34] Misdiagnosis can result in long, inappropriate hospital confinements for Deaf people; a few such cases of rescue from prolonged wrongful institutionalization make headlines each year. The culturally incompetent therapist can trigger feelings in the Deaf person related to previous experiences of oppression; at best, the therapist will be unable to explore this response with the patient; at worst, the therapist's behavior will confirm the patient's worst fears.[35]

The remedy for these problems in mental health research and services for Deaf people lies, in the first instance, in recruiting more Deaf people to programs in school, counseling, rehabilitation, and clinical psychology, since Deaf professionals would commonly have the language skills and cultural knowledge necessary for effective evaluation and treatment of Deaf clients. In 1990, there were only an estimated twenty Deaf psychologists in the United States! Many graduate psychology programs remain inaccessible to Deaf students; when a sample were asked if they would accept qualified Deaf interns, among the responses were these: "I can't believe President Bush would pass the Americans with Disabilities Act if it meant paying for interpreters"; "Don't all Deaf people read lips?"; "Patients are very disturbed already and having a hearing-impaired therapist would make them more so."[36]

Then, too, many more hearing mental health professionals are needed who know ASL and the culture of the DEAF–WORLD. A 1981 survey of mental health professionals working with Deaf students in the schools found that only fifteen percent had studied Deaf people as a focus in their own education. Only thirty percent rated their "sign language skills" as average or above, and fully half said they had no such skills whatever.[37] Such communication barriers prevent the clinician from doing a proper diagnostic interview and from providing effective counseling and psychotherapy. No wonder a 1995 study found Deaf clients less likely to go to community mental health centers and, once there, to receive less assessment and therapy and a more restricted range of diagnoses.[38]

A current directory of mental health services for Deaf people lists 109 private practitioners, an average of two per state! Only fifteen percent of these practitioners are Deaf. In addition, 261 programs are listed that provide at least some mental health services for Deaf people. Settings include community mental health centers, outpatient mental health facilities, schools, and merely twenty-six programs in psychiatric hospitals. Eight states have no such programs whatever.[39] Fewer resources combine with Deaf people's restricted access to commercial health insurance and restricted ability to pay; as a consequence, Deaf people are unfairly denied the mental health services they need.

According to the law, mental health facilities receiving federal funds must provide benefits and services in a way that does not limit the participation of Deaf people. Section 504 requires, as stated earlier, that programs receiving federal assistance may not discriminate against people with disabilities. Such facilities must provide interpreters, TTYs, etc.; Deaf people have brought several lawsuits seeking enforcement of this requirement. However, interpreters are not the full solution to the problem of providing appropriate mental health services for members of the DEAF–WORLD. Qualified interpreters are difficult to find for these assignments. The presence of an interpreter alters the dyadic relation between the therapist and the Deaf client. Many Deaf clients are reticent in the presence of an interpreter, whom they frequently know and whose discretion they frequently do not trust entirely. Moreover, much of importance to the therapy often gets lost in the process of interpretation: humor, sarcasm, and metaphors are all difficult to render appropriately in a second language.[40] Consequently, members of the DEAF–WORLD will not have equal access to mental health services until there are a great many more trained professionals who have a good command of the language of the Deaf and Deaf culture.

In recent decades, substance abuse has become a major public health issue in the United States and, naturally, the DEAF–WORLD has been affected too. One unit for the Deaf at a psychiatric hospital finds that seventeen percent of its patients over the last nine years have had a dual diagnosis of substance abuse and some other mental illness.[41] Ending chemical dependency is an enormous challenge for most people, but members of the DEAF–WORLD face some special barriers. There are few treatment services where personnel can communicate with Deaf clients and are knowledgeable about the DEAF–WORLD. The meetings of AA and other twelve-step programs that are interpreted tend to be in larger metropolitan areas only. Deaf clients are particularly concerned for confidentiality in the tight-knit DEAF–WORLD. Family and friends are often excessively protective of Deaf people and substance abuse aggravates that problem. Assessment and treatment are expensive and members of the DEAF–WORLD frequently lack the funds. Options for making new and sober Deaf friends are limited by the small numbers of Deaf people outside metropolitan areas, while establishing new friendships with hearing people brings up differences in language and culture.[42] There is a national information clearinghouse addressing alcohol and substance abuse among Deaf and hard-of-hearing people, located at the Minnesota Chemical Dependency Program in St. Paul; the National Technical Institute for the Deaf sponsors an addiction prevention program; and there have been several national conferences in recent years for professionals and recovering Deaf people.

Legal services

The Bilingual, Hearing and Speech-Impaired Court Interpreter Act of 1979 requires U.S. courts to appoint qualified interpreters for Deaf people in any criminal or civil action initiated by the federal government. In addition, the Department of Justice interprets Section 504 as requiring provision of interpreters when Deaf people are involved and the court receives federal funds. Finally, the Americans with Disabilities Act requires all state and local courts to be accessible to Deaf individuals and requires the provision of interpreters and appropriate auxiliary aids.[43] Nevertheless, lawyers and doctors frequently fail to provide interpreters, and Deaf clients must choose between alienating the professional on whom they rely by insisting on their right to an interpreter, or resignedly placing their interests at risk without one. To make matters worse, there is a severe shortage of qualified legal interpreters for the Deaf: in Massachusetts, for example, the courts filed over twelve hundred requests for signed-language interpreters in the 1995 fiscal year, but only half of those could be filled by the state referral agency.[44]

As in the case of mental health services, the provision of interpreters for legal proceedings is only a partial solution to the problem of nondiscrimination against Deaf people. In the first place, it is essential to have *qualified* interpreters, particularly for technical legal discourse and when liberty and even life are at stake. Moreover, when Deaf people are taken into custody and read their constitutional rights, as required by law, an interpreter is frequently not available. The written *Miranda* warning is beyond the reading level of many Deaf accused. Even when an interpreter is secured, there are substantial conceptual and linguistic difficulties in the way of rendering an effective translation. The *Guide* of the National Center for Law and Deafness at Gallaudet University states that some accused Deaf people are unfamiliar with the notion of a right, with the import of the constitution, and with the functions that a lawyer might fulfill.[45] While the same may be true of many hearing persons apprehended by the police, the problem is compounded by language barriers in the case of Deaf people.

A recent Maryland case illustrates the problem of safeguarding the rights of Deaf defendants. David Barker was charged with murder in 1975, but the charges were dropped. A year later, he was in custody on an unrelated matter, but police grilled him in writing about the murder. Barker had a third-grade reading ability. In the end, he signed the *Miranda* waiver of rights as well as a confession. When Barker was asked a month later through an interpreter if he had understood the waiver he had signed, he answered "a little bit." He also claimed that the police promised he wouldn't go to jail for his crime but rather to a hospital. And he signed another confession. The court threw out the first confession as involuntary and discarded the second confession on the grounds that the promise of hospitalization influenced him. There was testimony that Barker may have misunderstood "You have the right to an attorney present" as "It is all right to have an attorney present."[46]

Every accused person has the right to have an attorney, but no attorney can represent a client effectively without ample ability to communicate with the client. As with mental health services for Deaf people, attorneys who are Deaf and some coda lawyers commonly are the most qualified in language and culture to assist a Deaf client. There is a growing but small cadre of such attorneys, and there are several legal advocacy groups for the Deaf. The National Association of the Deaf created a Legal Defense Fund in 1976. This group of lawyers, located at NAD headquarters in Silver Spring, Maryland, brings lawsuits defending the rights of Deaf people. The cities of Sacramento and Oakland, California, and the metropolitan region of New York also have legal advocacy projects for Deaf people, and there is a Legal Network for the Deaf that lists 150 attorneys who specialize in serving Deaf and hard-of-hearing clients. Because these resources are small compared to the size and needs of the DEAF–WORLD, and because hearing attorneys fluent in ASL are rare indeed, Deaf clients must have recourse, once again, to interpreters in most legal matters. If Deaf defendants are found guilty and go to prison, it is very likely they will find their basic rights abrogated. Deaf prisoners are commonly left out of rehabilitation programs, and even denied exercise and medical care, because prison staff cannot communicate with them. This is the case of a group of Deaf prisoners in New York who have sued the state for violations of the ADA.

If members of the DEAF–WORLD are to enjoy their full rights within our legal system, they must be accorded the same protections as members of any other language minority. The states must provide interpreters to any Deaf party in any judicial action. Interpreters must be present during police interrogation and during all civil and administrative procedures, such as juvenile hearings, parole and probation. Then, too, much more needs to be done to encourage Deaf students to enter the legal profession, and hearing professionals in law and criminal justice to learn about the language and culture of the DEAF–WORLD. Because culturally Deaf people in the criminal justice system are a tiny minority, there need to be more centralized programs with a critical mass that would justify the assignment of specially trained personnel.

Interpreter services

Deaf and hearing people have been using interpreters to communicate across language barriers for centuries. Frequently those who served as interpreters were hearing children or other hearing relatives of Deaf people, or they were teachers of Deaf children. The DEAF–WORLD wants access to information and services in the larger society and wants to contribute its own information and services to that society, so it places high priority on the provision of skilled interpreters. However, interpreters are also part of the hearing agenda for Deaf people; their provision is indeed required by several laws. For this reason, and because it is hearing people who, for the most part, educate interpreters and govern their profession, some discussion of this social service is appropriate here.

The ADA requires agencies of state and local government and places of public accommodation to furnish appropriate aids and services, including qualified interpreters when necessary, to ensure effective communication. The Justice Department defines a qualified interpreter as someone who can "interpret effectively, accurately, and impartially." Unfortunately, many unqualified interpreters are engaged in interpreting in the United States. Employers hire such people because the employers are ignorant about the DEAF–WORLD, because they are trying to save money, or because unqualified interpreters are available when it would be more difficult to seek out qualified ones. In chapter 8 we discussed the monumental demand for interpreters created by the mainstreaming and inclusion movements in Deaf education and the unwillingness or inability of many schools to recruit qualified interpreters. We saw how the Deaf child in a hearing class has to struggle not only with the many difficulties inherent in using a classroom interpreter, but with the additional burden of using one who is inadequately skilled. The NAD and the Registry of Interpreters for the Deaf (RID) declared a nationwide crisis in 1994 in the delivery of qualified interpreter services.

The RID was established as recently as 1964, when participants at a conference on the shortage of interpreters agreed that there was a need for maintaining a list of qualified interpreters and for evaluating their competencies. Local RID chapters proliferated around the country, there were national biennial conventions, and a Code of Ethics was developed to ensure impartiality, confidentiality, and appropriate dress and professional behavior. With the mushrooming study of ASL in the following decades, many young people, frequently without the traditional ties to the Deaf community, turned toward interpreting as a career. The first pilot educational programs for interpreters were established in 1973. In the '70s, there were few recognized standards or accreditation procedures, however, and the competence of graduates from these programs varied widely.

If the 1960s were the infancy of the profession, and the '70s its childhood, then the 1980s brought the predictable adolescent search for identity. The profession had been implicitly guided at first by a "helper model": The interpreter not only worked between two languages, she (most are women) also explained things to the Deaf person that had been said in English and that might be unclear, and she readily advocated the Deaf client's position vis-à-vis the hearing client. If there was a heated disagreement, the interpreter might explain to the two parties how (in her bicultural view) the disagreement arose. For all its good intentions, however, this way of behaving proved paternalistic and disempowering for Deaf people.

The next stage of the profession's identity development was in part a reaction to those failings. The interpreter was now to conceptualize her role as a conduit or translating machine, a communication link, something like a sophisticated telephone. In interpreter education programs, issues such as this were debated: If the psychotherapist leaves the room for a moment and the Deaf patient climbs onto the window ledge, should the interpreter intervene? Or suppose a Deaf prisoner is asked if he understood his *Miranda* rights. Is it part of the interpreter's role to explain what *Miranda* rights are? During this period many interpreters rendered the English source language not in ASL but in contact sign, with its English word order. Some Deaf clients, particularly those with a good command of English, request such transliteration rather than ASL, especially if they are interested in how the English speaker expressed himself *in English.*

With the flourishing of linguistic and cultural research concerning Deaf communities around the world, interpreter education inevitably evolved in the direction of informing and empowering interpreters more. The conduit model was replaced by a view of the interpreter as a facilitator of communication, someone who took on significant responsibility for ensuring that the two parties understood each other.

Finally, beginning in the 1980s, the model of the interpreter as a linguistic and cultural mediator gained prominence. The interpreter should be bilingual and bicultural, allowing her to extract the profound message in the source language and to convey it, frequently in radically different form, in the target language.[47]

Linguist and interpreter-educator Charlotte Baker-Shenk has argued forcefully that all these models are inappropriate, because all ignore the power relations at work when the interpreter plies her trade. The interpreter has power as a hearing person and has the means for the Deaf person to secure what he seeks. Moreover, the interpreter can make the Deaf person appear smart or dumb, depending on her skill, choice of vocabulary, and the way she voices the Deaf person's message. Further, all parties know that the Deaf and hearing participants are rarely on an equal footing. To return to the *Miranda* example: suppose the interpreter simply fingerspells "M-I-R-A-N-D-A." Hasn't she participated in the oppression of the Deaf person? Baker-Shenk appeals to interpreters to recognize the power inequalities and to attempt to redress them, within the limits of their role. She calls this model, the *ally interpreter*.[48]

Speech and hearing services

The profession of speech-language pathology/audiology serves primarily the large population of Americans who have speech, language or hearing impairments. Because of the increasing average age of hearing society, and thus an increase in the numbers of people with hearing losses from aging and language disorders resulting from stroke, there is a growing demand for these professionals. According to a 1994 estimate, there are as many as twenty-three million Americans with significant hearing loss, but nearly nine out of ten of them have mild to moderate loss and are acculturated to mainstream hearing culture.[49] Naturally, the needs of such people shape the conception and provision of professional services.

Adult members of the DEAF–WORLD rarely seek such services, since speech and hearing are matters of marginal significance to the visual people in Deaf culture. Moreover, there is no rigorous evidence that oral and aural training actually enhance communication in Deaf children and adults.[50] Nevertheless, hearing parents of Deaf children and the schools those children attend seek the intervention of these professionals with their Deaf children. There are approximately 70,000 youths receiving special education services for the hearing-impaired, and about two-thirds of these children have mild to moderate hearing loss.[51]

Speech-language-hearing professionals offer a range of services that is as wide as human ailments in these areas are variegated. Some of the disorders of production that they treat are: apraxia (disorder of speech planning), aphasia (disordered manipulation of symbols due to brain damage), developmental language delay, articulation disorders, stuttering and other disorders of rate, and voice disorders, including those arising from laryngectomy. Speech-language-hearing professionals measure the intelligibility and other characteristics of disordered speech with various tests, participate in diagnosis, and offer training in language, communication strategies, articulation, and phonation. Frequently their efforts are aided by technology, which is discussed below.

These professionals also treat disorders of reception, including conductive hearing loss (arising from damage to the middle ear caused by disease, trauma and aging), and sensorineural hearing loss (arising from damage to the endings of the auditory nerve caused by aging, prolonged exposure to loud noise, misadministration of drugs, and disease). With various tests, they identify patients' language disorders and execute a program of therapy. However, there seems to be no interest in the profession in diagnosing signed language disorders and in developing therapies to improve mastery of ASL. Using audiometry of various kinds, they measure and diagnose hearing loss, provide hearing aid selection and fitting, train patients in speechreading (lipreading that also takes account of other facial and bodily clues), and provide auditory training.

The professional organization of most speech and language therapists and audiologists is the American Speech-Language-Hearing Association (known by its acronym, ASHA). It has about forty thousand members; nine out of ten are women, and seven in ten deliver services in schools and health clinics.[52]

The Communication Technology Sector

In our "hi-tech" society, a substantial industry has developed in recent years selling high technology equipment to government and individuals that is designed to enhance the lives and participation in the work force of people with disabilities. Power-driven wheelchairs, vans and buses with lifts, cars controlled by hand, and electronic prostheses (such as artificial limbs) provide just a few examples.[53] A considerable array of specialized devices is sold, mostly by hearing people, to or for members of the DEAF–WORLD. They include: TTYs; closed-caption television decoders; hearing aids; cochlear implants; visual doorbell signaling devices; sound and motion detectors; baby cry-signaling devices; vibrating alarm clocks; smoke and fire detectors with visual alarms; personal pagers; siren detectors; computer modems; answering machines; fax machines; electronic mail and bulletin boards; loud-ring signals; loud buzzers; strobe lights; and devices that convey information through vibration.[54] Some of these devices are modern versions of traditional artifacts of DEAF–WORLD culture. Mechanical clocks rigged so that a weight falls at the appointed hour and awakens the Deaf sleeper have been replaced by electronic bed vibrators. A stack of books placed next to a bedridden Deaf child, who can knock it over to summon a parent with the vibration, has been replaced by the baby cry signaler (a sound-activated flasher). The most widely used device, the TTY, was invented in the 1960s by Robert Weitbrecht, a Deaf astronomer, physicist and electrical engineer.

If you sorted the various kinds of technology that are sold for use by Deaf people into those devices that present visual information, like the TTY, and those that present auditory information, like the hearing aid, you would discover (it should be no surprise) that the former receive, in general, a warm welcome in the DEAF–WORLD, while the latter do not. Telecommunications technology, including the TTY and captioning, are important parts of the technology agenda that the DEAF–WORLD has established for itself; they will be discussed in chapter 15. High on the list of hearing agenda technology that is not well received by many members of the DEAF–WORLD is hearing aids. A more recent and controversial development in hearing technology is the cochlear implant, hailed as a miracle cure by some, called a dangerous experiment by others. The hearing agenda for the use of these devices concerns the DEAF–WORLD mainly when it comes to Deaf children. Most teachers of the Deaf commonly insist that their pupils wear hearing aids all the time (whether or not the child derives any obvious benefit or wishes to wear them); and cochlear implant teams generally do not perform implant surgery on adults in the DEAF–WORLD, since results with culturally Deaf adults have generally been poor and most do not desire it. Instead, they seek to implant Deaf children at ever earlier ages. Although various motives have been given for fitting Deaf children with hearing aids or with implants, the primary reason for the focus on hearing technology in childhood is the hope that improved hearing might assist the child in learning a spoken language—English, in the United States.[55]

Given that English is the language of the larger society in which the U.S. DEAF–WORLD is embedded, and that it is frequently the language of the Deaf child's parents, you might expect that the DEAF–WORLD would endorse efforts to assist the Deaf child in learning English, including the provision of hearing aids and cochlear implants. This is not totally accurate. There is indeed considerable consensus in the DEAF–WORLD, as in other American language minorities, that a command of written English is a valuable skill. Where the DEAF–WORLD and other American language minorities differ, however, is in the importance attached to spoken English. The DEAF–WORLD is definitely guarded when it comes to focusing on speech and on the technology designed to assist Deaf oral communication. It is our impression that most (but not all) Deaf leaders favor a measured effort to develop speech in Deaf children who have not learned the skill. However, they believe that that effort should never displace education, and it should be abandoned when it no longer proves fruitful.

The reason for this guarded position concerning speech and speech technology is that, in general, attempts to teach speech and speechreading fail with most Deaf children, while making great demands on their time and effort. Most adult members of the DEAF–WORLD were once Deaf children themselves, so they have a personal memory of that failure. Most, like Ben, and like Henry and Laurel from the Metro Silent Club, recall the experience as a painful and unprofitable ordeal. The vast majority of members of the DEAF–WORLD do not speak English intelligibly; no doubt because most of them were born Deaf.[56] Never having heard spoken English, these Deaf people are not familiar with its pronunciation, vocabulary and grammar, and thus they are not able to speech-read well either.[57]

The picture is quite different when it comes to the small minority of children who become Deaf *after* learning spoken English. Most such children go on speaking for many years, with or without therapy, and they have a distinct advantage in lipreading, since they have mastered the sound system of the language, as well its vocabulary and grammar. In evaluating methods for teaching speech to the Deaf, it has been exceedingly common, ever since the sixteenth century, to present the achievements of the minority of Deaf pupils who knew a spoken language before the therapy as representative of what could be achieved with the majority, who did not. This is not necessarily chicanery: frequently, neither the Deaf child nor the therapist or teacher is certain at what age the child's hearing loss began, and for many children no precise age can be given because their hearing declined gradually. Also, it is only in relatively recent times that speech teachers have known the extent of their pupil's residual hearing thanks to audiology. In the end, it is frequently unclear how much of a Deaf child's oral fluency should be attributed to natural language acquisition and how much to laborious tutoring. This ambiguity has contributed to the conflict between, on the one hand, hearing parents and specialists who are committed to what speech and speech technology can offer and, on the other, Deaf people who frequently find the effort largely fruitless, with its few fruits overvalued.

The conflict between the DEAF–WORLD and the profession of speech therapy is centuries old. You will recall that in 1779 the Deaf writer, Pierre Desloges, defended signed language against the oralist claims of a speech teacher. In the same era, the abbé de l'Epée and the most renowned "demutiser" in Europe, Jacob Pereire, were arch rivals. A century later, the Milan Congress pitted hearing professionals who advocated "pure oralism" against the DEAF–WORLD. The conflict is so old and widespread it might seem unavoidable, but speech-language pathologists at the National Technical Institute for the Deaf have argued that it is possible for the members of their profession to have a culturally sensitive approach to the DEAF–WORLD. Here is their prescription. They refuse to adopt a pathological model of the members of the DEAF–WORLD. They do not view Deaf people with intelligible speech as more successful. They do not believe that all Deaf people require their services. Rather, they are interested in providing those services only to Deaf people who seek them. They do not view culturally Deaf people as hearing impaired. They do look for their client's skills and gifts, particularly in visual/manual communication. They do seek collaboration with Deaf professionals. And, like all hearing professionals who work successfully with the members of the DEAF–WORLD, they keep a watchful eye on their own language and behavior so that it is not unwittingly oppressive.[58]

Hearing aids

Well over a million hearing aids are sold annually in the United States but few adult members of the DEAF–WORLD use them, since such Deaf people are primarily visual people.[59] On the other hand, virtually all Deaf children wear them because they are obliged to do so by their school and parents, who place great value on whatever ability the child may have to respond to sound and particularly to speech. Some children, like Laurel, rebel, but most are compliant under the watchful eyes of their parents and teachers.

Hearing aids are expensive. The average cost was five hundred dollars in 1990—and the average device must be replaced in under five years. In addition to the technology, the consumer also purchases services from an audiologist and a hearing aid prosthetist.

There are several different types of hearing aids in use. *Body aids* are worn in a case strapped to the chest or belt; a cord connects the aid to a miniature speaker snapped onto a plastic ear mold that fits into the ear canal. This type of aid can generate high (indeed, even harmful) signal levels and was widely used in the post-war era in schools for Deaf children. The most common aids are *behind-the-ear*: microphone, amplifier, and speaker all fit in a small plastic case that rides on the external ear, or is incorporated in the frames of eyeglasses. The aid is connected to the ear mold by a plastic tube. *In-the-ear* aids fit in the outer ear bowl, and *canal aids*, the newest design, fit into the ear canal itself. Both of these two aids are appropriate for mild to moderate hearing losses only and are appealing to many hard-of-hearing people for their small size.[60] Conventional hearing aids have many limitations. They are essentially amplifiers, so they cannot assist hearing at those frequencies at which the ear has no sensitivity. At very high amplification, they tend to squeal and they severely distort sound, rendering it less intelligible. Aids amplify noise as well as speech, since they lack the noise-canceling ability of normal binaural hearing. Scientists are at work on all these limitations. Newly developed all-digital hearing aids promise some advantages, including better control of squealing and better noise reduction. The trade-off between size and power remains a problem, however.[61]

Tactile aids

The sense of touch is capable of remarkably rapid and fine discriminations. Research has shown that Deaf-Blind subjects can follow speakers well at rates up to three-fourths of the normal speaking rate. One way they achieve this, we have been told, is by holding their hands, palm down, lightly over the hands of an interpreter speaking ASL. In another method, named *Tadoma* (after the two children with whom it was first used in the U.S.), the Deaf-Blind person places a hand on the face and neck of the talker and attends to lip and jaw movements, oral air flow, and laryngeal vibration accompanying speech. Because these people can understand rapid speech using the sense of touch, it ought to be possible to design a tactile aid that would convert sound into patterns of vibration on the skin, and would allow Deaf and Deaf-Blind people to follow rapid conversation. This has not yet been achieved. The tactile aids that are available offer little benefit to people at either extreme of hearing loss, those who can hear very little speech, and those who can hear a lot of speech. The tactile aid helps primarily the in-between group, particularly when supplemented by lipreading and aided by a native knowledge of English.[62] The most common design of tactile aid involves a microphone connected to an amplifier that splits the speech signal into two or more channels based on frequency; each signal is sent to its own vibrator in an array located on the wrist, arm, chest or abdomen.[63] The Tickle Talker delivers tactile signals electrically through eight small rings worn on the fingers.

Speech aids

Teaching Deaf children to speak is very high on the hearing agenda for the DEAF–WORLD. Well over one hundred electronic aids have been developed with the goal of assisting Deaf persons to learn or use speech, but none has been sufficiently successful to come into wide use. Visual displays of voice intensity and pitch have been used for some time in the clinic, but such progress as the student makes there commonly fails to transfer to the outside world. Efforts at the Bell Telephone Laboratories after World War II to develop a visual display of speech for hearing-impaired telephone users led to a device, the sound spectrograph, that proved of value only in speech research. Nearly half a century later, we still do not know what features to extract from the complex speech wave uttered by native speakers of English (or any other spoken language), and how to present those information-bearing elements of speech visually. It is even more uncertain what features should be extracted, and how to extract them with speech that has been disordered by hearing impairment. Even displays of normal speech vary widely from one speaker to the next and when a single speaker repeats an utterance. It follows that efforts have not proven successful to use visual displays of speech as targets that the hearing-impaired speaker should attempt to match in order to acquire good speech habits.[64]

It is probably fair to say that hearing provisions for mitigating the disability of members of the DEAF–WORLD, as hearing people perceive it, fail to reach their goals. Special education seeks to graduate informed citizens well-prepared for a rewarding career but, as we have seen, the majority of Deaf students leave school ill-informed, illiterate, and increasingly unprepared for the technological workplace. Vocational rehabilitation seeks to place Deaf people in trades and professions where they can fully put their talents and interests to work, but Deaf people are notoriously underemployed and only a tiny fraction complete higher education. Social work aims to provide a safety net for people with disabilities but ends up luring Deaf people who can work out of the work force. The mental health professions want to assist Deaf people in coping with emotional challenges and mental illness, but few members of the DEAF–WORLD are prepared to seek the services of professionals who do not know their culture and cannot communicate with them. Legal services also fall far short of their goal. The goals of speech-and-hearing services, and the associated technology to enable Deaf people to communicate more like hearing people, are not remotely achieved, both because of limitations in methods and equipment, and because those goals are antithetical to the values of the DEAF–WORLD.

Even interpreter services, which are predicated on a knowledge of ASL and Deaf culture, have come under severe criticism by the leadership of the DEAF–WORLD in America. For one thing, the disability model requires enormous numbers of highly skilled interpreters throughout the school systems of America; as a nation we are not remotely in a position to provide them, and so countless Deaf children rely on incompetent interpreters or none at all.

Thus, hearing professionals' interventions to mitigate the perceived disability of members of the DEAF–WORLD have proven unsatisfactory despite major efforts in education, social services and technology. One strategy that flows naturally from this disappointing outcome is to reexamine the principles on which hearing intervention in Deaf lives is predicated. That has barely begun. Another strategy is to redouble preventive measures in order to reduce the numbers of people entering the DEAF–WORLD, including eugenic measures and childhood implant surgery. Such a strategy naturally puts hearing professionals and the members of the DEAF–WORLD on a collision course. It shapes the political agenda of each party. And it obliges us to reexamine our thinking about disability, normalcy, acculturation, parenting, language rights and ethics. Our journey into the DEAF–WORLD has brought us to the place where worlds collide and where our moral compass no longer surely points the way.

❦

Part III

When Two Worlds Collide

Chapter 13

The Future of the DEAF-WORLD

IN the first part of this book, we explored the DEAF–WORLD, who its members are, its language and culture, customs and ethos. In part 2, we focused on the interface between the hearing world and the DEAF–WORLD, in particular on the education of the Deaf and the consequences for the DEAF–WORLD of the hearing world's conception of Deaf people as disabled. Now we turn explicitly to matters of politics and power and the future of the DEAF–WORLD itself. In particular, we will talk about the differences, the "points of collision," if you will, between the goals that hearing people have for Deaf people and the goals that members of the DEAF–WORLD have for themselves.

As we saw in part 2, much effort among the professionals (mostly hearing) who deal with the Deaf is aimed at the mitigation of the effects of what they perceive to be the disability arising from hearing-impairment. As we also saw, from the perspective of the DEAF–WORLD, many of these efforts have produced, and continue to produce, results contrary to this aim. In fact, especially in the area of education, they have been profoundly disabling for Deaf people, essentially depriving the majority of them in childhood of that most essential of human attributes, language and the ability to communicate, and thus severely limiting their opportunities in a society rushing into the information age.

Why should such well-meaning efforts produce these results?

Fundamentally, we have argued, because of the disability model on which these efforts are based. Here we consider what happens when the disability model is carried to its logical conclusion.

With any disability, the logical way to proceed is commonly considered to be to seek to avoid it, and to cure it if possible when it occurs. Thus the ultimate goal of those who perceive Deaf people as disabled is more than mere mitigation. It is the cure and/or prevention of deafness—in other words, the elimination of Deaf people, and, as an inevitable consequence, the eradication of the DEAF-WORLD.

Historically, the drive to cure deafness had much to do with the notion that the defining characteristic of human beings is their ability to speak; those who do not do so are not fully human. Now such attitudes, if they exist, are not articulated, and a more likely justification for intervention is: "This is a hearing world." But of course it is a DEAF-WORLD, too. So we must ask, who seeks to override the judgment of Deaf people about their own best interests and why do they do it? To many hearing people it is utterly obvious that it is better to be hearing than Deaf. They have only a subtractive understanding of deafness, and they count the things they suppose they would lose if they or their child had a profound hearing loss, from the melodious works of Bach to the chirps of a songbird to the warning blast of an onrushing truck's horn. But, as we hope our journey together thus far has made clear, subtracting features possessed by hearing people will not allow one to approximate a Deaf person. On the contrary, what this book bears witness to is the necessity of recognizing all that is *added* to the child who becomes culturally Deaf: language, heritage, artistic expression, social solidarity, and more.

Consider this analogy: Suppose you grew up in a country where people had never had television and had never been exposed to one. Then one day, your country's leader informed the nation that television was banned. You would wonder what the fuss was about. But if you grew up in a country where television was an important part of your life and the life of almost everyone in the land, and suddenly it was prohibited, and all TVs were confiscated, then you would surely miss it. You would probably move heaven and earth to get the prohibition lifted. Deaf people find themselves with a foot in each camp, for while they are the ones without television, they are surrounded by devotees of the tube. How can Deaf people respond? They can either be instilled with the wish to have TV (by their parents and teachers and doctors) and hence envy those who have it; or they can say, "Hey, we are fine without television." The latter attitude, with respect to hearing, is that of the DEAF–WORLD.

In short, when hearing people think about Deaf people, they project their concerns and subtractive perspective onto Deaf people. The result is an inevitable collision with the values of the DEAF–WORLD, whose goal is to promote the unique heritage of Deaf language and culture. The disparity in decision-making power between the hearing world and the DEAF–WORLD renders this collision frightening for Deaf people.

The power of the hearing world vis-à-vis the DEAF–WORLD is nowhere more frightening than in the application of medical science to Deaf people. Medical interventions aimed at the cure of deafness have a long history. It is a history that includes cruel and worse-than-useless experiments with Deaf children: fracturing their skulls, puncturing their eardrums, pouring bizarre liquids in their ears. It is a history that includes eugenic undertakings, among them sterilization, with Deaf children and adults. Today, as the DEAF–WORLD sees it, this torch has been passed to those who would "cure" Deaf children by implanting electronic devices in their skulls and those who would prevent their birth in the first place by genetic testing and counseling and, when feasible one day, genetic engineering.

Medical science is revered in our society and is well-funded by government and industry; the DEAF–WORLD is little known, and there is no one to promote and protect its values and views except Deaf people themselves and their hearing allies. It is also doubtless true, and members of the DEAF–WORLD acknowledge this, that in general, the mission of medical science to improve the lot of humanity is undertaken in all sincerity. As the next chapter documents, however, doctors and other professionals have commonly locked Deaf people out of the councils where decisions vitally affecting them are made. "Since when does the doctor consult the patient?" seems to be their policy.

Of all the forms that medical intervention in the DEAF–WORLD has taken, none has aroused deeper concern than cochlear implants, which have rightly been called "oralism with a scalpel." You will recall that oralism was a method of education in which Deaf children were to be taught above all to speak, and by means of speech; that oralists seized control of the education of the Deaf in the late nineteenth century; that for a hundred years thereafter the visual language of the Deaf was banished from their schools; and that oralism was discredited finally by its utter failure to produce the results it sought. Now it seems, just as oralism was discredited at last, and recognition has begun accruing to the language and culture of the DEAF–WORLD, as we saw especially in chapter 5, the oralist philosophy has reappeared in a new guise—one backed by all the authority of the modern medical establishment. Once again, the parents of Deaf children are advised not to let their Deaf children sign, if they are to be or have been implanted. The oral schools, like the one Laurel from the Metro Silent Club attended, have received a new lease on life. Yet, as we shall see in chapter 14, the implants do not give Deaf children access to the hearing world. Most children who receive them, the experimenters themselves acknowledge, remain "severely hearing impaired," and in need of long-term therapy. Once again, Deaf children are being deprived of access to natural language for years, in violation of their basic human rights, by those whose professed aim is to cure them of their disability by enabling them to speak the language of their hearing parents. We will consider these matters in detail in the next chapter. We raise them here to focus on the consequences for relations between the hearing world and the DEAF–WORLD: the potential for disaster through mistrust and misunderstanding as the two worlds collide at the place where the future of Deaf language and culture inevitably resides—because of the sheer force of numbers, among the Deaf children of hearing parents.

If the hearing parents of a hearing child deprived their child of the opportunity to learn language, whatever their intentions, we would all protest, probably accusing them of child abuse. Likewise, whatever the intentions of the hearing parents of a Deaf child, when they deprive that child of the same opportunity, it appears to many members of the DEAF–WORLD as child abuse. The term used in the DEAF–WORLD is *communication violence*,[1] and most Deaf people have been victims of it in one form or another, as we saw in part 2. Deaf parents certainly sympathize with hearing parents' desire to use their own language with their child and, more generally, to have a child in their own image. Deaf parents have the same desires. But members of the DEAF–WORLD, most of whom, remember, were themselves the children of hearing parents, know from personal and from cultural experience that the Deaf child's welfare is best served by embracing signed language and Deaf culture, not by rejecting them.

Many hearing parents find the Deaf point of view difficult to credit. They say to themselves, "Imagine this. Deaf people do not desire to hear and even wish their own children were Deaf." "Yes that's right," members of the DEAF–WORLD reply, and as self-evident as that proposition seems to the Deaf, it is utterly confounding to the hearing. It does not seem to matter if the Deaf say again and again that they value their culture, their language, and their world. The hearing remain perplexed. This, of course, perplexes the DEAF–WORLD. The gulf between the two worlds engenders accusations and recriminations. The DEAF–WORLD is accused of resisting cochlear implants because it wants to "steal" the Deaf child. Some Deaf people, afraid that the hearing world is out to destroy their culture, tend to see hearing people who make overtures as threats, potential Trojan horses. And yet we know that it is possible to bridge the divide. Encounters like Gloria Cosgrove's with the members of the Metro Silent Club are one way. We hope this book will prove to be another. Communication is vital. And there are many hearing parents in the U.S. and abroad who have learned some signed language, who have come to know Deaf culture and, in the end, to see the coming of their Deaf child as an event that has enriched their lives and their understanding of humanity.

AT THE METRO SILENT CLUB III

It was evening at the Metro Silent Club and the place had come alive. People were signing everywhere in the clubroom. Gloria wondered whether any of them were hearing. She glanced down at her notes, then said, "I've heard that some Deaf people feel strongly that hearing people shouldn't be involved in the DEAF–WORLD. What's your feeling about it?"

Jake shrugged. "It's true there are Deaf people who feel this way, but not everyone does."

"I do," said Henry emphatically. "Don't be offended, Gloria. You asked for the truth, after all. But my perspective is that hearing people should stay out of my world. When I was working, I spent all day with

hearing people, and when I was done I wanted to go home to my own people. Spanish-speaking people like Roberto's family, who go to work in a factory where most people are Anglo, go home to their culture at the end of the day. I'd rather go home to my DEAF-WORLD, to be with my people."

"But what about hearing people who sign well?"

Henry shook his head. "There's still a difference. Hearing people may learn to sign to be able to communicate with Deaf people, but is the DEAF-WORLD their world?"

Gloria wasn't sure she understood the question. Laurel sensed her confusion and explained. "I think what Henry is saying is that even hearing people who speak ASL very well still have the option of leaving the DEAF-WORLD any time they want and going back to their hearing world. It's not that Deaf people don't want to mingle with hearing people, it's that we make this world our place. Hearing people are like visitors who can stay a while, but not live here. Right?" Laurel glanced at Henry.

"Sort of," Henry replied. "I'm really asking, Where do hearing people feel their home is?"

Gloria wasn't offended; if that was the way Henry felt, so be it. But her gut-level reaction was negative. Henry's argument seemed not so different from the rationale behind every selective club in the world: We're not prejudiced, we just want to be with our own kind. *She glanced at the other three. "Do you agree with him?" she asked.*

Laurel said, "Generally, yes. The DEAF-WORLD is a social network. Take the Gay community, for example."

Now, Roberto shook his head in disagreement, and Laurel said quickly, "I am not comparing Deaf people with Gay people, but there is a parallel. Look, straight people can mingle with Gays if they want to, but then Gays prefer to socialize with each other, because they have a lot of things in common. I know because one of my roommates is Gay, and I have been involved with the community. They share customs and values and concerns. Well, so do Deaf people. And there's no way hearing people can walk in their shoes. That's just a fact."

"I agree with that," Roberto said.

But now Jake was shaking his head. "What about codas? They're hearing, but they're part of the DEAF-WORLD, aren't they?"

"Well, are they?" Henry asked.

Jake nodded. "I think they are. I think whether you're Deaf or hearing is irrelevant. What's important is understanding and valuing Deaf culture and ASL competency. If one is able to act in ways that fit the DEAF–WORLD, and to communicate, then you can socialize without a problem, and you should be able to if you want to, whether you are Deaf or hearing."

Henry countered, "I see your point, but I still disagree. The bottom line is that hearing people, whether they're codas or not, are still able to jump off the DEAF–WORLD boat and get on the hearing-world boat whenever they want to."

"So what?" Roberto said. "My problem about hearing people in the DEAF–WORLD has nothing to do with whether they're hearing or not, or welcome or not. It has to do with them thinking they can come in and take control of our lives."

"Can you give me some examples?" Gloria asked. "What do you mean?"

Roberto replied, "Okay, in schools where there are Deaf children, hearing people are in charge. For example, where I was mainstreamed, there were no Deaf teachers except for one in junior high school. All the other teachers and the principal were hearing and didn't communicate very well with Deaf children. In the residential schools, you'd expect to find more Deaf people running things, but it isn't true. For example, a school for the Deaf near here had an opening for a superintendent recently. Some Deaf people applied, but guess who they chose? A hearing person. Seven years after the Gallaudet Revolution!"

"But what if this person was the most qualified?" Gloria asked.

"Come on, Gloria, are you suggesting that there is no qualified Deaf person around? As the students at Gallaudet said, 'If that's true, then there must be something wrong with the way hearing people have run Deaf education.' If it isn't able to produce any qualified Deaf people, something is definitely wrong."

"So you wouldn't consider a hearing person at all, even if she or he was qualified in every way?" asked Gloria.

This time it was Jake who answered. "You're putting us on the hot spot there, Gloria. We're inclined to say yes, choose the Deaf person, even though we know that there are many qualified hearing people out there. But there are many qualified Deaf people out there, too. If this hearing person is pro-Deaf—that is, if he or she is able to see that Deaf language and DEAF–WORLD values should be an integral part of the school life of Deaf children, then that person might be great for the job. But Roberto and Henry are right, too. Something needs to be done to change the institutional arrangements that create a bias, always, in favor of those who are hearing."

Laurel added, "I want to make sure you understand what we're talking about. We want to work together with hearing people and share the decision-making. So far it hasn't been shared. I get the feeling we are leaving you with the impression we want to throw all hearing people out of the schools for the Deaf and prevent them from having anything to do with Deaf people and children."

"That's not far off," Gloria said wryly. "Is it true?"

"How could it be?" Henry said. "Obviously we can't throw away hearing people. Most of our parents are hearing. But what we find happening is that nobody bothers to ask for Deaf people's input on anything that affects our lives, from medical practice to kindergarten schooling. We want a piece of the action. If we have to seize control to get it, as we did at Gallaudet, we will."

"You mentioned medical practice," Gloria said. "Were you thinking about cochlear implants? Where do you stand on that?"

"It's a sensitive issue," said Jake. "If I may speak for most of us, we don't have a problem with cochlear implants for adults. But for children who were born Deaf, No! It's exposing children to an invasive experimental surgical procedure for dubious reasons and even more dubious results."

"My parents have asked me to consider getting a cochlear implant," Laurel said. "Can you believe it? I refused to talk to them for weeks after they suggested it. It made me realize that they still do not accept me for what I am. My mother is on the board of the oral school I went to, and they now have a huge program for implant children. So naturally my mother feels there is something that could still be done to me. But the fact that I understand where she's coming from doesn't make me want to forgive her."

"If more and more Deaf children get cochlear implants and are kept away from the DEAF–WORLD, that would mean the end of Deaf culture," Henry said.

"I don't think that's going to happen," Jake said. "It's my under-

standing that though the procedure is very invasive, an implant is just another kind of hearing aid, a built-in hearing aid. When hearing aids came into vogue, Deaf culture never faded away. Instead, we threw away the hearing aids. I think that when these implanted kids get older, they may get angry at their parents for making the implant decision for them when they were young. Look how angry Laurel is, and she could always take off her hearing aid. Or flush it down the toilet. With a cochlear implant, what can you do? Flush your head down the toilet?"

Everyone except Gloria laughed. "But would any of you have one?" she persisted.

"No!" They were all agreed, though Laurel said she knew of a few former classmates who were either totally in the hearing world or marginally in the Deaf, and they would do it.

Gloria glanced at her watch. "It's almost time for me to leave," she said, "but I want to come back to one issue. Jake said earlier that I would eventually understand it, but I still don't. It's about Deaf children. You would really like to have more of them?"

Henry glanced at the others. "Hearing people have so much trouble with this," he said. "It would sound better to them if we said we don't want Deaf children."

Gloria nodded in assent, but wondered if that really made any more sense.

"Well, I know I want Deaf children," Laurel said. "Anyway, it's codas who have a rough time of it. Of course, you can't be sure in marrying a Deaf person that it will work out the way it did for Henry. But there's a place you can go to get genetic counseling.

"Gloria, look," Henry said. "I'm happy my kids are like me. I know what to do for them, and we can share the same experiences, the same world. Why is that so difficult to understand?"

"Besides," Jake said, "Deaf kids are the future of the DEAF–WORLD. They will carry our language, our culture, our society into the next generation. I know what the problem is: You still see the Deaf child as a victim, someone who can't hear and who will have a rough time of it in a hearing world. But it's no more a hearing world than a white world or a man's world. We have our place in it."

"Of course, I agree. It's not that," Gloria said. "It's just that, if you

ask hearing people to understand that you want children like yourself and you want to see the continuation of your culture, then you must see that hearing parents want the same things and cannot have them with a Deaf child. So no matter how much they accept the DEAF–WORLD and their child's role in it, they are bound to have a regret."

"Well, then, let them have their regret and get on with it," Laurel said, visibly annoyed. "If I have a hearing child, I'm not going to dwell for long on what might have been. I'm going to love that child and do my best to help her learn about the hearing world and the DEAF–WORLD."

"You know," Roberto said, "in these changing times, I sometimes wonder about the future of our DEAF–WORLD. I wonder if hearing people will ever understand us. Do you see any hope?" he asked Gloria.

Gloria nodded. "I believe so," she said. "Some of us are trying."

"We'll see how your article turns out. It had better be good," Henry said, smiling. "Most reporters think they understand us when they write about our views and our world. But then it turns out they really don't."

"It's a challenge," Gloria said, glancing at Jake.

"You'll get it right," he said. "You know, many Deaf people believe we are made this way for a reason. Some say, God's will. One hears Deaf people say that 'God gave me this gift.' I myself think the gift lies in the blessings bestowed on us through having a close-knit DEAF–WORLD, where every member is like a member of a huge extended family. I hope you can make your readers see that. I mean the gift."

❦

Chapter 14

The Hearing Agenda II: Eradicating the DEAF-WORLD

BECAUSE the hearing agenda for Deaf people is constructed on the principle that members of the DEAF–WORLD have a disability, and because our society seeks to reduce the numbers of people with disabilities through preventive measures, hearing people have long sought ways to reduce the numbers of Deaf people, ultimately eliminating this form of human variation and with it the DEAF–WORLD. The chairman of a National Institutes of Health planning group acknowledged this in a 1993 interview with *The New York Times*: "I am dedicated to curing deafness. That puts me on a collision course with those who are culturally Deaf. That is interpreted as genocide of the Deaf."[1] Two measures that would reduce the numbers of Deaf people and are actively pursued today in many lands are eugenics and cochlear implant surgery on young Deaf children.

REPRODUCTIVE CONTROL OF DEAF PEOPLE

Hearing efforts to regulate childbearing by Deaf people have a long history which has not yet ended. Prior to the Enlightenment, Deaf scions of wealthy families, especially women, were frequently sequestered in religious institutions; this not only ensured their chastity, it kept them out of sight: if one child was known to be Deaf, other children would be less marriageable. Indeed, it was this practice of sequestering Deaf children in religious institutions in sixteenth century Spain that led Ponce de León to develop, at the monastery of Oña, the first recorded method of teaching the Deaf to speak.[2] With the beginnings of education for Deaf people as a group in eighteenth century France, Deaf boys and girls were not only strictly segregated in schools (a common, if less rigorous, practice with hearing children), but also Deaf girls were sent, on graduation, to special asylums with the explicit purpose of preventing their circulation in society at large.[3] Laws refusing primogeniture to Deaf-mutes, laws restricting consanguineous marriage, and laws specifically prohibiting or discouraging Deaf marriage, all had the effect of discouraging Deaf people from marrying and reproducing.[4] Such laws reflected values in society at large and presumably reinforced efforts by hearing parents to discourage their Deaf children from marrying and reproducing.

Before the advent of residential schools for the Deaf, marriages of Deaf people were relatively rare.[5] When scattered Deaf children gathered in residential schools, Deaf marriages were facilitated through increased contacts. Many educators were vigorously opposed to Deaf marriages, however, and they vigilantly kept boys and girls separated, while urging celibacy on the pupils.[6]

The stated goal of the movement for oral education of Deaf children that arose and flourished in the second half of the nineteenth century was not so much to enable Deaf people to speak with their neighbors, shopkeepers and the like; nor was it to facilitate their learning written English. In fact, the stated goal was not primarily educational at all. It was to discourage reproduction by Deaf people by discouraging their socializing and marriage.[7] The founder of this movement in the U.S., Samuel Gridley Howe, superintendent of the Perkins Institution for the Blind, appeared before a Massachusetts Legislative Commission in 1867 to support the establishment of the first oral school for the Deaf in America, the Clarke School. Howe assailed the network of state residential schools for the Deaf, which, he contended, fomented intermarriage of these defectives. "You would discountenance association between deaf-mutes?" the commission chairman asked. "Entirely," Howe replied, "but mind you, I would not discountenance association between them and other persons. I would endeavor to prevent the effects of their infirmity by bringing them into relations as close as possible with ordinary persons so that their infirmity should be, so to speak, wiped out of sight."[8]

In the following decades, more oral schools were founded while others abandoned ASL in favor of spoken English. Again, an explicit motive was the regulation of Deaf reproduction. For example, in the heated debate over a Nebraska law, which required the state residential school for the Deaf to use oral methods only, the president of the National Education Association weighed in with this support of oralism: Deaf people who sign "tend to segregate themselves from society—to intermarry. [They are] freaks, dummies."[9]

However, Deaf schoolmates intermarried whether their residential school used ASL or English. More stringent means of separation would be required to keep them apart. That meant boarding them at home and instructing them in small classes to minimize contact. This was the aim of the day-school movement, which began in Wisconsin in the late 1800s and was championed and funded in part by Alexander Graham Bell.[10] Day schools, Bell told Wisconsin lawmakers, allow "keeping deaf-mutes separated from one another as much as possible."[11] He warned of the dangers of Deaf congregation at the state residential school. An 1894 attempt by educators to expand the day-school law and reduce class size to four or five Deaf pupils provided that "congenital deaf-mutes of opposite sexes shall be kept apart as much as possible and marriage between them discouraged."[12] The next major day-school movement began in Chicago. The Chicago Board of Education similarly declared that day schools were valuable because they prevented Deaf intermarriage and the production of Deaf offspring.[13]

Hearing people have embarked on direct as well as indirect programs to restrict Deaf reproduction. In this century, there have been movements in the United States and in Germany, for example, to sterilize Deaf people by law and to encourage Deaf people in voluntary sterilization. The legal initiative in the United States had limited success, but its well-publicized pursuit led untold numbers of Deaf people to abandon plans for marriage and reproduction or to submit to voluntary sterilization, and untold numbers of hearing parents to have their Deaf children sterilized.[14] Alexander Graham Bell, head of the Eugenics Section of the American Breeders Association (later the American Genetics Association), laid the groundwork for such efforts in his numerous statistical studies and censuses of the Deaf population in the United States and, especially, in his 1883 *Memoir Upon the Formation of a Deaf Variety of the Human Race,* which he printed privately and distributed widely. Moreover, he presented this broadside against Deaf culture and Deaf intermarriage to the National Academy of Sciences on his election to that body, giving the false impression that it was sanctioned by the academy and was scientifically valid. In *Memoir*, Bell warned that "the congenital deaf-mutes of the country are increasing at a greater rate than the population at large; and the deaf-mute children of deaf-mutes at a greater rate than the congenital deaf-mute population."[15] Bell attributed the problem to signed language, which "causes the intermarriage of deaf-mutes and the propagation of their physical defect."[16] The Eugenics Section prepared a model sterilization law and promoted it in the nation's state legislatures; it called for sterilization of feebleminded, insane, criminalistic, deaf, and other "socially unfit" classes.[17] By the time of the German sterilization program, some thirty states in the U.S. had sterilization laws in force. However, none of them specifically included Deaf people.

It is difficult to find a rationale for Bell's actions, and for those of other advocates for reproductive regulation of Deaf people, if they are taken at face value. The tables of data in *Memoir* show that only one percent of the pupils in Bell's sample had two Deaf parents; hence it was evident that if all Deaf couples in the U.S. stopped reproducing entirely, either through birth control or sterilization, there would be an insignificant reduction in the Deaf population. For the same reason, it must have been evident to him and other advocates of day schools, oral education, and other measures to discourage Deaf socialization, that such measures, even if totally successful, would have a trivial impact. A statistical study of the Deaf population conducted with funding from Bell showed that there was no greater likelihood of a Deaf child if both parents were Deaf than if only one was, and that Deaf married Deaf three-fourths of the time no matter whether the partners attended manual or oral schools, residential or day schools.[18] All of this must have been known by Bell and other eugenicists.

Consequently, the purpose of the eugenics movement with respect to Deaf people, of the measures aimed at discouraging their socialization, intermarriage and reproduction, could not have truly been to achieve those goals, which were largely unachievable and would be ineffective if achieved. Instead, the purpose must have been to reinforce a certain social construction of Deaf people, one that was linked to the construction of people with impairments such as feeblemindedness and to a particular non-infirm establishment with its own authorities, legislation, institutions and professions. Moreover, the eugenics campaign marked the DEAF–WORLD as an important social problem requiring expertise, one that had been previously overlooked, much to the danger of society. In this respect, the claims-making closely paralleled the movement to awaken society to the dangers of mentally retarded people in our midst. We may surmise that, as psychologists and superintendents of institutions for the feebleminded stood to gain from the recognition of the newly discovered social problem of mild retardation, so a competent authority that stood to gain from the construction of Deaf people as a newly-discovered menace was the burgeoning organization Bell had founded, the American Association to Promote the Teaching of Speech to the Deaf. In 1969, this association, now known as the Alexander Graham Bell Association for the Deaf, republished Bell's *Memoir* without disclaimers, still warning stridently of the "calamitous results to their offspring" of Deaf intermarriage.[19]

The eugenics movement as it concerned Deaf people worldwide has received regrettably little study.[20] When National Socialism came to power in Germany, fully forty organizations of the Deaf in Berlin were combined into two; the treasuries of the original organizations were confiscated; the Jewish Deaf Association was prohibited, and Jewish members of all other Deaf organizations were expelled. Teachers of the Deaf advocated adherence to the hereditary purity laws, including the sterilization of congenitally Deaf people. Deaf school children were required to prepare family trees, and the school reported those who were congenitally Deaf or who had a Deaf relative to the Department of Health for possible sterilization. Leaders of the unified Deaf organization and the Deaf newspaper, themselves late-deafened, endorsed the sterilization campaign.[21]

The German sterilization law that went into effect in 1934 provided that: "Those hereditarily sick may be made unfruitful (sterilized) through surgical intervention . . . [Among] hereditary sick, in the sense of this law, is the person who suffers from . . . hereditary deafness. . . ."[22] The census of 1933 showed forty-five thousand "deaf and dumb" persons in a total population of over sixty-six million. An estimated seventeen thousand of these Deaf Germans, a third of them minors, were sterilized. In nine percent of the cases, sterilization was accompanied by forced abortion. An additional sixteen hundred Deaf people were exterminated in concentration camps in the 1940s; they were considered "useless eaters," with lives unworthy of being lived.[23] As in the United States, the medical profession was the certifying authority for forced sterilization. And as in the United States, the overriding purpose may have been to reinforce their authority in the solution of perceived social problems.

In 1992, researchers at Boston University announced that they had identified the "genetic error responsible for the most common type of inherited deafness."[24] The director of the National Institute on Deafness and Other Communication Disorders (NIDCD, one of the National Institutes of Health) called the finding a "major breakthrough that will improve diagnosis and genetic counseling and ultimately lead to substitution therapy or gene transfer therapy." Thus a new form of medical eugenics applied to Deaf people was envisioned, in this case by an agency of the U.S. government. The primary characteristics of Deaf people with this genetic background are numerous Deaf relatives, signed language fluency, facial features such as widely spaced eyebrows, and coloring features such as a white forelock and freckling.[25] For such characteristics to be viewed primarily not as normal human variation in physiognomy, coloring, etc., but as a "genetic error," some of the common features must clearly be construed as signs of a disease or infirmity. In fact, according to a leading medical geneticist, the "sole detrimental feature" of the syndrome is that some of these people are Deaf.[26] Within the culture of the DEAF-WORLD, then, this cannot be a disease.

In the director's statement to the press, there were several explicit claims. In short, he claimed a major breakthrough that would enhance diagnosis and genetic counseling and lead to genetic engineering. There are further claims implied by his statement: this human variation is a disease and hence should be avoided; society's interest in avoiding it outweighs any individual or group's desire to continue it; medical research such as the institute supports has led to this achievement, and the public's investment in its research is justified in part by these developments; the competent authority in these matters is medical authority.

In its *National Strategic Research Plan* issued the same year, the NIDCD points out that at least half of all children born Deaf or who become so early in life are Deaf by virtue of heredity. The strategic plan continues: "The insertion of genetic material into cells to prevent or ameliorate hereditary hearing impairment may soon become a possible treatment option."[27] The foundation of the hearing agenda for the DEAF–WORLD on a disability model could not be clearer. Since all forms of human variation are genetically determined, but the genetic causes for only some of these are actively sought, the pursuit of such genetic causes tells much about how that variation is construed as a social problem. Federally funded research in the U.S. is currently seeking to uncover the hereditary basis for some people being Gay, others Deaf, and for an alleged intellectual inferiority of Black Americans. Research on the genetics of heterosexuality, hearing, and Caucasian intelligence, such as it is, reflects quite a different construction of those social groups.

The NIDCD explicitly addresses this issue in its strategic plan, where it acknowledges that "many Deaf individuals believe that deafness is not a disorder but a culturally defining condition."[28] Because the statement makes this a matter of individual belief among Deaf people (whereas it is a tenet of Deaf culture), and because the statement makes no mention of what hearing people believe, there is the implication that the authors of the statement and other such authorities have a different and perhaps more objective view of the matter. The statement goes on to say, however, that the NIDCD respects "the cultural integrity of Deaf society." What construction of Deaf people would allow the institute logically to support eugenic measures for limiting the membership of the DEAF–WORLD, all the while respecting the cultural integrity of Deaf society? The institute planners were willing to acknowledge, it seems, that there was a problem, but that was as far as they were prepared to go. Elsewhere in the report, the institute's commitment to a single, underlying construction of all people with limited hearing is as clear as its name: It calls for genetic research to improve diagnosis, counseling, and gene therapy, all with a view to reducing the numbers of children who enter the DEAF–WORLD. On the face of it, it is unethical to seek to prevent a "culturally defining condition." Is genetic counseling available for mixed-race couples? For homosexual prospective parents? For what culturally defining conditions is it available?

The main reason that issues like gene therapy generate strong feelings and invite pronouncements by various leaders and organizations is not because of direct practical consequences. Rather, they reveal underlying and conflicting constructions of Deaf people. Similarly, surgeons and audiologists in the lead to surgically implant young Deaf children (see below) discourage parents from allowing their children to use signed language. For example, a 1992 manual on the management of implanted Deaf children steers parents away from schools that use Total Communication as follows: "Most implanted children who used TC prior to implantation will always depend on sign to some degree and many will never develop the skills to communicate without it."[29] Such advice is given not because of any evidence that signed language would detract from the child's learning English (indeed, the available evidence points to the contrary), but because the child with a surgically implanted prosthesis is the archetype of a certain construction of Deaf people, while the signer is the archetype of a diametrically opposed construction. Thus to sign is symbolically to negate the construction of Deaf people that has motivated the costly surgery, and the efforts of the surgeons, audiologists, speech therapists, special educators, and others.

COCHLEAR IMPLANT SURGERY ON DEAF CHILDREN

The most sorely contested issue in the collision between the DEAF-WORLD and medical professionals is the growing practice of surgically implanting cochlear implants in Deaf children. The box on page 388 shows the components of a cochlear implant and describes the implantation surgery and the way the device works.

Concise history of cochlear implants

The first cochlear implant was implanted in a late-deafened adult in Paris by Dr. Charles Eyries. The patient terminated use one year later. In 1961, the first American implants were done by Dr. William House, inspired by the French. In general, the reaction of the scientific community was negative. Ear specialists protested that the basic scientific research hadn't been done. The inner ear of the patient was being destroyed in what amounted to an experimental procedure with no reason to expect that such a crude device would work and every reason to think that it would not, since the original implant recipient had stopped using the device.

In the 1970s, the French, undeterred by the initial negative results, resumed their experiments, to media acclaim (see below), and the first children were implanted by Dr. Claude-Henri Chouard in Paris. The French association of the parents of Deaf children protested that their children were being used as guinea pigs, and the French scientific community also reacted negatively. Nevertheless, Australian and Austrian implant programs began, using improved technology. The original implant had been a "single channel" device. The newest device, the Australian Nucleus-22 implant, contained twenty-two bands on the wire, which allowed the positioning of some of the components of speech sounds in distinctive places in the inner ear. Manufacturing agreements were reached with commercial firms.

In 1985, the U.S. Food and Drug Administration (FDA) approved the marketing of the Nucleus-22 implant for adults who had been deafened after learning to speak, and the *experimental* implanting of the device in children as young as two. The procedure continued to be used on children as well as adults in other countries, despite the resistance of organizations of parents in Great Britain, the Netherlands, and Sweden. In the U.S., the first protest from the DEAF–WORLD at the implantation of children came in 1985 from the Greater Los Angeles Council of the Deaf. The World Federation of the Deaf also condemned "experimentation on Deaf children." By the end of 1990, however, approximately 600 children worldwide had been implanted with the Australian Nucleus-22 device.

In 1990, the FDA approved the marketing of the Nucleus-22 implant for children two years old and older, stating that there were 166 implant centers in the U.S. The Canadian government followed suit. The protests of the Canadian, Danish, Dutch, German, Norwegian, Swedish, and American national associations of the Deaf received wide media coverage, but the implants continued. Harlan's book, *The Mask of Benevolence*, published in 1992, criticized the practice of implanting young children, especially children who were born Deaf or had been deafened before learning to speak, and raised numerous ethical issues. In the same year, the Alexander Graham Bell Association published a book on the "management" of the implanted child.[33]

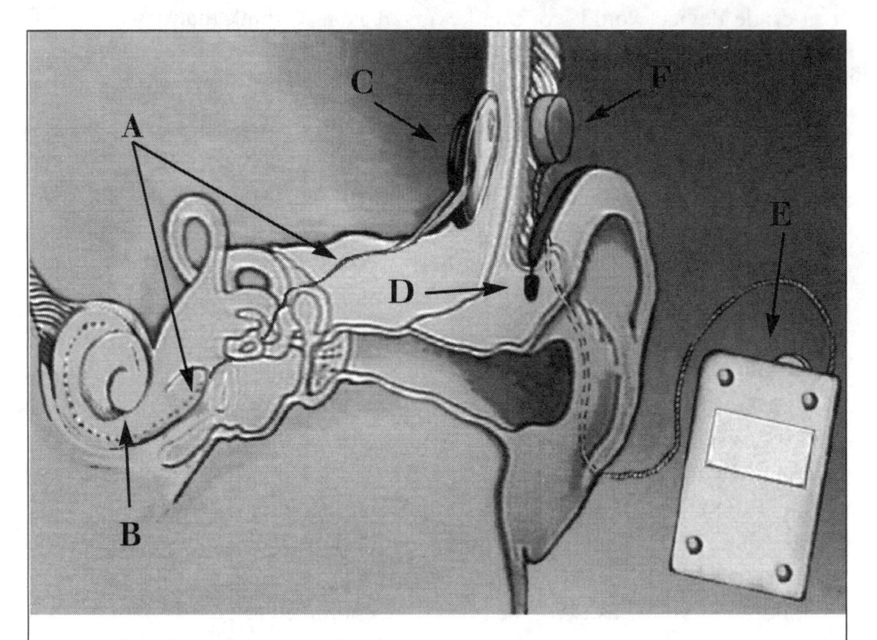

Fig. 14-1. **A cochlear implant**

Implantation of a Multichannel Implant

The hospitalized child is placed under general anesthesia for three to four hours. The surgeon cuts the skin behind the ear, raises the flap, and drills a hole in the bone. Then a wire carrying electrodes (A) is pushed some twenty-five millimeters into the coiled inner ear (B). The tiny endings of the auditory nerve are destroyed and electrical fields from the wire stimulate the auditory nerve directly. A small receiver coil connected to the wire is sutured to the skull (C) and the skin is sewn over it. A small microphone worn on an ear piece (D) picks up sound and sends signals to a processor (E) worn on a belt or in a pocket. The processor sends electrical signals back to the implanted receiver via a transmitter mounted behind the ear (F), and those signals stimulate the auditory nerve.

Deaf opposition

Organizations of Deaf people around the world have vigorously protested the practice of childhood cochlear implant surgery. A national demonstration against childhood cochlear implants was conducted by Swiss Deaf people in March of 1993. A few months later, eight hundred people demonstrated in Lyons, France, where hearing advocates of cochlear implants for children were conducting the First National Information Day for Parents. Refused admission to the congress hall despite their having registered by mail, the organization *Sourds en Colère* (Deaf Anger) gained access only after three hours, when a television crew arrived. Refused permission to address the meeting, the demonstrators blocked exits from the congress hall with human chains and engaged small groups of congress-goers in discussion as they were trying to leave. The Deaf demands: a stop to childhood implants and a broad-based commission of inquiry (they would ultimately get their official commission of inquiry). Between one and two thousand demonstrators turned out in Paris in November of that year under the leadership of *Sourds en Colère* to bring their demands to national attention. Refused admission to the national welfare offices despite an appointment, the demonstrators marched to the National Institute for Young Deaf, which many had attended as students and where now several ranks of riot police awaited them. Some of the demonstrators went on to the Saint Antoine Hospital and sought to engage the French implant pioneer, otosurgeon Claude-Henri Chouard, in discussion. A few weeks later, *Sourds en Colère* brought their case before an open meeting of the French National Committee on Ethics. During the discussion time, Deaf leaders unfurled banners and described the ethical issues to the assembly. Some of the delegates stated that the surgery appeared to violate laws on the protection of human subjects in medical research.

In January of 1994, representatives of the Ontario, Canada Deaf community demonstrated at entrances to legislative and hospital buildings to protest a recent government decision to launch a 1.7 million dollar childhood cochlear implant program. They called for an end to "experimental cochlear implant surgery on children," and the establishment of a commission of inquiry. The Canadian Association of the Deaf, calling for a moratorium on cochlear implants for Deaf children, sponsored rallies in several cities in May, 1994. A Toronto Star headline the next day read: "People Born Deaf Have Right to Keep their 'Silent but Rich Culture,' say 100 at Noisy Demonstration."

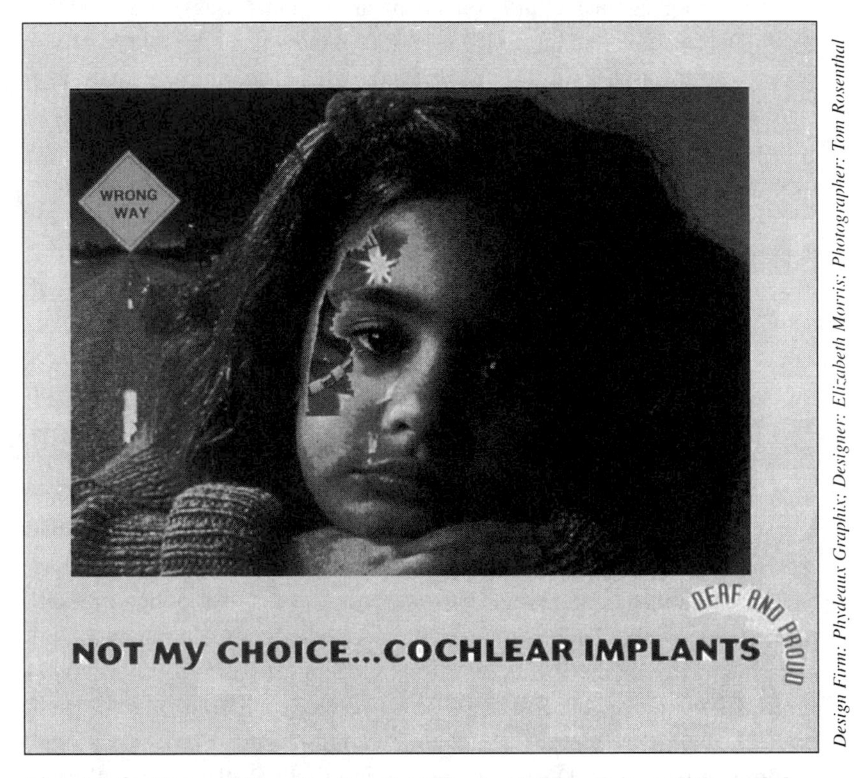

Design Firm: Phydeaux Graphix; Designer: Elizabeth Morris; Photographer: Tom Rosenthal

Fig. 14-2. ***Wrong Way*; Deaf artist Elizabeth Morris' rendition of the DEAF–WORLD perspective on childhood cochlear implants**

Fourteen national associations of the Deaf around the world have published position papers disapproving of implant surgery on Deaf children. The U.S. National Association of the Deaf condemned unrestricted marketing of cochlear implants for children down to the age of two as "unsound scientifically, procedurally, and ethically." In its 1991 position paper, the NAD stated that the surgery remains highly experimental, without evidence of significant benefit, and without evaluation of long-term risks, social, psychological, linguistic, and medical.[34] It criticized the Food and Drug Administration for failing to involve Deaf people in decisions concerning Deaf children and the implant. And it questioned whether it is ethical to use surgery in an attempt to move a child out of a linguistic and cultural minority and into the majority culture.

The 1993 position paper of *Sourds en Colère* lists twelve demands, among them: recognition of the Deaf community, its language and its culture, and dissemination of information about the community in the schools; a halt to government subsidized childhood implants; access to full information about implants and the right to participate in conferences and counseling of parents.[35] A position paper the same year by the Canadian Cultural Society of the Deaf concludes that the surgery is not justified in view of "the psychological trauma, the confusion of identity, and the loss of self-esteem it might foster in profoundly Deaf children."[36] The position paper of the Canadian Association of the Deaf affirms: "Cochlear implants do not restore hearing . . . [We] question whether an increase in hearing . . . for environmental sounds is worth the risk, expense . . . [Implant surgery] perpetuates the view of deafness as a pathological condition . . . [There is] no proof that the device improves the educational achievement of Deaf children . . . It does not justify the emotional, physical and psychological suffering that the implanted child undergoes in the years before he/she recognizes and accepts his/her identity as a member of the Deaf community."[37]

The Danish Deaf Association in its position paper the same year states that the operation should not be performed on Deaf children. They find a lack of research into the sociological and psychological consequences of the surgery, and a lack of information concerning Deaf culture on the part of parents considering the implants.[38] The Netherlands Deaf Association disapproves of childhood implant surgery as long as the patient has no say in the decision. The Austrian Deaf Association describes the position of its membership as "very negative" on childhood implant surgery. The Swedish Deaf Association states: "[Our organization, as well as] the Association of Parents of Deaf, Hard-of-Hearing and Speech-Impaired Children, and the Association of the Hard-of-Hearing do not approve of cochlear implants for children under the age of 18." The Norwegian Deaf Association has taken the following position: "The parents' section is against cochlear implants for children under the age of 18, but accepts the operation for deafened people over the age of 18." The position paper of the German Deaf Association concludes: "[We] reject cochlear implantation of Deaf children when this procedure leads to separating the implanted children from other Deaf children and is associated with an exclusively oral language orientation." The British Deaf Association "does not accept the negative model of deafness as a pathological defect to be cured or eradicated"; it calls for extended research on the consequences of childhood implants and is "unable to recommend" them for children. The World Federation of the Deaf resolved at its 1995 World Congress that "the congress does not recommend cochlear implant operations for Deaf children because cochlear implants will not help the language acquisition of a Deaf child and can harm the emotional/psychological personality development and physical development."[39]

Positions of medical organizations

In the United States, a 1988 medical conference aimed at creating a consensus on cochlear implant surgery (no Deaf people participated) concluded that the usual implant candidate is a healthy adult who lost hearing after learning spoken language and who does not get any benefit in lipreading from a hearing aid. The conference concluded that the most common benefit of cochlear implants is some improvement in lipreading. It found, furthermore, that it is not possible to predict who will benefit from an implant and that patients with implants must avoid contact sports, magnetic resonance imagery (MRI) and some other medical procedures. The conference recommended that children should receive implants only after a six-month trial of hearing aids with no success. And it cautioned that "children with implants still must be regarded as hearing-impaired [and] will continue to require educational, audiological, and speech and language support services for long periods of time."[40] Perhaps initiated in part because of the vigorous protests against childhood implants coming from the DEAF–WORLD and disseminated in the media, or by the reservations of some audiologists and otosurgeons, a second consensus conference was held by the National Institutes of Health in 1995. To many of those present, the consensus seemed assured beforehand. There were no formal presentations by Deaf scholars (although public interest groups, including the NAD, were invited to address the meeting for five minutes), nor by hearing professionals who had expressed grave reservations. Four of twenty-five presentations, including the report on speech perception benefit in children born Deaf, listed an implant manufacturer as their professional affiliation; approximately eighty percent of the remaining presentations were by surgeons or paramedical professionals who were supported by NIH in their programs of cochlear implantation. The conference concluded that adults who became deaf after learning spoken language demonstrate significantly enhanced lipreading with an implant. Adults deafened before learning spoken language show little improvement. Improvements in children's speech perception and production are often reported. The language and educational outcomes of childhood implants are not well known, but oral language development remains slow and training intensive.[41]

The 1989 position statement of the American Academy of Otolaryngology–Head and Neck Surgery finds "implants an acceptable procedure in prelingual children when approved [by regulatory agencies]."[42] (A *prelingual* child is one who lost hearing before mastering oral language.) A leading implant surgeon has defended to his colleagues the ethics of cochlear implant surgery on children. His article in the January 1994 issue of the *American Journal of Otology* finds childhood implants ethical since (1) to be Deaf is to have "a handicap and a disability," (2) the question of their effectiveness "should no longer be asked," and (3) Deaf children of hearing parents are not members of the Deaf community.[43]

Many otosurgeons are now performing cochlear implant surgery on children. By one estimate, nearly two thousand Deaf children have received implants. Many of these children have been implanted at specialized centers organized for this purpose with an extensive staff that includes, in addition to the surgeon, audiologists, speech-language therapists, hearing therapists, and special educators, administrators, and access to radiologists and social workers. The Nucleus-22 implant costs about fifteen thousand dollars. Additional medical expenses and post-operative training can cost another fifteen thousand. In the United States, as in many other countries, contributions toward the expense come from government research funds, health insurance, charities, and the child's family.

The media and the "miracle"

The advent of cochlear implant surgery for Deaf children was widely heralded in the media as a miracle. Some headlines from the British press include: "Upton Boy Can Hear At Last!"; "Girl with a New Song in Her Heart"; "Children Head Queue for Bionic Ears." The term *bionic ear* suggests to many not only a cure for hearing loss but actually an improvement over normal hearing.[44] Headlines in the U.S. included: "New Hope for Deaf Children: Implant Gives Them Hearing and Speech" (*American Health*); "Breaking the Sound Barrier" (*Boston Herald*); "Sweet Music for the Deaf" (*Newsweek*); "With Implant and Hard Work, Deaf People Can Hear, Speak" (*L.A. Life*); "Ears for the Deaf, Eyes for the Blind" (*John Hopkins Medical News*).

The opposition of Deaf organizations and individuals to childhood implant surgery has also received extensive media coverage. With rare exception, however, the coverage of the DEAF–WORLD position compares unfavorably with that announcing the "miracle" of implants. In some cases the reporting is openly hostile, as in the French headline, "The Deaf: Those Who Refuse to Listen." In others, the bias is more subtle, leaving the reader with the impression that Deaf people are anti-social and their demands unreasonable. Even in the most sincere attempts at neutrality on the issues, the hearing author's or commentator's conviction that to be Deaf is not merely another way to be, but a tragic impairment, seems to surface. This is why Jake and the others at the Metro Silent Club are wary of being interviewed by Gloria Cosgrove. They fear that she will misrepresent them as they have characteristically been misrepresented.

In the U.S., several nationally televised news magazines covered the story. In Great Britain, in 1994, the BBC aired a debate on the topic. At least two televised programs on the controversy were shown in Canada. A Canadian newspaper headline reads: "Ontario Deaf Community Opposes Experimental Ear Implant for Kids." Recent French headlines, in translation, include: "Deaf People Opposed to Artificial Ears"; "The Debate between the Deaf and the Doctors on Ear Implants"; "Deaf People Raising a Ruckus." And in the U.S.: "Deaf Denounce Cochlear Implants"; "Deaf Conference on Controversy Draws Crowds"; "Some Deaf Won't Join the Hearing"; "Deaf Say Hearing Aid Collides with

Their Culture"; "Implant Alarms Many of the Deaf"; "Two Ways of Looking at Deafness."

Research on language benefit

The overriding goal of programs of childhood cochlear implantation is to enable Deaf children to communicate orally. The scientific research to assess whether this goal is achieved is extremely limited.[45] Most of the studies have serious methodological limitations, such as pooling results from distinct groups, selective reporting, neglecting statistical tests of the reliability of findings, and following procedures that allow experimenter-bias to influence results. Therefore, all conclusions must remain tentative for some time to come. There is not a single published case, after a decade of experimentation with the multichannel implant and more than a thousand implanted children, of a child acquiring oral language with an implant.

In general, there are striking differences in performance, using multichannel implants, between the minority of Deaf children who had acquired spoken language by ear before losing their hearing—a mere three percent[46]—and the majority who had not.[47] The Cochlear Corporation (and collaborating research centers) administered several vocabulary tests to a large group of children implanted with the Nucleus-22 multichannel prosthesis. (These were 'open-set' tests, in which the children identified the spoken words without choosing from a set of alternatives.) They found that those children who could recognize at least some words had lost their hearing on the average when they were five years four months old, whereas those who could not recognize words at all using the device had lost their hearing on the average at age one year six months.[48] Audiologists call the former group *postlingual* and the latter *prelingual*. (This distinction rides only on the child's ability to use oral language.) The upper limit of "prelingual" is generally set rather arbitrarily at three years of age, so the grouping includes the vast majority of implant candidates, eighty-six percent of whom are born Deaf, but also a small minority, seven percent of implant candidates, who lost hearing during the first three years of life and may have acquired a little or a lot of English beforehand.

The Cochlear Corporation scientists found that prelingually Deaf children scored only eight percent correct on a particularly easy test of word recognition. Two independent studies using the same test found a median of six percent correct[49] and zero percent correct.[50] * Investigators at the Indiana University Medical School found that prelingually Deaf children had a median score of zero on two other tests of unprompted word recognition.[51] A New York University study administered one of those tests to children who had used their implant for up to three years. Many of the children were unable to do the test. If we assign those children a score of zero, then the median speech recognition score in this study was zero, confirming the Indiana result.[52] Investigators at the University of Iowa confirmed a median score of zero on one of those tests using their own group of prelingually Deaf children, and also found a median score of zero on a different test of unprompted word recognition.[53] Implanted children achieve higher scores in word recognition when prompted with the correct answers visually by pictures or by lipreading. However, most investigators believe that it is not possible to acquire a spoken language using lipreading or pictures. The children's ability to correctly perceive spoken language without prompting is probably the best gauge of their language learning in the absence of direct measures. By that criterion, there is no published evidence as yet that children who have not mastered spoken language by ear will be able to do so using an implant.

A survey in progress of children with implants in sixty-four U.S. residential schools for the Deaf found seventy-five such children in the first thirty schools responding to the survey. Seventy-three percent of those children are no longer using their implants. The disuse rate might be lower if the survey were restricted to oral schools and further restricted to users of the implants with the latest technology; on the other hand, the disuse rate might be higher if there was a representative mix of pre- and postlingually Deaf children in the sample (the preliminary report does not specify devices or ages at onset of hearing loss).[54]

---

* Because an average score can be misleading with small numbers of subjects, many scientists prefer to report the median—the middle score in a rank ordering of the scores. The only studies cited here are those for which the median score obtained by prelingually deaf children could be determined.

In general, the less demanding the definition of "benefit," the greater the percent of implanted children who receive that benefit. Thus, nearly all implanted children can detect environmental sound. A large number can identify many of those sounds. Many implanted children can distinguish some properties of speech sounds even if they cannot identify those sounds. Some children achieve higher lipreading scores with an implant than without one and a few can understand spoken language; these tend to be late-deafened, as we have seen. Some experts believe, however, that the nine out of ten early-deafened children benefit as much from a tactile aid (see chapter 12) as from an implant.[55] Compared with an equally effective implant, the tactile aid presents many advantages: It is relatively cheap, requires no surgery, and is easy to remove. (There is much clearer evidence of perceptual benefit from cochlear implants when it comes to late-deafened adults. For example, one study of recognition of words in sentences found forty-four percent correct by lipreading alone, thirty-one percent using the implant only, and seventy-six percent using both. A second set of sentences, somewhat harder, yielded scores of eighteen, thirteen and fifty-seven percent correct, respectively.[56] There is also reasonable consensus when it comes to teen-agers and adults Deaf since birth or infancy; many implant teams do not consider them appropriate candidates for implantation because of the poor perceptual benefit usually obtained.)

Despite the poor results, however, increasing numbers of Deaf children are being implanted. The consensus that only children with total hearing loss who had tried amplification for six months should be implanted is no longer honored. As implant technology improves and more children are implanted, there may eventually be published evidence that a Deaf child has acquired spoken language using an implant. If so, interpreting that evidence will require information about all the methodological issues raised, especially age at onset of profound hearing loss, language abilities prior to implantation, and artifacts of testing and scoring. If at least one Deaf child has acquired spoken language mediated by the implant, oral advocates will need to know next what conditions favor that acquisition and what percent of children born Deaf can achieve it. It seems to be a relatively rare achievement, since the median speech perception benefit in study after study has been zero, and there are no published cases of a Deaf child acquiring spoken language to date.

Critical periods and cochlear implants

An important force in the growing practice of surgically implanting Deaf children as young as possible is the belief that the ability to acquire language wanes rapidly with age. Chapter 3 discussed this critical period hypothesis in connection with the acquisition of ASL. In brief, children who begin learning ASL in infancy achieve greater mastery than those who begin at school age, and the latter are more proficient, in turn, than those who start in adolescence. In a related finding, Deaf teenagers and adults who were born Deaf are no longer implanted in many medical centers because the results have been so disappointing. Although they are able to learn ASL, they are apparently unable to learn to recognize a significant number of spoken words using the implant. The discouraging results also obtained from children who were born Deaf and implanted at school age, have led many audiologists to speculate that the critical period is over by then and to urge implantation as early as allowed by the FDA (age two). However, there is no research that reveals whether implanting Deaf children as early as possible improves results. The critical period hypothesis for language acquisition may well not apply to aural rehabilitation, with its repetition, feedback, and correction, as these are not a normal part of biologically regulated first-language acquisition.

Although it seems clear that people master languages more readily earlier in life, it is surprising how little can be said with certainty about the critical period hypothesis. It is not clear when the period begins and ends, or if there is a period at all, or if it is critical. The critical period for learning language may be over by age two, at which age hearing and Deaf children are speaking their first sentences (in spoken or signed languages) and have mastered considerable vocabulary. In that event, there is no reason to hasten the surgery since, according to FDA rules, it cannot be conducted before the child has reached two years of age. Since Deaf children do learn ASL later in life, it may be a mistake to think there is a single period; there may be a gradual decline in capacity, starting in infancy, but not ending until adolescence. Or perhaps normal mastery requires starting language learning at birth: Perhaps language mastery progresses in relatively fixed stages, beginning with babbling in the first year of life. Deaf children who acquire ASL as a native language start out with manual babbling, as we have seen. Babbling may reflect a stage in the maturation of the brain for language. To end up with normal language, the child may need to board the nonstop train before it leaves the station.[57] In that case, there is no period in the critical period.

Some advocates for cochlear implants, particularly in Europe, would like to see cochlear-implant surgery conducted much earlier than age two. They argue that the auditory area of the brain degenerates as long as the infant is Deaf, but early stimulation, such as an implant could provide, would slow or reverse that degeneration so that the child with an early implant would have greater capacity to learn spoken language by ear. However, this is all speculation. It is based on research with neonatal mice, rats and gerbils; destroying their hearing reduces neuron number and size in the auditory pathway and area of their brains, and stimulating their hearing with implants slows or reverses degeneration somewhat. However, this has not been demonstrated in humans, nor do we know whether the modest reductions in neuron numbers and size really matter for hearing. For example, the brain might have more than it needs for this purpose, or it may mobilize some other area to offset the loss. In fact, stimulation from an implant could be harmful, for it does not undo the effects of destroying hearing in the laboratory animals; rather, it creates a unique pattern in their nervous tissue, one that is neither that associated with normal hearing nor that associated with deafness. Moreover, there is evidence that, in people who grow up Deaf, some brain tissue used for hearing in hearing people has been reallocated for visual information processing.[58] A little auditory stimulation might block this reorganization of the brain without providing usable hearing, so the child would not acquire spoken language and would be hampered in acquiring signed language.[59] In light of all this uncertainty and speculation by the experts on when to implant Deaf children—if at all—it is perhaps clearer why the World Federation of the Deaf was moved to condemn "experimentation on Deaf children."

Ethical problems with cochlear implant surgery

It must be an unparalleled event in medical history for organizations of adults to raise such an outcry against medical intervention for children like themselves. Cochlear implant surgery on young Deaf children encounters serious ethical problems that have not received widespread discussion and thoughtful exploration. We want to focus on the ethics of cochlear implant surgery with, specifically, children born Deaf, because they comprise about nine out of ten children who could be cochlear implant candidates, as we have seen, and because the issues are more sharply drawn in their case.[60]

The challenges to ethical decisions about surgically implanting children born Deaf cluster around four themes. These are risk/benefit ratio; cultural values in conflict; surrogate decision-making; and ethnocide (that is, cultural genocide):

Risk/Benefit ratio: Apart from the risks associated with surgery and anesthesia, cochlear implantation of children poses several primary risks: The combination of implant surgery and post-surgical oral/aural rehabilitation may leave the implanted child substantially languageless for several years.[61] The medium and long-term effects of cochlear implants on the child's language acquisition, social identity, psychological adjustment and mental health are unknown, and these may be compromised in varying degrees. Full participation in the language and culture of the DEAF–WORLD will undoubtedly elude many implanted children as they develop, but they may also be unable to participate fully in spoken language and hearing culture. We simply do not know the outcome of the implantation. When it comes to potential benefit oral advocates agree that, with children born Deaf, acquisition of spoken language is the significant benefit desired. However, there is *no* conclusive evidence yet of that benefit, and if it exists, we are unable to predict which children will receive it. Consequently, although more than a thousand children have been implanted, the treatment remains highly experimental. If experimental medical treatments of children can be justified ethically at all, it is only in the setting of a small, highly controlled long-term study.

Cultural values in conflict: As implants are perfected and more research is conducted, the risk/benefit ratio seems likely to improve. We want to consider the ethical issues if the implant did, in fact, offer a substantial opportunity to acquire spoken language. Three serious ethical challenges to implantation of children born Deaf remain. Is the possibility of acquiring some spoken language a benefit that would justify the surgery? Suppose one viewed children born Deaf as suffering from a gravely disabling condition; then the potential benefits loom large compared to the risks. Now suppose one viewed children born Deaf as exhibiting merely another form of human variation, like small stature; then the risks loom large and the benefits small. The opposing perspectives on Deaf people were nicely drawn by the founder of Gallaudet University, Edward Miner Gallaudet, and by Alexander Graham Bell. Addressing a professional conference, Gallaudet stated that education had transformed being Deaf from a calamity to "little more than a serious inconvenience" and, stopping to brush his bald pate, he added, "something like baldness in fly time." Bell, on the other hand, when challenged on the importance of speech to the Deaf, replied: "I am astonished. I am pained. To ask the value of speech? It is like asking the value of life!"[62]

It is a tenet of Deaf culture that Deaf people do not have an impairment merely by virtue of limited hearing. Deaf children in general are healthy, and it is unethical to operate on healthy children. The hearing parents and professionals insist that the Deaf child is not healthy and has a major impairment; it is a tenet of their culture that it is bad to be Deaf. How do we decide the ethical dispute when two cultures disagree on the wisdom of a surgical procedure because of fundamentally opposed values? Under certain restricted conditions, it does seem possible for one culture to ethically overrule the other. Thus, members of one culture might intercede when torture or murder is permitted in another culture. Is American culture thereby justified in interceding in Deaf culture? Implants are not a life or death matter. Nor are Deaf children caused suffering by the failure to provide them with implants. No one claims that Deaf parents are guilty of neglect of their Deaf children by refusing them implants. Since these special conditions do not apply, shouldn't the parents and medical personnel respect the values of Deaf culture as they demand that the members of the DEAF–WORLD respect their values? If so, how can they justify implant surgery on their born-Deaf child?

If the young Deaf child has not yet had an opportunity to acquire the language and values of Deaf culture, do the values of Deaf culture have standing in this matter? We have argued in chapter 5 that a child born Deaf is as surely a member of the Deaf cultural minority as a child born Black is a member of the Black cultural minority. That is, their life trajectories can be deflected, but the potential they have to enter into their respective cultures travels with them. If the child born Deaf is in principle a member of the DEAF–WORLD at birth, then do the parents have a moral obligation to respect the wishes of the DEAF–WORLD in this matter, even if they disagree with them given their own cultural background? How much of an obligation to respect the values of the Black community do white parents incur who have adopted a Black child?

Surrogate decision-making: The decision to perform implant surgery on the Deaf child is made *for* the child who, as a minor, is considered temporarily incompetent to make that decision. It is the surrogate's responsibility to make decisions which will promote the patient's well-being, as that well-being would be understood by the patient.[63] Parents cannot know with certainty what their individual child would decide if able to make the implant decision but they do know the next best thing—what adults born Deaf like their child would decide. Such adults refuse the implant for themselves and protest its use with children.

There are, moreover, three considerations that challenge surrogate decision-making by hearing parents for their Deaf children. First, there is the problem of communication. The presumption for parents to be surrogates is that they care deeply about their children and know them and their needs better than others do.[64] No one doubts that parents of Deaf children are devoted to them. However, it is primarily young, largely languageless children who are implanted, so there are uncommon obstacles in the way of parents satisfying the presumption that they know their Deaf child's character and needs well. With older children who were born Deaf, parents might try to determine their child's wishes, but their inability to communicate in signed language and the natural desire of children to please their parents are serious obstacles.

Second, there is the problem of conflicting values. Parents should be especially cautious in weighting their views of childhood implantation more heavily than the views of the DEAF–WORLD, because they are naturally advocates for their language and culture, but their child, when adult, will likely be an advocate for the language and culture of the DEAF–WORLD.

Third, there is the problem of informed consent. Parents frequently cannot give informed consent to the operation because they know no Deaf adults and have no information about what growing up Deaf, with or without an implant, involves. They neither know the alternatives to surgery, nor the likely outcome of the surgery. Given these facts, it is unclear how their consent can be informed. Yet to perform the surgery requires the child or the surrogate to give genuinely informed consent.

It would seem, then, that the parents have an ethical obligation to give great weight to the negative views of the DEAF–WORLD about childhood implants. However, they also have an obligation to do what they believe to be in the best interests of their child. Which should weigh more heavily in their choice, the belief that a certain surgical procedure is in the best interests of the child, or the knowledge that the child, as an adult, would likely disapprove of the surgery? Because parents are making the decision for someone else, the benefits of the surgery must outweigh the risks by a larger margin than if adults were making that decision for themselves.[65]

Ethnocide: The program of childhood implantation has as a primary goal to permit Deaf children to acquire the majority spoken language in place of the minority signed language they would have acquired. If this goal could bc achieved on a wide scale, the consequence, however unintended, would be *ethnocide*, the systematic blocking of a language minority from coming into its own and from pursuing its way of life. Such actions are widely considered to be unethical. Contemporary ethical standards with regard to the treatment of such minorities are captured in part in the United Nations Declaration of the Rights of Persons Belonging to National or Ethnic, Religious and Linguistic Minorities. Article 1 calls on states to protect and foster the existence and identity of linguistic minorities (among others). Article 2 affirms the right of such minorities to enjoy their culture and use their language, and to participate in decisions on the national level affecting their minority. Article 4 asks that states take measures to ensure that persons belonging to minorities have adequate opportunities to learn the minority language. In addition, as several Deaf organizations have pointed out, the United Nations Convention on the Crime of Genocide prohibits forcibly transferring children from a minority group to another group.

A member of a cochlear implant team who wrote to the *Atlantic Monthly* after its September, 1993, cover story on "Deaf: The New Ethnicity" acknowledged that ethnocide is indeed the likely consequence of programs of cochlear implantation and that he (or she) is contributing to ethnocide: "The cochlear prosthesis on which I have worked for years with many other scientists, engineers and clinicians, will lead inevitably to the extinction of the alternative culture of the Deaf, probably within a decade."[66] The author likens Deaf culture to Yiddish culture and concludes, "Both are unsustainable." Is it self-indulgent nostalgia to want to protect Deaf culture and Yiddish culture, or do we all have an ethical obligation to do so? If ASL speakers or Yiddish speakers want to protect their culture, but other groups have an interest in seeing them disappear, how do we decide the ethical dispute?

It may clarify our ethical thinking on this issue to examine the arguments while supposing cochlear implants were able to do what they cannot do now, namely deliver close to normal hearing for most patients. In that case, the risk/benefit ratio would be more favorable (for example, the risk of remaining languageless would be smaller); the assumption that the implanted child would disapprove as an adult would likely be false, since the formerly Deaf child would probably be acculturated to his or her parents' culture; and the interests of the child, as parent and child would see them, would be pitted against the interests of the language minority. Do parents have an obligation to consider the rights of the concerned minority as well as the interests of their own child? Are parents acting ethically if they promote school desegregation by busing but refuse to have their child bused? Suppose these are white parents who have adopted a Black child? Are the parents required ethically to consider not only the interests of the community and their child, but also the views that Black parents of a Black child would have in the same situation? Suppose the parents believe that Black parents might give even more weight than they do to desegregation. Should they allow that to tip the balance in favor of busing their child?

Leading audiologists and otologists state that they respect and wish to preserve Deaf minority language and culture. Thus, for example, the director of childhood implant research at New York University Medical Center, Dr. Noel Cohen, has written: "We have uppermost in our minds not to harm let alone destroy the deaf community; not to do damage to deaf culture. . . ."[67] Otology and audiology want to provide implants to Deaf children who they believe need them, but also to protect Deaf culture. Are these two goals compatible?

Here's our view on these issues. Our experiences with Deaf people have led us to view being born Deaf as a form of human variation that does not require medical intervention. More important, Deaf people themselves, who surely must know whether they have a grave impairment, say they do not. Consequently, the risks of childhood implantation would have to be much smaller than they are, and the benefits much larger, before the risk/benefit ratio would ethically justify surgery (and post-surgical rehabilitation). We know of no acultural set of values (unless it be a value on reducing human suffering or death) that one can use to choose between competing cultural claims with regard to the ethics of some surgery. Therefore, we believe that the values of Deaf culture should be decisive in childhood implantation of Deaf children. We expect that Deaf children have many of those values, such as being attuned to the visual world and preferring signed language, and will acquire many more as they mature. Thus parents who make a surrogate decision for them should choose in accord with the values of Deaf culture. Finally, we believe it is unethical to restrict a language minority from coming into its own. Each cultural group demands that others give it their moral backing in defending the flourishing of its language and culture, and thus its members should feel obliged to reciprocate.

As we have seen, Deaf groups and hearing parents and professionals frequently have different views about the wisdom of cochlear implants for young Deaf children, even though they share the same principal goal—to contribute to the welfare of the child. The fundamentals of this disagreement on the means by which to assure the Deaf child a fulfilling life in hearing society is centuries old. U.S. Deaf scholar Tom Humphries has summarized it as follows: "There is no room within the culture of Deaf people for an ideology that all Deaf people are deficient. It simply does not compute. There is no 'handicap' to overcome . . . Deaf people have a vision of integration [in the hearing world] that is different from what hearing people envision for them. Deaf people see a grounding in the culture and signed language of the Deaf community in which they live as the most important factor in their lives. Integration comes more easily and more effectively from these roots."[68]

The insistence of culturally Deaf people on their normalcy, and their resistance to using a prosthesis, oblige those who still view Deaf people only in a pathological light to take account of Deaf language, culture, and pride. To avoid this, some implant advocates have sought to dismiss the

Deaf point of view by attributing devious motivations to Deaf people's protests against implant surgery on children.[69] More subtly, however, the advocates of implantation merely exclude Deaf people from the discussion. The message is: The parents have the rights, and the hearing professionals have the knowledge, so the views of Deaf people are simply of no concern. For example, although there is wide agreement that most implanted children will remain "severely hearing-impaired" and will continue to rely on manual communication, none of the five childhood implant conferences to date in the U.S. has had a single Deaf speaker.*

How are Deaf organizations to respond to this exclusion while acting in the best interests of the child and the community that child will likely join? Deaf leaders understand that their discourse of normalcy is marginalized by the more dominant discourse of medical authority. They rarely have an opportunity to talk with decision-making parents, while doctors and audiologists have privileged access. They do not have an opportunity to talk to doctors, who systematically exclude them from their programs. Speeches at Deaf congresses affirming the normalcy of Deaf culture are not reported in the national presses. These Deaf communities therefore have faced a choice: to remain silenced, or to force others to listen.

What is the purpose of implant manufacturing and of childhood implant surgery? We are told that it is to remedy a serious social problem or set of problems. There is the problem of the child acquiring language, the problem of communication and special education, the problem of the child's learning a trade or profession, and so on. However, it is instructive to observe how people who are intimately familiar with growing up Deaf in a hearing world raise a Deaf child. They are not normally organized toward the solution of problems more than any other parents; they simply expect that their child will acquire language, communicate with them, go to school, and acquire a trade or profession and so on. They do not seek the services of professionals such as audiologists and ear surgeons. This contrast calls our attention to the source of the claim that a social problem exists: It is the very professionals devoted to remedying the problem who promote the claim. Does the implant then exist for the problem, or the problem for the implant? Note how the very existence of

* Ben Bahan addressed the Sixth Symposium on Cochlear Implants in Children as this book went to press.

implant surgery creates a link that has not existed before, between the ear surgeon and the Deaf child.

Hearing parents could (and some do) construe the advent of their Deaf child in quite a different light, not as a social problem, but as a joyful event that makes an unexpected language demand of them. All children, Deaf and hearing, are able to acquire a full language naturally. They are apparently best able to do it in the first years of life, when caretakers need merely expose them to an accessible language. The hearing parents of a Deaf child usually cannot fulfill this parental role without first learning a manual language, or introducing into the family people who know a manual language, such as Deaf friends or employees. Later, parents may seek help in socializing their child from teachers, child-care workers, scout leaders, clergymen, and relatives; at this early stage they can benefit from the help of culturally Deaf people.

Even parents who are decided on implantation for their child might be wise to follow this strategy, thus avoiding formative years in their child's life during which there is no substantive communication and no exposure to language structure. There is reason to think that children who are given a rich signed language environment may have an advantage learning some spoken language with or without an implant. Perhaps the very limited achievement in language learning of prelingually Deaf children with implants is partly the result of their being deprived of language during the first two years or more of life. This matter has not yet been studied. Nor, as we have said, are there studies in progress concerning the long-term risks and benefits of childhood implantation. These should have high priority. More research and better implants, which are certain to come in time, may bring all concerned parties closer to agreement on the scientific issues. What will remain, however, is the profound difference between Deaf and hearing cultures in the construction of being Deaf, and therefore disagreement on the ethics of childhood implant surgery.

Chapter 15

The Deaf Agenda: Enriching the Deaf-World

IN most of the world's cultures, which are overwhelmingly comprised of hearing people, hearing itself and its associated activities, such as singing and listening to music, are highly valued. They are, indeed, embedded in everyday life, from the *Star-Spangled Banner* to rock n' roll, from the sermon in the church to the call of the muezzin. Naturally enough, hearing people (and especially many hearing professionals who serve hearing people with hearing loss), commonly see Deaf people as seriously disabled. "When deafness is total, it is a catastrophe," writes the eminent French ear surgeon and cochlear implant pioneer, Claude-Henri Chouard, referring to children born Deaf.[1]

By the same token, in the cultures of the Deaf–Worlds all over the globe, vision and its associated activities, such as visual/manual language and attentiveness to the visual environment, are highly valued. They are, indeed, embedded in everyday life, from conversations with Deaf co-workers to socializing at the Deaf club, from formal lectures in signed language at a university to face recognition at a large party. Naturally enough, members of the Deaf–World in the U.S. frequently view hearing people, with their more limited capacities in visual perception and manual language, and their misbegotten attitudes toward visual people, as possessing some serious limitations. Deaf people decry the many hearing professionals who claim to serve the DEAF–WORLD, but who are handicapped by their inability to communicate fluently with its members. Most handicapping, however, are hearing people's attitudes toward Deaf people. Hearing people find it so difficult to conceive of any legitimate physical organization other than their own, that they value what Deaf people disparage and disparage what is in fact valuable. Thus hearing people often place a greater value on being hard-of-hearing than on being Deaf, thereby preferring what is commonly a no-man's-land between the hearing mainstream and the Deaf minority to a rich language and culture. And hearing people disparage the greatest eloquence in ASL in favor of the feeblest short-lived oral efforts. In brief, members of the DEAF–WORLD think "it's dandy to be Deaf," as a U.S. Deaf leader explained on the television magazine, *Sixty Minutes*. As it is grand to be a Gypsy, and nice to be a Navaho (though not always easy, mind you), it is a reason for pride and pleasure.

Whereas the hearing agenda for Deaf people is founded on the premise that Deaf people are disabled, the DEAF–WORLD agenda for Deaf people is founded on the premise that Deaf people are members of a linguistic and cultural minority. At the top of the hearing agenda for Deaf people is to reduce the number of Deaf people and make Deaf people more like hearing people (through prosthesis, surgery, training, and education). Such goals are not on the Deaf agenda at all. On the contrary, to be hearing is to be other. One of the four student leaders who led the Gallaudet Revolution explained to *USA Today* the significance of the Revolution as it relates to the construction of Deaf people: "Hearing people sometimes call us handicapped. But most—maybe all Deaf people—feel that we're more of an ethnic group because we speak a different language . . . We also have our own culture . . . There's more of an ethnic difference than a handicap difference between us and hearing people."[2]

Before contrasting the agendas of the DEAF–WORLD and of people with disabilities, let's start by acknowledging that there is great heterogeneity in each of those groups. We will comment on the varying points of view within the DEAF–WORLD below. With regard to disabilities, there are many kinds, both physical and intellectual, that give rise to quite different demands. People who have the same type of disability may, and frequently do, disagree strongly on the right political agenda to follow. Nevertheless, there are some commonalities that are the foundation of the

Disability Rights movement. When we examine those commonalities and compare them to the values and goals of people in the DEAF–WORLD, we find Deaf priorities so radically different from those of people with disabilities that it is hard to imagine anything useful being achieved when neglecting those differences and conflating the two groups.

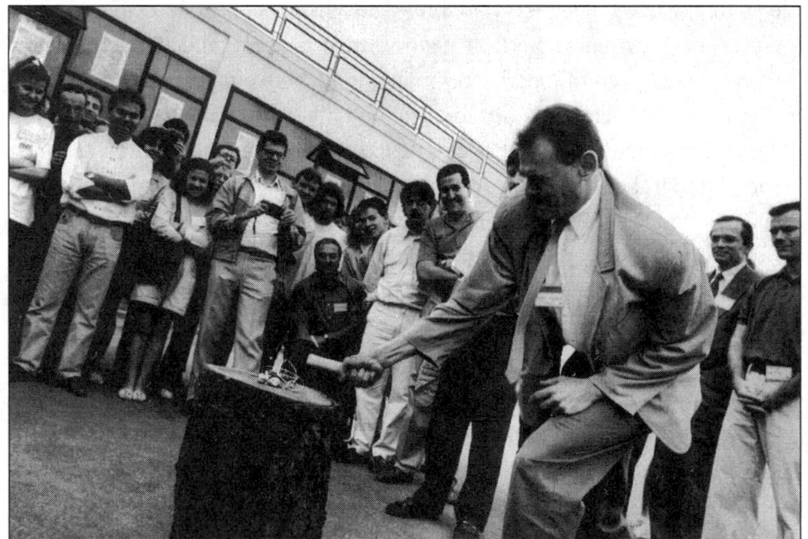

Dominique Bordier

Fig. 15-1. **French Deaf leader J. -F. Mercurio takes a sledgehammer to a hearing aid at the opening of the International Symposium on Sign Language, Poitiers, France, 1990.**

Start with this observation: Deaf people themselves, who surely should know whether they have a disability or not, typically find they do not have a disability. Now that's an odd position for people with a disability to take! Shall we conclude that millions of Deaf people around the world are mistaken about their identity, as you might say about some mentally ill people who have a disability without knowing it? Clearly not. Then, too, people with disabilities tend to be ambivalent about their impairment; individually they want it valued, as a part of who they are. At the same time, it is the result of poverty, war, disease, and accident, so they ask that we regret the impairment and try to prevent it.[3] The DEAF–WORLD is not ambivalent, however; its members commonly think it is a good thing to be Deaf and would like to see more of it. Unlike expectant parents with disabilities, expectant Deaf parents, like those in any other language minority, commonly hope to have children just like themselves, with whom they can share their language, culture and unique experiences. That is, they hope to have Deaf children, as we have said before.

Next consider what people with disabilities around the world are striving for. What are their goals? According to the United Nations, people with disabilities seek, above all, better medical care, rehabilitation services, personal assistance services (commonly, help with personal hygiene, dressing and eating) and independence.[4] However, Deaf people do not attach particular importance to medical care, or place any special value on rehabilitation or personal assistance services; nor do they have any more concern with autonomy and independent living than people in general. (Proponents of a disability construction of the DEAF–WORLD have said that signed language interpreters are personal assistants. But, the services of these highly trained professionals are frequently not personal, since they are usually provided in settings involving large audiences, and "assist" the hearing people present as well as, and at the same time as, the Deaf people. Nor is interpreting between any other two languages, for example, at the United Nations, considered personal assistance.) Instead, like other language minorities (for example, Hispanic-Americans), Deaf people campaign for acceptance of their language and its broader use in the schools, the workplace, and in public events.

Because of the unique language and culture of the DEAF–WORLD, further differences arise between the Deaf agenda and the disability agenda. We are told that integration, in the classroom, the work force, and the community, "has become a primary goal of today's disability movement."[5] But school integration is anathema to the DEAF–WORLD. Because most Deaf children have hearing parents, they can only acquire full language and socialization in specialized schools, in particular the prized network of residential schools. As we have contended, Deaf children are drowning in the mainstream schools. Whereas advocates for people with disabilities recoil in horror at segregated institutions, many Deaf alumni of residential schools return to their Deaf alma maters repeatedly over the years, contribute to their support, send their Deaf children to them, and vigorously protest the efforts of well-meaning but misguided members of the Disability Rights movement to close them down. These disability advocates fail to take account of language and culture, and therefore of the difference between imposed and elective separateness. Where people with disabilities cherish independence, culturally Deaf people cherish interdependence. People with disabilities may gather for political action; Deaf people traditionally gather primarily for socializing. Indeed, Deaf people marry Deaf people ninety percent of the time in the U.S., as we mentioned earlier.[6]

It seems that people with disabilities and the members of the DEAF–WORLD could scarcely have more disparate agendas. Please do not misunderstand us: The DEAF–WORLD has good reason to support the Disability Rights movement. Both endeavor to promote their construction of their identity, in competition with the interested (and generally better-funded) efforts of professionals to promote *their* constructions of their clients' identities. Both the DEAF–WORLD and the Disability Rights movement struggle for control of their destiny with the *troubled-persons industries*—the professions that, in the words of sociologist Joseph Gusfield, "bestow benevolence on people defined as in need."[7] The Deaf struggle with special education and audiology, for example. People with visual impairments struggle with the American Association of Workers with the Blind. People with motor impairments struggle with orthopedics, etc.[8] Both Deaf people and those with disabilities pay the price of social stigma. Finally, Deaf people have special reasons for solidarity with people whose primary acculturation is to the hearing society and who have hearing losses; their combined numbers have created services, commissions and laws that the DEAF–WORLD alone probably could not have achieved. Solidarity, yes. But when culturally Deaf people allow their special identity to be subsumed under the construct of disability, they set themselves up for wrong solutions and bitter disappointments. They relinquish the Deaf agenda for Deaf people, and watch it supplanted by an alien disability agenda for Deaf people, which they come to resent bitterly. For example, there is a movement to close specialized schools for children with disabilities and to educate them, fully integrated, with their able-bodied peers, as we discussed in chapter 8. For most Deaf children, this is the wrong solution. The DEAF–WORLD is indeed bitter about mainstreaming and full inclusion, but Deaf children and schools have been swept up in this movement largely because the members of the DEAF–WORLD are subsumed under the category of people with disabilities.

Lately, some advocates for people with disabilities have been emphasizing the bonds that unite people with disabilities to the rest of society, with whom they generally share not only culture, but also ranges of capacities and incapacities.[9] More than twenty percent of the non-institutionalized population of the United States has a disability, we are told, and over 7.7 million Americans report that hearing is their primary functional limitation.[10] This universalizing view, according to which most people have some disability at least some of the time, is strikingly at odds with the facts of the DEAF–WORLD, which is small, tightly knit, and possesses its own language and culture. There is no continuum between Deaf and hearing. Recall NAD President Olof Hanson's remark that Deaf people are foreigners. Indeed, members of the DEAF–WORLD commonly refer to themselves as *the Deaf,* in conversation and in the names of their organizations (NAD, WFD, etc.). It seems right to speak of *the Deaf* as we speak of *the French* or *the British*; by this we do not imply that all culturally Deaf people or French people are alike, merely that they have some defining characteristic in common. It is alien to Deaf culture for several reasons to speak of its members as *people with hearing-impairment.* First, it is the troubled-persons industry that invented and promoted the label in English *hearing-impaired;*[11] it is transparently and exclusively based on a disability construction of Deaf people. Second, the members of the DEAF–WORLD generally see their difference as natural human variation, not as impairment. Third, the *people with* construction (*people with hearing impairment*) implies that the trait is incidental rather than defining, but one's culture is never an incidental trait. It seems to be an error in ordinary language to say, *I happen to be Hispanic*, or *I happen to be Deaf,* because these are features that define identity; who would you be, after all, if you were you and yet not Hispanic, or not a member of the DEAF–WORLD? On the other hand, in reference to disabilities, it is acceptable to say, *I happen to have a spinal cord injury.*

On all these different counts, then, hearing people's view of Deaf people as disabled just does not square with what we expect from a group of people with a disability: Deaf people do not see themselves as being disabled; Deaf people value their Deaf identity and culture and wish to see the DEAF–WORLD grow; Deaf people seek language acceptance, not personal assistance; Deaf people seek voluntary separation, not forced integration. Of course, all these matters are quite otherwise for people acculturated to hearing society who have hearing loss. Organizations of those people do share aims and values with the disability rights movement. They affirm that they have hearing impairment. They regret the fact, or are at least ambivalent. They want measures to mitigate hearing impairment for themselves and to prevent it in others. Thus, they are keenly interested in treatments and prostheses. Their organizations include: The American Association of Late-Deafened Adults (approximately 2,000 members); Self Help for Hard of Hearing People (13,000); Cochlear Implant Club International (1,000); Alexander Graham Bell Association for the Deaf, Oral Deaf Section (400).

CULTURE VS. DISABILITY AND THE DEAF AGENDA

The Deaf agenda for Deaf people has bilingualism and biculturalism as its mainstay. The agenda can be conveniently organized around four themes. The first is winning fundamental human rights that are guaranteed under international covenant, such as the right to use one's minority language. Second, securing an education for Deaf children that uses their primary signed language, but teaches them the majority language. Next, improving Deaf people's access to information through both the signed language and the majority language. And finally, enhancing Deaf culture and social life.

Before we turn to the specifics of the Deaf agenda, let us note that what Deaf people want for one another is, overall, informed by their view of themselves as a linguistic and cultural minority. Most of the practices that the Deaf agenda seeks to reform arise because hearing people do not view Deaf people as the Deaf view themselves. Much of the Deaf battle for human rights—better education, more access to information, and an enriched culture—would be won if hearing people and governments could be persuaded to construe Deaf people as they do themselves, in terms of language and culture. Imagine it for a moment. How would things change?[12] When society changes its construction of a social issue:

- The legitimate authority changes. In many areas, such as schooling, the authority would become Deaf adults, linguists and sociologists among others. There would be many more service providers from the minority. Deaf people would be prominent as teachers, foster and adoptive parents, information officers, social workers, advocates. Non Deaf service providers would be expected to know the language, history, and culture of the Deaf linguistic minority.

- Behavior is construed differently. Deaf people would be expected to use ASL (in the U.S.) and to have interpreters available. Hearing and Deaf people would expect to have conversations through interpreters that were substantive and fluent; laborious communication in the speakers' secondary languages would be seen as inappropriate.

- The legal status of the social issue changes. Most Deaf people would no longer claim disability benefits or services under the present legislation for disabled people. The services to which the Deaf linguistic minority has a right in order to obtain equal treatment under the law would be provided by other legislation and bureaucracies. Deaf people would receive greater protection against employment discrimination under civil rights laws and rulings. Where there are special provisions to assist the education of linguistic minority children, Deaf children would be eligible.

- The arena where identification and labeling take place also changes. In the disability construction, being Deaf is medicalized and labeled in the audiologist's clinic. In the construction as linguistic minority, being Deaf is viewed as a social variety and would be labeled in the peer group.

- Types of intervention change. The Deaf child would not be operated on because he or she is Deaf, but would be brought together with other Deaf children and Deaf adults. The disability construction orients hearing parents to the question, What can be done to mitigate my child's impairment? The linguistic minority construction presents them with the challenge of ensuring that their child has language and role models from the minority.[13]

Each language minority differs from the others in important ways. Members of the Chinese-American community are increasingly marrying outside their linguistic minorities, but this is rare for ASL speakers. Many Native American languages are dying out or have disappeared, but this is not true of ASL. Spanish-speaking Americans are so diverse a group that it may not be appropriate to speak of *Hispanics*, a term that reflects bureaucratic convenience more than underlying commonalities.[14] ASL speakers also comprise a language minority that is unique in some respects. Deaf people cannot learn English as a second language as easily as other minorities. Second- and third-generation Deaf children find learning English no easier than their forebears, but second and third generation immigrants to the U.S. frequently learn English before entering school. The language of the DEAF–WORLD is not usually passed on from generation to generation; instead, it is commonly transmitted by peers or associates. Normally, Deaf people are not proficient in this native language until they reach school age. Deaf people are more scattered geographically than many linguistic minorities. The availability of interpreters is even more vital for Deaf people than for many other linguistic minorities, because there are so few Deaf lawyers, doctors, accountants and the like. Relatively few Deaf people are in high-status public positions in our society (in contrast with, say, Hispanics), and this has hindered the legitimation of ASL use.[15]

At the outset of our journey into the DEAF–WORLD, we cited the growing perception of that world in the U.S. as a "new ethnicity." However, the characteristics of the DEAF–WORLD we have just listed that set it apart from ethnic groups such as Chinese Americans or Hispanic Americans, challenge that description. Perhaps most fundamentally, members of the DEAF–WORLD are different from these other ethnic minorities in that they do not usually receive their DEAF–WORLD heritage from their parents and pass it on to *their* children in turn (sociolinguist Joshua Fishman has called this a difference in degree of 'historicity'[16]). Then, too, the DEAF–WORLD has rather limited autonomy compared to many ethnic groups. It does not control its own institutions, such as school, church, and workplace. On the other hand, the family is not the only means of maintaining historical continuity: language, the arts, recorded history and storytelling, customs, and institutions such as schools and clubs, all transmit culture from generation to generation. And ethnic minorities in most lands have limited if any autonomy. It is significant that enhancing historicity and autonomy are central to the agenda of the DEAF–WORLD, which seeks to reform and reinforce the residential schools as an important vehicle for transmitting Deaf culture from generation to generation and for increasing Deaf self-determination.

Not all members of the DEAF–WORLD seek change based on recognition of their language and culture, and not all disown the disability construction. Just as there is language diversity in the DEAF–WORLD, as we have seen, so there are diverse views on the centrality of ASL to the Deaf experience. Moreover, some Deaf people want to reinforce ties to the powerful Disability Rights movement, if only as a matter of political expediency, especially in the present political climate in the U.S. The general secretary of the World Federation of the Deaf has pointed out that, while many Deaf organizations view the DEAF–WORLD in their region or nation as a linguistic and cultural minority, such minorities frequently lack strong international networks and umbrella organizations. Since international organizations like the United Nations are working for the empowerment of people with disabilities worldwide, doesn't it make sense for organizations of the Deaf to avail themselves of that advocacy? For example, the U.N. Standard Rules on the Equalization of Opportunities for Persons with Disabilities mention, as a result of Deaf activism, signed language courses for parents and the use of signed language in the schools; separate schools for Deaf persons; interpreter services and access to information; and self-determination.[17] "Taking part actively in disability movements," the general secretary has affirmed, "is not inconsistent with being a linguistic and cultural minority."[18]

Deaf cultures do not exist in a vacuum. Members of the DEAF–WORLD in the U.S. embrace many cultural values, attitudes, beliefs and behaviors that are part of the larger American culture and, in some instances, that are part of ethnic minority cultures, such as Hispanic-American and African-American culture, as we have discussed. The embedding of the DEAF–WORLD within a larger culture raises the question of whether Deaf culture is best described as a subculture. If by calling the culture of the DEAF–WORLD in the U.S., for example, a *subculture,* we mean to recognize an imbalance of power that is clearly accurate and applies as well to the cultures of other language minorities such as French-Americans, Hispanic-Americans and Native Americans. The term *subculture* does not apply, however, if we mean by it that the members of the DEAF–WORLD are more like an interest group, people acculturated to the dominant culture but organized in a more-or-less structured way, perhaps over a period of time, to address problems of shared concern. In some ways, the boundaries of the DEAF–WORLD are less permeable to majority culture than those of other language minorities. Members of those minorities are exposed to the mainstream culture in both their primary language and in the national language—as they master it—from early childhood on, through the school years, and into adulthood, when they may marry out of the minority and even assimilate into the mainstream. As we indicated above, relatively few members of the DEAF–WORLD master English as a second language and assimilate into the mainstream culture. Deaf children are given limited access to the majority culture and Deaf people generally marry other Deaf people.

Because hearing people have obliged Deaf people to interact with the larger hearing society in terms of a disability model, that model has left its mark on Deaf culture. In particular, Deaf people frequently have found themselves recipients of unwanted special services provided by hearing people. The DEAF–WORLD can be viewed as a colony when it comes to certain facets of its relations with hearing society, including political, economic, and social areas.[19] As with colonized peoples, some Deaf people have internalized the "other's" construction of themselves (in this case, the disability construction), alongside their own cultural construction.[20] For example, some Deaf people are active in their Deaf club and yet denigrate skilled use of ASL as "low sign." The Deaf person who uses a variety of ASL marked by English word order frequently has greater access to wider resources such as education and employment. Knowing when to use which variety is an important part of being Deaf.[21] But granted that culturally Deaf people must take account of the disability model of their way of being, that they sometimes internalize it, and that it leaves its mark on the culture of the DEAF–WORLD—all this does not mean that the model is legitimate. After all, we can grant that African-Americans had to take account of the construction of the slave-as-property, that they sometimes internalized that construction, and that their culture has been marked by it, without then concluding that those facts support a construction of their ethnic group as property.

Thus, there are all sorts of people in the DEAF–WORLD in the U.S., and there are all sorts of DEAF–WORLDS to be found on the planet. Nevertheless, each Deaf society has values embedded in it, and each has a more or less structured agenda for promoting those values. To take an analogy, the Hispanic-American minority in the U.S. is proud of its linguistic and cultural heritage. Not all Hispanic-Americans, however, are interested in preserving their heritage; some wish to set it aside and, as members of other minorities have done, assimilate into the mainstream. Indeed, there is certain to be dissent in any minority. In stating what we believe to be the Deaf agenda for Deaf people, we generally draw on (and cite) the views and actions of national and international organizations of Deaf people. Every now and then a disgruntled person will accuse some organization of being out of touch with the views of the "real," or "grassroots" Deaf people. Of course, an organization can stray from the values of its core membership, but we are impressed with all the safeguards to prevent this happening often in the DEAF–WORLD. Many national Deaf organizations are comprised of local Deaf clubs with a direct say at the national level. All such organizations have regional and national meetings, and many have publications in which opposing views can be expressed. In most cases, leadership is democratically elected for limited terms.

WINNING FUNDAMENTAL HUMAN RIGHTS

The right to dignity

It is shocking and unacceptable to realize that Deaf people around the world, in the United States as elsewhere, are deprived of fundamental human rights; and yet it is true. The World Federation of the Deaf and the national organizations of Deaf people that are its members, are engaged in a ceaseless struggle to gain fundamental human rights for Deaf people. Such rights are guaranteed by, among other documents in international law, the 1948 Universal Declaration of Human Rights. Article I of that declaration states that all human beings are born equal in dignity and rights. However, in a 1994 presentation to the assistant secretary general for human rights of the United Nations, the WFD affirmed that Deaf people are not accorded equal dignity and "there are even many who want to get rid of us."[22] Practices of genetic counseling and genetic research are commonly aimed at reducing the numbers of, or eliminating, Deaf people, and this goal has been explicitly championed by some scientists and government research institutes in the United States as elsewhere. The secretary-general responded that "for me and my colleagues, Deaf people are not a disability group [but] a linguistic minority. And I understand that recognizing Deaf people as a linguistic minority goes hand in hand with respect for the Deaf community."[23] In an effort to make more progress in securing human rights for Deaf children and adults, the WFD made "Toward Human Rights" the theme of its quadrennial congress held in Vienna in 1995.

The right to language

The second article of the Universal Declaration of Human Rights prohibits discrimination against people based on language. Language minorities are severely discriminated against all over the world, and signed language minorities are no exception. This problem has been so persistent and widespread that in 1992 the United Nations General Assembly adopted a Declaration of the Rights of Persons Belonging to National or Ethnic, Religious and Linguistic Minorities. Precisely because minorities are so imperiled by majority oppression, this document charges all states with protecting them and their linguistic identity, and with taking steps to promote that identity. Deaf societies have an additional reason for putting language rights at the head of their agenda; they know that efforts to supplant their minority language with the majority spoken language will never succeed, and that such efforts can only deprive them of their education, employment, and participation in the life of the nation. Thus numerous Deaf organizations have made securing language rights a primary policy objective; they seek, in the words of the Finnish Association of the Deaf, "to attain equality in society by improving linguistic rights."[24]

Some steps have been taken in the United States and elsewhere to protect and encourage the identity of signed-language speaking minorities. For example, Deaf activism in the U.S. has led to laws in more than half the states that acknowledge the legitimacy of ASL.[25] However, as this book amply testifies, our educational policies, like those in a great many countries, are hostile to ASL and prevent Deaf children from mastering the language (and Deaf culture) in the primary way available to most of them—in educational programs for Deaf children. This directly contravenes Article 3 of the U.N. declaration on the rights of minorities, cited above, which states that persons belonging to language minorities should have adequate opportunities to learn the language of their minority. United Nations Secretary General Boutros Boutros-Ghali has affirmed that "Deaf people should have the right to use Sign Language as the medium of communication."[26] According to the WFD, "The first three years of life are the most important ones for child language development. Therefore, children under school age must have the opportunity to grow up in an environment using sign language and hearing parents must be provided counseling services and instruction in the use of sign language."[27] A 1985 UNESCO report on Deaf education states as a principle that "We must recognize the legitimacy of the signed languages [and] they should be accorded the same status as other languages . . . It is no longer admissible to overlook them or to fail to encourage their integration into Deaf education."[28] The European Parliament made a similar proclamation in 1987, urging its member states to value their signed languages and encourage their development, but the violations of these fundamental human rights continue.[29] In Germany, for example, German Sign Language is tolerated in only one educational program for Deaf children in the entire nation. The situation is similar in Japan, obliging the Japanese Association of the Deaf to establish signed language classes for Deaf school leavers, so that they can communicate with other members of the DEAF–WORLD, including their future spouses. ASL is extensively used in only a handful of American schools; BSL in only one or two British schools; Kenyan Sign Language is not used to instruct Deaf children in a single school, and so on around the globe (with a few notable exceptions, such as Sweden, which we spoke of earlier).

Some hearing parents may object that the preeminent Deaf agenda of ensuring that Deaf children have early access to signed language is in conflict with their own language rights. Do they not have the right, even the obligation, to ensure that their child acquires their own language, culture and traditions? However, the conflict here is more apparent than real. For most Deaf children, if they are to acquire any full natural language during the first years of life, it must be a signed language, since spoken language is inaccessible to them. In the United States, for example, some nine out of ten Deaf children become Deaf at birth or so shortly afterward that they never have the opportunity to acquire spoken language naturally from their hearing parents. If a signed language such as ASL has been acquired instead, and thus the language instinct has been allowed to develop normally, there is a foundation on which a mastery of other languages can be erected. Some hearing parents might prefer it the other way around—mastery of their spoken language first, mastery of signed language later. But that is simply not a biological possibility for most Deaf children, so in the end, the language agendas for the Deaf child of the DEAF–WORLD and of the child's parents ought to coincide.

The rights guaranteed to language minorities by Article 4 of the U.N. declaration are almost universally violated when it comes to signed language minorities: states should take measures in education to promote a knowledge of the history, traditions, language and culture of its minorities. In most countries in the world, Deaf children have no opportunity to study their minority language and culture, although the national language and culture are a required subject for all children every single term of their educational program. In very few nations can Deaf children learn about the language and culture of the DEAF–WORLD.

Article 2 of the declaration on the rights of minorities affirms that persons belonging to minorities have the right to enjoy their own culture and to use their own language in private and public freely, without any form of discrimination. In most countries in the world, it is not possible for Deaf people to use their signed language in many public places, for example, in the schools, in addressing various audiences, in employment interviews, on the job, in court, in medical facilities and so on. Moreover, most Deaf children are unable to use their minority language and enjoy their culture in the privacy of their own homes, because their parents have been unable or unwilling to make a place for that language and culture.

The right to marry and found a family

Returning to the Universal Declaration of Human Rights, Article 16 guarantees to all adults the right to marry. The WFD *Survey of Deaf People in the Developing World* confirmed that there are still countries in which Deaf people are deprived of this human right, and others in which Deaf women are married without their approval.[30]

The right to drive

Article 13 guarantees the right of movement and residence within the borders of each state. Twenty-six of the countries surveyed reported that Deaf people cannot have a driver's license because of prejudice and misinformation.

The right to social services

Article 25 guarantees the right to medical care and other social services. Deaf people are routinely deprived of these rights by the absence of internists, psychiatrists, and other medical specialists and the absence of lawyers and other professionals who know their language and culture. Qualified interpreters are a partial remedy for this neglect, but most Deaf people do not have access to qualified interpreters. A survey of southern and eastern Africa found no professional interpreters whatsoever! How are Deaf Africans to defend themselves in court, for example, or to give informed consent to medical treatment or surgery? Many South American countries have one or no professional interpreters. Most countries do not have interpreter education programs, not to mention certification standards. In the United States, there are interpreter education programs and certification standards, and the ADA and other laws affirm the right of Deaf clients to interpreters in specific circumstances. However, in practice Deaf people are commonly deprived of access to social services because of unavailable or poorly qualified interpreters and unenforced laws. To illustrate: In 1994, the Massachusetts Commission on the Deaf and Hard of Hearing filled only sixty-two percent of requests for interpreter services because of shortages of interpreters and funding. Numerous schools in the U.S. that would never hire an uncertified audiologist, for example, have taken on unqualified interpreters, using whatever job titles could be conveniently assigned, such as "library assistant."

The right to work

Article 23 of the Universal Declaration of Human Rights guarantees to everyone the right to work, free choice of employment, favorable conditions of work, and absence of discrimination. Deaf people's rights in this regard are violated routinely throughout the world. The absence of education for Deaf children or unsuccessful education, deprives those citizens of free choice of employment and thus, frequently, of the means to earn a decent living. In post-industrial societies, Deaf people are being left behind as large segments of the work force develop the skills and knowledge required for positions that process information and deliver technical services. Employer prejudices against Deaf workers and the shortage or absence of interpreters often deprive the Deaf worker of an even chance at a job opening. Some employers hire Deaf people, especially in developing nations, because they have found they can get assiduous labor at well below the market rates for that labor.

Women and minorities

Deaf women in developing countries have suffered greatly. They have been particularly deprived of their right to dignity, to their own language and culture, to marry and found a family, to drive, to obtain social services, and to work. Deaf women are at a much greater risk than their hearing counterparts of sexual abuse and physical abuse. Pregnant Deaf women are required to undergo prenatal tests in some countries. Deaf women in developing countries have fewer educational opportunities than hearing women and they encounter severe employment discrimination.[31] Likewise, Deaf people who are members of national minorities (for example, Deaf African-Americans) have suffered a double oppression and a double measure of deprivation of fundamental human rights. On a worldwide scale, organizations such as the WFD are giving renewed attention to these groups of doubly oppressed people, always seeking to involve them in creating national organizations, regional secretariats, and long-term plans. In the U.S., as we saw in chapter 5, these doubly oppressed groups have spawned organizations to advocate their interests and assist their members.

Securing Effective Education for Deaf Children

Minorities often give priority to seeking effective education for their children. They look to education to provide their children not only with a richer appreciation of the natural, social and aesthetic world and their place within it, but also with a practical livelihood and upward social mobility, ultimately giving them a greater measure of empowerment than their parents had enjoyed. The DEAF–WORLD, however, attaches even more importance to schools and the school years than the great importance typically accorded them by other minorities. No doubt the reason is this: Throughout Deaf history, the language and culture of this minority could not be transmitted through the home, so it was done primarily through the schools. Since most Deaf children have hearing parents, it has traditionally been in the residential schools that Deaf children were put in possession of their proud heritage—especially, of course, their minority language. The United Nations has recognized this principle, affirming in a 1994 guideline, "Owing to the particular communication needs of Deaf and Deaf-Blind persons, their education may be more suitably provided in schools for such persons [and] special attention needs to be focused on culturally sensitive instruction. . . . "[32]

In view of the critical importance of Deaf education, it is especially dismaying, then, to read in the WFD survey of developing nations that primary education remains a privilege accorded very few Deaf children. Moreover, such schools as exist are small, of uneven quality, and frequently staffed by unqualified teachers; they commonly award diplomas that have no official standing in the national educational system.

The educational situation for Deaf people in the United States and in many other nations called "First World" is also, as we saw in part 2, grievously lacking. A recent commission of the U.S. Congress found, after much inquiry: "The present status of education for persons who are Deaf in the United States, is unsatisfactory. Unacceptably so."[33]

The National Association of the Deaf presented to Congress in 1992 the following agenda for improvements: Deaf children need appropriate early intervention so they receive full access to language; they need valid tests of their strengths and weaknesses; they must have access to top-quality residential schools, and no Deaf child should be isolated in a classroom with few or no other Deaf children; Deaf pupils need teachers and other professionals who can communicate with them fluently, and they need qualified interpreters. To meet many of these needs, the field of Deaf education must do much more than it does at present to improve the training and hiring of Deaf professionals as teachers, counselors and administrators at every educational level. In addition, the government must do much more to implement the recommendations of the 1988 Commission on the Education of the Deaf, especially those concerning primary and secondary education. Several position papers of the NAD, and articles in its newspaper and magazine, flesh out this Deaf agenda for Deaf education.

Residential schools and a continuum of placements

Many leaders in the DEAF–WORLD want to reform the residential schools for Deaf children and to reintroduce signed language and Deaf teachers in their classrooms. These practices proved successful in the last century, when most Deaf children in the U.S. studied all their subjects in their most fluent language, ASL. "In a school where signed language is used," Deaf leaders reason from their own experience, "the Deaf student is able not only to understand and respond to the instruction, but also to get help after class with course work; to discuss local, national, and international events; to participate in student activities; to develop friendships with other Deaf students; to emulate older students and Deaf teachers; to acquire self-respect as a Deaf person; and to come to know hearing people and relate to them effectively." In the words of the WFD, "Deaf children need schools of their own. The mainstream system does not offer the deaf child the interaction with deaf persons he/she needs. In the mainstream system, the Deaf child becomes marginalized [and] learning results will be poor."[34]

Because of the widespread abuses of mainstreaming, which have left many Deaf students stranded in classrooms where they cannot understand the instruction, and the instructor and hearing classmates cannot understand them, and because of agitation for reform by Deaf groups in several states, the federal Office of Special Education and Rehabilitation Services issued its policy guidance, mentioned in chapter 8, reminding teachers and administrators that a classroom failing to meet the communication needs of the Deaf child is not the Least Restrictive Environment for that child.

The NAD wants the Individuals with Disabilities Education Act revised to require a "continuum of alternative educational placements" for Deaf children.[35] This would ensure residential schools for Deaf children as one option. It would also provide for *magnet schools*, which would gather scattered Deaf children into a single school or program, providing a critical mass that would allow them many—though not all—of the advantages of residential schools. A continuum of placements would also include classrooms with interpreters, and even some classrooms without interpreters, for those rare Deaf students who flourish in that environment. By 1995, Deaf activism in the U.S. had led three states (Louisiana, South Dakota and California) to pass a Deaf education bill of rights that helps to ensure the survival of specialized schools and programs for Deaf children by requiring that those children's communicative needs be respected, including access to peers and teachers who are proficient in the child's primary language, signed language.

The antithesis of a continuum of educational placements for Deaf children is *full inclusion*—a popular movement that, as we have seen, aims at the placement of all children with disabilities in their neighborhood schools. Such a practice would clearly be disastrous for most Deaf children, and the NAD is vehemently opposed. Advocates for children with disabilities, however, seem to believe that they dare not make an exception to "full inclusion" for Deaf children, lest it set a precedent for the segregation of many other specialized groups, thus undermining their cherished goal of integration. The graft of Deaf educational goals to the disability tree is bearing some bitter fruit indeed.

At the same time as they are endeavoring to replace the disability model of Deaf people, leaders in the DEAF–WORLD have been working internationally within the disability framework to obtain special provisions for Deaf children. They have had two recent successes at the level of policy. A 1994 UNESCO world conference on special needs education stated that provision should be made "to ensure that all Deaf persons have access to education in their national sign language" and acknowledged that special schools or classes for Deaf and Deaf-Blind children are thus necessary.[36] Furthermore, the Standard Rules on the Equalization of Opportunities for Persons with Disabilities, adopted by the United Nations in 1993, affirms, as we noted earlier, that Deaf and Deaf-Blind children have particular communication needs that make their education in special schools or classes more suitable.[37]

Teachers who can communicate with their pupils

Around the world, where education is available to Deaf children it is often available only nominally, because instruction is conducted in a language which most Deaf children have not mastered (the national, or official, spoken language) and which many know scarcely at all. Indeed, frequently the Deaf child's parents and many times the child's teachers as well have not mastered the language used in instruction. In many developing nations, for example, the Deaf child's most familiar communication is comprised of home sign; then comes the manual language of broader communication (there may be more than one); the Deaf child may have some slight familiarity with the tribal language of his or her parents and with a spoken language of broader communication in the region (again, there may be more than one); finally, there are the official national languages, commonly including the language of the former colonizer, which is often the primary language of instruction!

Take Deaf Hispanic-American children, like Roberto Rivera from the Metro Silent Club. Roberto comes from a home where Spanish is spoken, his best language is ASL, and his teachers know neither language. The communication barrier is also insurmountable, however, for Deaf children in general, since they cannot grasp the teacher's oral language (whether it be written or spoken, supported with the occasional sign or not), and the teacher cannot grasp the child's manual one. High on the agenda of the U.S. DEAF–WORLD, as with its counterparts around the globe, is restoring signed language and Deaf teachers to education, and requiring hearing teachers of Deaf children to study the language and culture of the

DEAF–WORLD. We have seen that in the U.S., most teachers of the Deaf acknowledge that they cannot understand ASL and only a tiny fraction use ASL (less than one percent, according to one estimate).[38]

In recent years, the NAD came to believe that the way to improve language practices in the classroom was to change the curriculum that future teachers of the Deaf must follow to receive a degree. The current standards for accrediting some forty college and university programs that prepare teachers and administrators for careers in Deaf education in the United States are dominated by a disability construction of the Deaf child; they emphasize audiology, speech science, and language disorders; and they barely mention "sign language" (never ASL), along with fingerspelling and lipreading, as "modes of communication." These accreditation standards are set collaboratively by four national organizations comprised largely of hearing professionals. However, in 1994, NAD was admitted to membership in the accrediting group, so it may now prove to be in a better position to make progress in behalf of this important objective on the Deaf agenda: teachers who can communicate fluently with their students.[39]

There was a time in U.S. history when nearly half of all teachers of the Deaf were Deaf themselves. The other half commonly had personal ties to the DEAF–WORLD and were knowledgeable about its language and culture. However, hearing teachers of the Deaf changed all that, beginning with the Milan Congress of 1880. Securing an end to the lockout of Deaf teachers in Deaf education faces formidable obstacles. In the U.S., as in many other lands, there is the underlying obstacle that current educational practices with Deaf children prepare very few for professional careers. Then there is the reluctance of many graduate programs in special education to admit Deaf students (because of the cost of interpreters; because of incompatible philosophies of education; because of the difficulties Deaf graduates would have obtaining certification and employment—see chapter 8). Next there are states (and nations) where it just happens that special education teachers must first teach in general education and, as it happens, people with disabilities (Deaf are included) are not permitted to teach in general education. Many states (and nations) also administer language competency tests, which have the paradoxical result that the teacher-candidates most able to communicate with their Deaf students often fail (because English, for example, is their second language). Those unable to communicate with their Deaf students (because they are monolingual English speakers) often succeed. Finally, school superintendents must be willing (and able) to hire Deaf teachers, and the teachers must frequently be willing to go to rural communities where they are the sole Deaf person, or one of a very small number.

Bilingual/bicultural education of Deaf children

Educating Deaf children on the model of education of children from other language minorities is an idea whose time has come. Spurred by national Deaf organizations, by the inadequacy of present educational achievement, and by reports of its success in Sweden and other countries, it is sweeping many nations. The WFD seeks reforms that will allow signed language to be the language of instruction for Deaf children throughout the world.[40] The NAD has issued a position paper on ASL and bilingual education which states, in part, that ASL must be the primary language of instruction for Deaf students. It should also be an academic subject in their curriculum. Hence, teachers of the Deaf must be fluent in ASL.[41] The organization has been vigorously pursuing, with the federal Office of Bilingual Affairs, the recommendation on bilingual/bicultural education made by the 1986 Congressional Commission on the Education of the Deaf:

> The Department of Education should take positive action to encourage practices under the Bilingual Education Act that seek to enhance the quality of education received by limited-English-proficiency children whose native (primary) language is American Sign Language.

The commission found that children whose primary language is ASL, "like those who speak other minority languages such as Spanish or Navaho, are at a severe educational disadvantage in a system that disbars, denigrates and denies their primary language." The Commission urged the Department of Education to apply to children who use ASL the existing laws and court rulings that require bilingual/bicultural education for language minority children.[42]

The DEAF–WORLD is thus making some headway, here and abroad, in introducing bilingual and bicultural education of Deaf children. We described earlier the progress of the last two decades in Sweden and the initiatives begun in France and culminating in a law guaranteeing bilingual/bicultural education as an educational choice for parents of Deaf children. Denmark's and Finland's bilingual programs for Deaf children got under way early in the 1990s.[43] Bilingual/bicultural education was formally adopted as the educational policy for Deaf children in the province of Ontario in 1989. Progress toward bilingual education has also been taking place as a matter of national policy in Uruguay and Venezuela. In the U.S., as of this writing, there are bilingual education programs for ASL-using children in seven states (the oldest is in Massachusetts), and the list grows longer as the months pass. In several states, organizations of Deaf people have established "charter schools" for Deaf children with bilingual/bicultural curricula. One such school opened in Minneapolis in 1993 and another was under development in Denver. If the negotiations of the NAD commission with the Office of Bilingual Affairs are successful, and federal aid is extended to schools with large numbers of ASL-speaking pupils, as it is to those with children speaking other minority languages, the growth of bilingual/bicultural programs will be considerably accelerated. In a further development facilitating the growth of bilingual education for children in the DEAF–WORLD, through 1995 three more states had followed California's example and passed a Deaf Child's Bill of Rights. These laws require an assessment of the child's primary language; a placement that takes account of that language and the child's social, emotional and cultural needs; and competency in ASL on the part of teachers of the Deaf.

IMPROVING DEAF ACCESS TO INFORMATION

Imagine you are a Deaf entrepreneur (or lawyer, or teacher, or whatever) living in Boston and planning to attend an important meeting in Dallas one chilly winter morning. It looks like it may snow, delaying or even canceling your flight. There is no point trying to call the airline—even if you could get through to the airline recording using the TTY relay service, there's a litany of choices and numbers to be pressed, and the whole process really would make you late. None of the cab companies has a TTY, but you hope to catch a taxi on the street. You hail a cab, the driver's Haitian, and you have no language in common. You also have no valises, so he's really skeptical that you mean "the airport" despite your dazzling impersonation of an airplane taking off. Still, he takes the right route. At Logan Airport they are announcing the delayed departure of an earlier flight to Dallas, but of course you don't know that. Too bad, because the monitors say your flight is canceled. You get in a long line, which lands you in front of a clerk who can't communicate with you. Somehow, the clerk books you on another flight, but then you need to find a TTY (where?) to alert your Dallas hosts. Eventually, you're in a plane sitting in the snow at Logan. Presumably the pilot has told the passengers something about why the engines are not running, but it's not for you to know. The safety procedures were apparently not for you to know either. And now there's an unintelligible movie. Have a nice flight and take a nap! New challenges await you at your hotel.

For the DEAF-WORLD, the big trouble with technology (in those societies that rely on it extensively) is that it first develops in a way that discriminates against various minorities, including the Deaf. Then there is a long and slow political and engineering process by which catch-up technology is added to lessen the discrimination. Television in the U.S. was long accessible only to people who knew spoken English; thanks to cable TV, multilingual broadcasting, and captioning, this has begun to change. Public transport has long been inaccessible to many people with disabilities; lately, our society has been modifying the transport at great cost, and discovering that many rider groups benefit. The moral for the future is to adopt universal design principles for new technology: information must be available in several modes simultaneously.[44] Until that glorious day, the DEAF-WORLD must rely on catch-up technology, especially the TTY and captioning.

The TTY and relay services

The relay services that link TTY users and those who do not have TTYs, newly mandated by the ADA, were mentioned earlier. Traditionally, members of the DEAF-WORLD did not have access to telecommunications. Consequently, personal visits and scheduled reunions, for example at the Deaf club, were occasions to receive and pass on information and to "stay in touch." Deaf people also asked their hearing children, hearing church members, and others to relay messages by telephone. Permanent relay services organized by Deaf groups grew out of these arrangements. The first such around-the-clock relay service was established by the Deaf community in California in 1987, and several other states soon followed suit. These services promptly became swamped with callers and funding limitations obliged many to restrict use. The California relay service, for example, handled fifty thousand calls during its first month of operation; the number has now surpassed a quarter of a million calls per month.[45] A national organization, Telecommunications for the Deaf, Inc. (TDI, 45,000 subscribers), promotes TTY use and improvements and publishes a national directory of TTY owners.

Despite their popularity for lack of anything better, the relay services present many inconveniences, some of them inherent in the TTY, others in the procedure of relay itself. TTYs are expensive and there are only about 200,000 in use in the U.S. About half the states distribute TTYs at reduced cost to qualified consumers, but they are rarely available in public places. Then, too, it is painfully slow to communicate through the relay. We ran a little test. One of us, Bob, who is hearing, ordered a pizza and timed it. He pressed the seven-digit number, waited for the store to answer, then placed his order. The store asked for his phone number (so they could call him back for confirmation) and his address, and they estimated the wait. The process took one minute and twenty-eight seconds. When Ben, who is Deaf, ordered from the same store shortly thereafter, using the relay, it took six minutes and twenty-five seconds—four and a half times as long. Here's why. First Ben dialed the relay service and, when the operator answered, told her the phone number of the pizzeria. She in turn called the store, asked the manager if he knew how to use the relay (he didn't), and explained that there would be long delays while she typed what the manager said and waited for the Deaf client's typewritten response. She typed to Ben that the manager was on the line and wanted the address; she waited while Ben provided it, then she read it to the manager. The manager asked for a call-back number; the operator typed that request to Ben, who explained, typing, that the manager would need to call the relay service before reaching him, and then gave him both telephone numbers. The operator read that information aloud, and then the manager asked why he had to do that—go through the relay. The operator typed his question, Ben explained, the operator voiced the explanation, and the manager said okay. Finally Ben got to state his order, which the operator read aloud . . . and so on and so on.

Slow speed means high cost in long distance calls, but speed is not the only drawback of the relay compared to hearing telecommunications. The English that many Deaf people use on the TTY frequently reflects their native ASL; the operator who is not well trained simply reads aloud to the hearing client what he or she sees, and it may not make much sense. On the other hand, the operator who recodes the message into grammatical English instead of just reading it verbatim sometimes misunderstands and conveys the wrong message. The only check available to the Deaf person using the relay is to judge whether the hearing person's response was appropriate; this is often quite an unsatisfactory check. Fairly often, telephone calls are answered by answering machines. By the time the relay operator has heard and typed the recorded message, it is too late for the caller to leave a message. So the operator must place a second call to the same number. When the Deaf caller reaches the desired party, he or she types the message in English and the operator voices it, so the Deaf caller's affect—whether he or she is happy, sleepy, angry, etc.—is not communicated; neither is the hearing person's affect communicated to the Deaf caller. Then, too, the private communication feels public because the operator is listening in. Some callers do not feel that they have adequate confidentiality using the relay.

The long distance telephone companies have hired substantial numbers of Deaf people in an effort to improve their services and compete for the business of relay calls. In this new market, there are many positions in sales, marketing, publicity, field testing, training and management, where Deaf employees offer particular advantages arising from their knowledge of the DEAF–WORLD. Deaf managers at the phone company object to the limited knowledge of the operators when it comes to the language and culture of the DEAF–WORLD. They point out that another language minority, the Hispanic community, is served by bilingual operators, and they ask why operators serving the DEAF–WORLD are not equally qualified. True,

Deaf people would be unsuitable as relay operators, since if Deaf and hearing people could converse, the relay would be unnecessary. But the hearing relay operators could be required to have language fluency and cultural knowledge of the DEAF–WORLD.

The decoder and captioning

In the era of silent films, members of the DEAF–WORLD not only attended this form of entertainment as hearing people did, they also acted in and produced movies, as we saw in chapter 5 on Deaf culture. With the advent of the "talkies," however, Deaf people were shut out of the enjoyment and the business of movies. In 1958, Congress passed a law creating a federal program that subtitled some 16mm films with "open captions," captions visible to all viewers without special decoding devices. Such films were shown at the Deaf club, at residential schools, and occasionally in private homes. About a decade later, the Caption Center was established with federal funds in Boston, at public television's flagship WGBH, and the first television program was open-captioned; it was Julia Child's *The French Chef.* The Center soon went on to caption the *ABC Evening News*. Because it was widely believed that hearing viewers would find open captions an unwelcome distraction, the news was broadcast without captions first, and then rebroadcast with captions on public service stations only, about five hours after the original broadcast.

If captions could be *closed*, that is, made invisible for broadcast and decoded by the Deaf consumer with special equipment, it would be possible for Deaf and hearing viewers to see the same program at the same time. Research during the 1970s solved this problem but encountered another one. Networks did not want to pay for closed-captioning because they felt the cost would not be recovered from the increase in the viewing audience. Thus the National Captioning Institute was created with federal funds and began with a commitment from the major networks to present closed-caption programming for fifteen hours per week; today that figure has risen to over 770 hours a week of captioned programming.[46] Increasingly, captioning has become "real time," with news, sports events, and special broadcasts captioned by court reporters at speeds up to 250 words per minute.

Sales of television decoders to display the closed captions, however, have proved to be slow. One reason is cost: the original device sold for about $250; by the mid 1990s, prices ranged up to $175 and it was estimated that 400,000 were in use in the U.S.. However, potential users include Deaf and hard-of-hearing people (an estimated 24 million), Americans for whom English is a second language (30 million), adults with limited literacy seeking to improve their literacy through practice (27 million), children with reading problems (3.7 million), and young children learning to read (12 million).[47] Consequently, in 1993, Congress passed the Television Decoder Circuitry Act, which requires U.S. manufacturers of all television sets thirteen inches or larger to install a decoder chip that, at the touch of a button, displays closed captions on the screen. Since twenty million sets of this size are sold every year, by the end of the decade it is probable that nearly all U.S. homes will be able to display closed captions.[48] Americans watch television outside their homes as well. The ADA requires, as we have seen, that businesses and public accommodations do not exclude people with disabilities. Hence hospitals and hotels, for example, must provide access to closed captions on request. Computer-assisted real-time captioning (CART) is also increasingly to be found in courtrooms, meetings, theaters and classrooms.

Thanks to the energetic lobbying of the DEAF–WORLD and other groups, captioning has made great strides: most new releases of high-budget Hollywood films have closed captions. However, nine out of ten videos for sale or rent do not have captions. The NAD seeks captioning of all new release (or re-released) home videos, all new programs on cable TV, and most reruns. Deaf societies in several lands also have national TV programs in their signed language with themes of particular interest to them. Some countries, such as France and Switzerland, present some news programs interpreted into the national signed language, with the interpreter image in a corner of the TV screen; its small size makes it rather difficult to follow the signed language, however. In the United States, there is limited cable access to ASL programming.

You may wonder why captioning is so high on the Deaf agenda, when so many Deaf people have difficulty reading English, especially English that rapidly disappears. We wondered too, so we asked some Deaf friends. The consensus seems to be, it's better than nothing. However, ASL would be much preferable. The future in the U.S. will no doubt hold more programming on cable channels with Deaf people speaking ASL, perhaps captioned in English for a larger audience.

Signed languages and access

For most Deaf people in the world, who live in non-industrialized nations, captioning, the TTY, computer e-mail, and other forms of technology hold little of hope of providing them with access to information concerning local, national and international events. If such Deaf citizens are to receive their rights, lead fulfilling lives, and contribute to the welfare of their society, they must have access through signed language not only at home and at school, but in the workplace and in communal life. Sports, religion, government services and so on must be made accessible. The main means available are creating a corps of interpreters and teaching signed language to service personnel. We have spoken earlier of the lack of qualified interpreters in many lands. Even in those few nations with a relatively mature profession of interpreting, such as the United States, there are acute shortages.

With the growing empowerment of members of the DEAF–WORLD in providing services to other Deaf people (see below), a battle royal has been developing in the U.S. over the control of interpreting services. Interpreters (many of them codas), have long been partners with Deaf people in their quest for equal access to information and services. Indeed, they have contributed importantly to the very empowerment of Deaf people that now challenges the management of their profession. Reform of interpreter services is high on the agenda of the DEAF–WORLD in the U.S. and the list of their complaints is long. When presidents of the state associations of the Deaf gathered at NAD headquarters to discuss interpreting problems, they formulated a list of twenty-two concerns! Here are some of them:

- Schools hire uncertified interpreters almost exclusively.
- There is a shortage of interpreters in rural areas, in community centers, and just about everywhere else.
- Interpreters charge too much for their services.
- Interpreters need to get more and better benefits.

- There is no consumer complaint procedure that works.
- Interpreter education is not practical enough and needs Deaf community involvement.[49]

The five-thousand member Registry of Interpreters for the Deaf and the NAD are working together to try and resolve some of these concerns. Nevertheless, interpreter reform remains high on the Deaf agenda, and we should expect growing Deaf involvement in the provision of interpreter services in the United States as in other lands.

ENHANCING DEAF CULTURE AND SOCIAL LIFE

"Deaf people's enduring concerns have been these," writes Tom Humphries: "Finding each other and staying together; preserving their language; and maintaining lines of transmittal of their culture."[50]

Staying together

In America's DEAF-WORLD, the pursuit of "staying together" has been carried out on several fronts. First, as we have already discussed, there is the continuing struggle to protect and preserve the residential schools, where Deaf language and culture have been acquired and transmitted, lifelong Deaf friendships have been formed, and Deaf youngsters have been trained in the many roles demanded of them in adult society.

A vital structure for staying together once school days are over is the Deaf club. In many countries, the national Deaf organization is comprised of the local Deaf clubs. Hence the welfare of the entire DEAF-WORLD and the pursuit of its dreams is founded on the strength of the local Deaf clubs. The local Deaf clubs support athletic events, and those are another important way that Deaf people pursue their agenda of staying together.

Nowadays, many young Deaf people in the U.S. attend mainstream schools where they have little or no opportunity to learn about Deaf culture, to acquire pride as Deaf people, to develop the social and language skills they will need as Deaf adults, or to practice leadership. Consequently, on graduation, many of these young Deaf adults are slow to get involved in their local Deaf club. Then, too, with the advent of television captioning, there is more home-entertainment available to club members than in the past. It is widely believed that these two forces have drawn down membership in many Deaf clubs. On the other hand, growing numbers of Deaf Americans, like their counterparts in other lands, are finding each other and staying together in recreation programs organized by and for Deaf people. [51] (See chapter 5.)

Another arena in which Deaf people find each other and stay together is the workplace. American Deaf professionals seek to play a larger role in providing services to Deaf people. Traditionally, Deaf people frequently found employment through contacts with Deaf friends. With large numbers of Deaf people unemployed today and a broader range of employment opportunities available, it seems likely that very few Deaf people will have Deaf co-workers in the years ahead, except in Deaf-run businesses and social service agencies. More Deaf professionals are engaged in providing services to Deaf people than in any other single occupation. The U.S. DEAF–WORLD believes deeply that the most successful services are *of, by, and for the Deaf.* This means that agencies staffed by Deaf people, like the one Jake, at the Metro Silent Club, works for, do a better job of providing services to Deaf people than governmental or other community-based organizations. In the U.S., that claim is almost a truism; we have come to believe as a nation that minorities generally know best how to guide their own development and, in any case, have the moral right to do so.

Social Services of, by, and for the Deaf

In 1969, two Deaf students from the National Leadership Training Program for the Deaf at California State University, Northridge, did a survey of the Deaf community in the Los Angeles area and recommended a coordinating council for the numerous Deaf clubs and other groups. The result was GLAD, the Greater Los Angeles Council on Deafness. GLAD began with a small budget and one volunteer staff person; it has grown to a budget of nearly three million annually and a staff of over sixty Deaf and hearing workers. GLAD runs six outreach programs, four adult employment development programs, an AIDS education and services program, a tobacco control program, a bookstore, and an active agenda of lobbying for Deaf interests.

(Adapted from Meyer, 1994.)

There are numerous Deaf-run social services agencies all over the United States providing communication access, mental health services, educational services, and employment opportunity. Deaf people are finding each other, staying together, and helping each other in ever-increasing numbers. Likewise, there are growing numbers of Deaf-run businesses and professional practices that serve the DEAF–WORLD. A 1982 survey of 1,735 Deaf people in professional jobs found four out of five of them working in the "Deaf sector," providing services to Deaf and hard-of-hearing people.[52]

Preserving the language and transmitting the culture

The DEAF–WORLD here and abroad gives top priority to preserving its language. We have discussed the profound commitment to this issue on the Deaf agenda under the heading of education, for it is in the schools that most Deaf children are first able to fulfill their capacity for acquiring a natural language. Deaf societies around the world have been pursuing the preservation of their language in the political as well as the educational sphere. Scandinavian countries have succeeded in having their signed languages recognized formally by government as minority languages; many other countries, from Austria to Uganda, have such initiatives under way. In the U.S., Deaf organizations have secured legislation acknowledging ASL in more than half the states, and, as we said earlier, negotiations are in progress with the federal government to secure the rights of ASL speaking children to the educational benefits of the Bilingual Education Act. ASL is taught in more than one thousand colleges and universities and in a small but growing number of high schools. Increasing numbers of universities are allowing the study of ASL to satisfy their requirement that students study a second language; more than a score already do so.[53]

Many Deaf groups are active in transmitting the culture in a variety of settings. Deaf theater, of, by and about the DEAF–WORLD, is flourishing, as are the Deaf arts. Deaf journalism is reaching larger audiences, with better coverage, greater independence, and more outspoken Deaf pride. An initiative to ensure that Deaf culture materials are available in America's libraries and to make libraries "Deaf friendly" has made important headway.[54] In many developing nations, the first step in awakening

Deaf consciousness has been the study of their signed language and the preparation of signed language dictionaries (and sometimes grammars), which ensures the transmission of knowledge about the language across the generations. Many national Deaf organizations sponsor Deaf culture festivals. In the United States, each September brings Deaf Awareness Week, when local groups across the nation put on cultural events and national organizations redouble their efforts to inform the Congress and other bodies of the Deaf presence and agenda in America.

A striking development in the U.S., which is bound to have an important impact on the preservation of the language and culture of the DEAF–WORLD, is the development of the field of Deaf Studies. Growing numbers of schools are offering Deaf studies classes, and Gallaudet University has established a Department of Deaf Studies. Much new material is available for conducting these courses, designed for people of all ages, from preschoolers to adults.

Just what is Deaf studies and who should study it? The field of Deaf studies has grown out of the avalanche of scholarship concerning the DEAF–WORLD in the United States and around the globe. In recent years, numerous works have appeared in linguistics, sociology and anthropology, history, and literature—to mention just a few disciplines—that have generated a rich scholarly knowledge-base concerning Deaf culture and society. The overriding goal of Deaf studies is to understand better the lives of Deaf people so as to improve their lot; just as the goal of women's studies is to understand and improve the lot of women, and the goal of Black studies to understand and improve the lot of Black people. In addition to righting wrongs, programs such as these also enrich our understanding of what it is to be human by broadening our awareness of the forms of human activity and values.

Each of these fields draws on the social sciences and humanities but has its own issues and theories. What are the central issues in Deaf studies? Since the field aims to redress a wrong, namely, the oppression of a minority, it follows that the principles of repression in general, and of oppression of Deaf people in particular, are at the very core of the field. Moreover, wherever you investigate Deaf studies, you will find evidence of oppression. If you study language, you will find here a language minority whose people find it impossible to use their language in many walks of life. If you study education, you will find a system that perpetuates a working underclass. If you study history, you will learn about the timeless yearning of Deaf people for a place of their own, and how hearing people displaced Deaf adults from their rightful roles in the lives of Deaf children. In the context of oppression, the DEAF–WORLD grapples with questions such as these: Shall Deaf people grasp the banner of "disabled," with all the short-term benefits that it brings, or does that banner mask, at too high a price, the unique language and culture of Deaf people? Shall Deaf people strive for more success on hearing terms, such as better English literacy, and wider acceptance in the job market, or shall they seek also to change those terms, working for better signed-language literacy and developing Deaf markets? Shall Deaf leaders aim to rally all the community in behalf of a few clearly stated reforms, or shall they recognize the enormous diversity of Deaf people by qualifying their goals, at the risk of qualifying their progress?

Thus, Deaf leaders are crucial consumers of Deaf studies, for they must provide the intellectual leadership of the Deaf minority. They must draw up the agenda for reform and they must carry it out. This will be done more intelligently and successfully if they are knowledgeable over the whole spectrum of Deaf studies and if they have, with that knowledge, analyzed and refined the great issues related to oppression that face their minority. Deaf scholars are not only consumers of Deaf studies, but they are also among its producers, and this is vital. Whether it be Deaf culture, Deaf language or Deaf arts, the Deaf scholar brings a unique insight, intuition and creative imagination to the process of discovery, theorizing, and dissemination.

The present shortage of Deaf scholars is a great limitation on the field of Deaf studies. Deaf people, like Black people, are hampered in their efforts to describe and overcome their oppression by the nature of the education they received. If all Deaf college students had the opportunity to learn about the history, the social and language structure, and the arts of their nation's Deaf community, the field of Deaf studies would win the commitment of more Deaf scholars. It would leap forward, and so would efforts to improve the lives of Deaf people.

Deaf college students, and Deaf adults in general, will also find it rewarding to pursue Deaf studies for some more personal reasons. In learning through Deaf history about the lives of Deaf people before them, they can imagine more possible lives for themselves. In learning about Deaf society, Deaf education and Deaf culture, they can better equip themselves to be advocates for Deaf people. In seeing their personal struggles projected onto the screen of the Deaf arts, they can better understand what is unique to them and what they share in their struggle with millions of other Deaf people. They can laugh and cry and rage and applaud as timeless Deaf themes touch them deeply. It is no simple matter, however, to bring Deaf studies to most Deaf adults. For reasons that lie at the heart of this field, the schools often failed them pitifully when they were young, and they know it. They know that hearing people set the agenda of instruction. They know that hearing people tried to teach them in a hearing way and with a spoken language. They will not soon forget the pain of being led blindfolded through a dense thicket of English along a path not of their own choosing. This problem is worthy of the deepest thought of Deaf leaders. How can we bring the enjoyment and liberation of Deaf studies to Deaf adults?

However great the need for Deaf adults to pursue Deaf studies, the need is even greater for the Deaf child and his or her parents. Rural Deaf children in some countries live far apart, and there are no schools to bring them together and into contact with Deaf adults. In other countries, Deaf children are actively discouraged from contact with each other and with Deaf adults, and they are flung pell-mell into the local hearing school. These children may be seriously harmed in their linguistic, psychological and educational development. Magazines, books, films, theater and other means of bringing Deaf studies to Deaf children could make a vital difference in their lives.

What does Deaf studies have to offer to the parents of a Deaf child? Communication. Insight. Empathy. Acceptance. Respect.

Another audience for Deaf studies is people in the professions serving the Deaf: teachers, interpreters, counselors, psychologists, and so on. None of these professional people can do their job effectively if they are ignorant of the language and culture of the people they profess to serve.

The largest potential audience of all for Deaf studies is hearing students pursuing a liberal education in high school and especially college. The universities have nurtured women's studies and Black studies, and they must nurture Deaf studies, too. After all, the accumulation of knowledge is largely carried out in the universities. What Deaf studies has to offer the average hearing student is one way of acquiring the most important knowledge of all in a liberal education—an awareness of one's own cultural assumptions.

Most people are not aware of the cultural premises that guide their lives; they are ethnocentric and naturally so, for social life would be impossible if every action required reflection. People have an unconscious mental model of their culture that makes most of their choices for them, leaving them free to grapple with the remaining choices. Their ideas about wealth, family, sexuality, and disability, for example, all seem more or less given. They know abstractly and vaguely that other people live in other ways; but they do not know the premises beneath those differences. They do not see the linkages among the differences, and they cannot make the empathic leap to see the world from another vantage point. Not seeing that there is a range of choices of how to live, they do not realize that they have made such choices themselves. Since they do not realize they have made choices, in fact they have not. To choose is an act of conscious volition. For many members of the dominant majority, the fundamental choices have been made for them, by their parents and most of all, by historical inevitability.

For such people, the study of another culture can be a revelation; it can liberate and empower them by helping them to imagine other premises and other ways of life. Liberated by cultural perspective, these fortunate people are more able to fashion their own lives and "to connect" with the lives of others. These are the masses of people who should study Deaf studies. Ordinary hearing people all over the world are now enriching their lives by learning signed languages. International bodies like the European Parliament and UNESCO proclaim the importance of this cultural discovery. Now an important challenge before the field of Deaf studies is to develop an enriched body of knowledge about Deaf culture and arts and to disseminate it to hearing people at large, as well as to Deaf people of all ages and to their hearing friends and relations.

THE COLLISION BETWEEN HEARING AND DEAF AGENDAS

The hearing and Deaf agendas have been colliding at least since the 1700s. You will recall Pierre Desloges' protest against oralism in favor of LSF cited in chapter 3. Severe collisions occurred in the U.S. in the 1860s, as we have seen, when hearing professionals, parents, and legislators combined to create schools for Deaf children that used only spoken English. The agendas collided again, this time on an international scale, after the Congress of Milan. The congress, combined with social forces at the end of the last century such as immigration, xenophobia and nationalism, drove the U.S. DEAF–WORLD and its agenda underground and assured an era marked more by surface tranquility than by substantive progress. With the arrival of the Civil Rights movement in the 1960s, however, and the subsequent linguistic discoveries concerning ASL, the American DEAF–WORLD began anew to promote its values and agenda stridently. DEAF–WORLD self-affirmation has been growing similarly in other lands, as we have seen, fueled and nourished by a renaissance in Deaf culture here and abroad.

Just at that period in history when the DEAF–WORLDS are closest to full recognition of their languages and cultures, hearing professions that would eradicate Deaf culture have taken up their most powerful arms against Deaf people—surgery on Deaf children and eugenics. The effect of these concurrent developments, in the direction both of reinforcing Deaf culture and undermining it, has been to create conditions for the severest conflicts yet to be encountered in Deaf history. Growing violence is evident not only in the language of charges and counter-charges, but also in actions. In 1995, as we have noted, the French riot police blocked a Deaf march, led by the Deaf group *Sourds en Colère*, to the Paris school for the Deaf, founded by the abbé de l'Epée. That same year, *Sourds en Colère* broke into a session of the Third Paris International Congress on Cochlear Implants and shut it down.

It is hard to see how the American DEAF–WORLD, once emancipated and in the wake of the Gallaudet Revolution, can ever be persuaded to embrace, or even tolerate, a hearing agenda based on disability that includes such provisions as mainstreaming, cochlear implants, and eugenics. Yet, the obstacles to replacing a disability construction of Deaf people with a language-minority construction are daunting. In the first place, people who have little familiarity with the DEAF–WORLD find the disability construction self-evident and the minority construction elusive. Hearing people, if they have some occasion to think about Deaf people, frequently begin by imagining themselves without hearing, which is, of course, to have a disability but not to be Deaf.

Another obstacle to reforming the construction of Deaf people is the troubled-persons industry. Advocates of the disability construction control teacher training programs, university research facilities, the process of peer review for federal grant monies, the presentations made at professional meetings, and publications in professional journals; they control promotions and, through promotions, salaries. They have privileged access to the media and to law-making bodies when Deaf people are at issue. Although they lack the credibility of Deaf people themselves, they have expert credentials and they are fluent in speaking and writing English, so policy makers and the media find it easier to consult them.

When a troubled-persons industry recasts social problems as private troubles it can treat, it is removing them from the social arena that invites political debate. The World Health Organization, for example, has medicalized and individualized what is social; services are based on an individualized view of disability and are designed by professionals in the disability industry.[55] The U.S. National Institute on Deafness and Other Communication Disorders proclaims in its very title the disability construction of Deaf people that it seeks to promote. Less than two percent of its budget in the current fiscal year is devoted to research of direct concern to culturally Deaf people. The American Speech-Language Hearing Association has the power of accrediting graduate programs for training professionals who work with Deaf people; a program that deviated too far from the disability construction could lose its accreditation; without accreditation its students would not be certified; without the promise of certification, no one would enter the training program.

Some of the gravest obstacles to broader acceptance of the linguistic-minority model come from members of the minority itself. Many members of the minority were socialized in part by professionals (and parents) to adopt a disabled role. Some Deaf people openly embrace the disability construction and thus undercut the efforts of other Deaf people to discredit it. Worse yet, many opportunities are provided to Deaf people (e.g., access to interpreters) on the condition that they subscribe to an alien classification of themselves based on disability. This double bind, to accept the hearing construction of your life or give up your access to equal citizenship, is a powerful form of oppression. Thus, many members of the DEAF–WORLD endorsed the Americans with Disabilities Act, with its provisions for Deaf people, all the while believing that they were not disabled but lending credence to the claim that they were. In a related double bind, Deaf adults who want to become part of the professions serving Deaf people, find that they must subscribe to oppressive views of rehabilitation, special education, etc.

Exponents of the linguistic-minority construction are at a further disadvantage because there is little built-in cultural transmission of their beliefs. The most persuasive advocates for Deaf children, their parents, must be taught generation after generation the counter-intuitive linguistic-minority construction, because most are neither Deaf themselves nor did they have Deaf parents.

Despite all the obstacles, there are powerful social forces to assist the efforts of the DEAF–WORLD to promote the linguistic-minority construction. The body of knowledge developed in linguistics, history, sociology, and anthropology (to mention just four disciplines) concerning DEAF–WORLDS has influenced Deaf leadership, bureaucratic decision-making, and legislation. The Civil Rights movement has given great impetus to the belief that minorities should define themselves and that minority leaders should have a significant say in the conduct of minority affairs. Moreover, the failure of the present predominant disability construction to deliver more able Deaf children is a source of professional and public embarrassment and promotes change. Then, too, Deaf children of Deaf parents are frequently insulated against the disability construction, at least to a degree, by their early acquisition of language and culture within the DEAF–WORLD. These native ASL-users have important allies among others in the DEAF–WORLD, among hearing children of Deaf parents, and among disaffected hearing professionals. The Gallaudet Revolution did not change the disability construction on a large scale, but it led to inroads against it.

COLLISIONS OR ALLIANCES?

Perhaps the greatest hope for avoiding damaging conflict is our mutual respect for human differences, the kind of respect that made this book possible, and that sustained you in reading it. When it comes to disputes like this, over contrasting beliefs and practices in two different cultures, there may be no reasonable alternative to mutual respect (even though we are convinced the other side is wrong). Who is right? Is the DEAF–WORLD a group of people with a disability, as mainstream (hearing) culture maintains, or is it a linguistic and cultural minority, as Deaf people themselves contend? The answer is: It depends on your cultural frame of reference; there is no culture-free vantage point from which we can look down on this issue and make the right choice. In such cross-cultural disputes, if it doesn't make sense to ask "Who is right?" perhaps we can ask, "What works best?" Probably what would most promote the interests of Deaf children, and therefore of their parents and the DEAF–WORLD, are alliances among the concerned parties: Deaf people, parents, professionals, politicians, other minorities (including people with disabilities), and scholars.

Many Deaf leaders and their hearing allies see in bilingual/bicultural education a model for the relations between the DEAF–WORLD and the larger hearing society. BiBi, as it is affectionately called, is premised on mutual respect for each other's languages and cultures. It is operationally an alliance between Deaf and hearing people to accomplish shared goals.

Deaf leaders have long been forging alliances with hearing people in the pursuit of the Deaf agenda. The alliance between the DEAF–WORLD and the parents' organization in Sweden made possible enormous strides toward the acceptance of Deaf language and culture, as it has in other lands. The DEAF–WORLD has every motive for collaborating with parents, for the parents are the guardians of the Deaf child's development and welfare; their decisions shape the future Deaf adult. At the same time, the DEAF–WORLD holds the key to that child's successful development, language and culture, and Deaf adults "have been there"—they know exactly what it means to grow up Deaf in a hearing world, and how to do it and succeed. Their counsel and support can be a priceless asset. Deaf people, in fact, desire this collaboration and, in our experience, are ready to meet hearing parents more than half way. The ASL poet Ella Mae Lentz, whose work we quoted in chapter 4, devoted a poem to this theme in Deaf culture; it appears below, translated from ASL (alas, the moving imagery does not translate). Admittedly, parents and professionals hear at times a shrill voice coming from the DEAF–WORLD. People become shrill when they feel they are being ignored, marginalized, excluded from decisions that vitally affect them. If parents also desire a collaboration, they should strive for the empowerment of Deaf adults today, as they would wish their own child to be empowered as an adult tomorrow. If both parties show their mutual respect for each other's languages and cultures, the road is wide open to collaboration.

To a Hearing Mother
by Ella Mae Lentz

You and I are different.
Different worlds, languages, life experiences.
You grew up ignorant of Deaf people though
You may have heard of a few
Here and there.
I grew up in the DEAF–WORLD, all too familiar with the
hearing and their oppressive ways.

Now you give birth to a boy. He's Deaf!
You're shocked! I'm surprised and delighted!

You struggle to make the boy like you.
However, he'll grow up to be like me.
He has your likeness.
However, he has my ears, soul, language and world view.
He's your son, but he's of my people.
Then, who does the boy belong to? You or me?
He's like a tree.
Without our people,
he would wither and be left with no soul, no sense of self.
But without you, there wouldn't be any trees.
Our great people and language would dwindle.

> Our struggles and fighting can be like a saw
> that brings down the tree.
> We must stop it, and share, and love, and accept
> and together be the ground to nourish the tree
> So it will grow tall, proud and strong.
> And seek the heavens.
>
> (Lentz, 1995. Based on a translation from the ASL by the author.)

The alliances between Deaf leaders and hearing politicians in many of the states of the U.S. and in Congress during the Gallaudet Revolution have made it possible for Deaf people to play a larger role in delivering services to Deaf children and adults. The National Association of the Deaf and the Registry of Interpreters for the Deaf in the U.S. are working to forge an alliance. Other professions in the social sector, such as rehabilitation, counseling, and mental health services, are aware as never before that alliances with the DEAF–WORLD are essential if professionals are to have proper training, a successful practice, and the confidence of their clientele.

We have seen that the DEAF–WORLD contains many members from ethnic minorities; moreover, it shares several focal concerns with those minorities and with the disability rights movement. Of course, parents and professionals must be part of those alliances, too. In recent years professions such as audiology, speech and language pathology, and Deaf education have made a major effort to forge alliances with ethnic minorities; perhaps that will facilitate forging alliances with the DEAF–WORLD. The president of Gallaudet University, I. King Jordan, has called for an alliance between geneticists and the DEAF–WORLD to educate each other, as well as parents, who need to understand the potential of a Deaf child to lead a rewarding and contributing life.[56]

Hearing scholars in many lands have gladly entered into alliances with the DEAF–WORLD because it was obvious to them, both ethically and practically, that they could not pursue their studies in the language, culture, history, etc., of the DEAF–WORLD without its active guidance and collaboration. Those scholars have brought greater recognition of Deaf culture, contributed to the exchange of ideas about improving the lot of

Deaf people, and in some cases aided Deaf people in advancing their own scholarship and professional standing. Indeed, this very book is the fruit of collaboration among a DEAF–WORLD publisher, a hearing editor, a Deaf scholar and leader, a coda educator, and a hearing scholar.

Vive la collaboration!

❦

Chapter 16

Journey's End

NOW we have reached the end of our journey into the DEAF–WORLD. In fact it is probably more like a beginning. We would like to say good-bye to you, the readers, who have spent time with us. We're optimistic that the great, universal issues we've raised, issues like diversity versus deviance, will help to guide you as you navigate your own journey into the sea of humanity. If you ever land in a harbor where there are Deaf people, you will know they sail on the seas of brotherhood just like you. Sometimes a brother has to tell you, "You are crowding me, give me some room." This has to happen in order for us to grow together and to make a place for everyone.

It is late at the club room. People are leaving gradually, in groups, in pairs, singly. Gloria scans her notes, then stacks the papers with finality. She has completed the interview. She thanks the group for their time and for sharing their intimate thoughts, feelings and lives. Then she thanks the interpreters. Laurel, Henry, Roberto and Jake stand and shake her hand, then resume their seats and their conversation. Gloria smiles good-bye, slips her bag over her shoulder, and waves a last time. She walks toward the door.

If we had only one thought to leave you with it would be this: that the best hope for alliances between Deaf and hearing people lies in the creation of bilingual and bicultural education for Deaf children. This model allows for both languages and cultures to be treated with equal respect. Imagine a world in which the Deaf child learns that hearing people value Deaf language and culture as they value their own; a world in which Deaf adults and hearing adults work alongside each other. This creates a lot of possibilities. And promise for succeeding generations. For the future.

Gloria reaches the door that leads to the hallway going downstairs to the street, turns, and looks back. The others are still at the table. Roberto has stood up and is laughing at something Henry has just said. Gloria waves, hoping they will see her, and turns to walk down the hall. The clubroom's light begins to flash on and off, signifying that it is closing time. The group now rises and walks slowly to the doorway. Roberto hugs Laurel good-bye. Jake shakes Henry's hand and comments that it was an interesting evening. They hope Gloria will be one of those reporters who "gets it."

A few years ago we heard a tale about a little Deaf boy, some seven years old, who went to a residential school. At school he was normally taciturn. At most residential schools the boarders go home on Fridays and return to school on Mondays. One Monday, this boy's teacher noticed that the boy had come to school quite changed. He had turned into a very active, outgoing kid over the weekend. The teacher, who was hearing, went over and asked him, "What makes you so happy this morning?" The boy replied, bubbling, "My mother is Deaf." The teacher was taken aback; she knew the boy's mother was hearing. Perhaps she'd had a tragic accident. It took the teacher a while to recoup and ask the boy, "How did your mother become Deaf?" The boy didn't really understand the question and said, smiling,"My mother is Deaf now!"

"I know she is Deaf now, but how did she become that way? Did she get sick?" asked the teacher again.

"No, she did not get sick. She can sign now!" the boy replied, beaming.

In this story, the Deaf boy saw the difference between what makes a person Deaf and what makes a person hearing: it is the use of signed language. So the hope for the future lies in more and more people using ASL, which then might reshape how we view and define the DEAF–WORLD. Perhaps one day the DEAF–WORLD will be called the *ASL–WORLD*.

Laurel hugs Jake and Roberto again at the door and reminds them that she really has to go. "Don't forget bingo night," Henry says. "I'll be there with Maggie." The manager of the club goes around the clubroom telling people to leave. Everyone is making his or her way gradually toward the door, but clusters of chatting people block the way. The manager goes over to the group and tells them to get going. Then he gives them a little push, until everyone gets out the door, and he closes it. Henry glances at his watch and remembers his promise to be home by eleven, gives them all a "thumbs-up," leave-taking signal, and turns to go down the hallway. Jake follows Henry and taps him on his shoulder, stopping him at the top of the staircase. Roberto and Laurel hug good-bye one more time, then meet the others at the stairs.

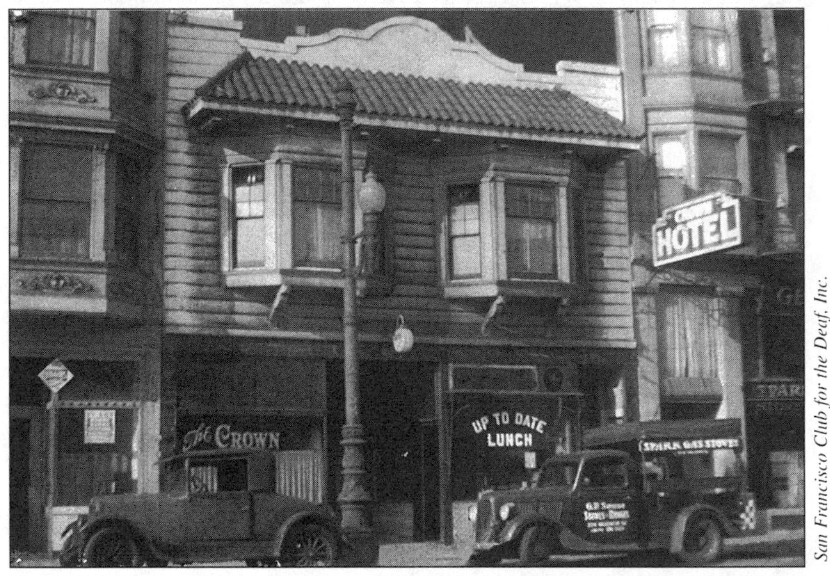

San Francisco Club for the Deaf, Inc.

Fig. 16-1. **Home of the San Francisco Club for the Deaf; the clubhall is on the second floor**

The story about the little boy and his mother offers another glimpse of hope for the future. We see the need for hearing parents and Deaf people to work together to create a better place for Deaf children. Ella Lentz, in her poem *To a Hearing Mother*, said it perfectly when she pointed out that "the Deaf child is your child, but he is my people." Lentz's poem offers a solution better than fighting over parents' rights and children's rights: Working together to foster the child's development.

Gloria is still outside; she's been waiting a long time for her streetcar. She sees the group finally come out the front door and gather in a circle under a bright street light. Henry tells Roberto and Laurel—for the fifth time—that he needs to go home, his wife is expecting him. Jake ignores Henry and continues to talk with the group. He glances over to the streetcar stop and notices Gloria standing there. He waves at her, she waves back. Then the car arrives and Gloria gets on and finds a seat by the window. She puts her briefcase down. As the streetcar moves off she looks back at the group one more time and sees them under the street light hugging and shaking hands, saying good-bye once more.

❦

Notes

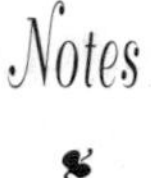

Chapter 1 Welcome to the DEAF–WORLD

1. Most of the information on the DEAF–WORLD in this chapter is extracted from Bahan, 1995.

Chapter 2 Families with Deaf Children

1. Lane, 1992, 1995.
2. Petitto & Marentette, 1991.
3. Reviews in: Israelite, Ewoldt & Hoffmeister 1989; Johnson, Liddell & Erting 1989; Mindel & Vernon, 1971; Vernon, 1969b. Also see, Brasel, 1975; Charrow & Fletcher, 1974; Corson, 1973; Geers & Schick, 1988; Hansen & Kjaer-Sorensen, 1976; Harris, 1978; Kourbetis, 1987; Moores, 1987; Weisel & Reichstein, 1987; Zweibel 1987.
4. Recounted by S. Supalla in Padden & Humphries, 1988.
5. Preston, 1994.
6. Schein, 1989.
7. Moores & Meadow-Orlans, 1990.
8. Scott, 1981.
9. Cf. review in Israeliste, Ewoldt & Hoffmeister, 1989; Rodda & Grove, 1987.
10. Freeman, Carbin, & Boese, 1975.
11. Tronick, Als, Adamson, Wise & Brazelton, 1978
12. Freeman, Boese, & Carbin, 1975; Lenneberg, 1967; Moores, 1987.
13. Harvey, 1989; Meadow, 1980.
14. Martin, 1994.
15. United Nations, 1994.
16. Tucker & Nolan, 1984.
17. Gjerdingen, 1987.
18. Jodoin & Hoffmeister, 1994.
19. Marlowe, 1987.
20. Ross, 1990.
21. Marlowe, 1987.
22. Hawkins & Baker-Hawkins, 1991.
23. Luterman, 1986.
24. Balkany, 1994.
25. Harris, 1978; Harvey, 1989; Hoffmeister, 1985; Mindel & Vernon, 1971.
26. Moores, 1987.
27. Schlesinger, 1972.
28. Freeman, Carbin & Boese, 1981; Freeman, Malkin & Hastings, 1975; Greenberg, 1980, 1983; Harris, 1978; Meadow, 1968; Schlesinger, 1972; Schlesinger & Meadow, 1972.
29. Swisher, 1983, 1984.
30. Gregory, 1976; Ross, 1990; Spradley & Spradley, 1978.
31. Luterman, 1986.
32. Newport & Gleitman, 1977.
33. Hoffmeister & Wilbur, 1980.
34. Goldin-Meadow, 1985.
35. Goldin-Meadow, 1985; Goldin-Meadow & Mylander, 1990a, b.
36. Chess and Fernandez, 1980.
37. Greenberg, 1980.
38. Swisher & Thompson, 1985.
39. Mindel & Vernon, 1971.
40. Harvey, 1989.

Chapter 3 The Language of the DEAF–WORLD

1. Schein, 1989.
2. Grosjean, 1982.
3. Fischer, 1982.
4. Pettito & Marentette, 1991.
5. Bonvillian, Orlansky & Folven, 1994; McIntire, 1977; Meier & Newport, 1990.
6. Newport & Meier, 1985.
7. Pizzuto, 1994.

Chapter 3 The Language of the Deaf-World (cont.)

8. Petitto & Bellugi, 1988.
9. Based on Israelite, Ewoldt & Hoffmeister, 1989; Newport & Meier, 1985.
10. Newport & Meier, 1985; Petitto, 1993.
11. Goldin-Meadow, 1985; Newport & Meier, 1985.
12. Gee & Mounty, 1991; Livingston, 1983; Supalla, 1986, 1991.
13. Gee & Mounty, 1991; Supalla, 1986.
14. Mayberry & Eichen, 1991; Newport, 1988, 1990.
15. Newport, 1990.
16. Mayberry & Eichen, 1991.
17. Moody, 1987.
18. Woodward, 1978.
19. Fischer, 1978.
20. Goldin-Meadow & Mylander, 1984.
21. Frishberg, 1975.
22. Congress On Deaf, 1878.
23. Lane, 1984.
24. Cited in Lane, 1984.
25. Schildroth & Hoto, 1991.
26. Woodward, 1973.
27. Woodward, 1974.
28. Shroyer & Shroyer, 1984.
29. Woodward, 1976.
30. Lucas & Valli, 1992.
31. Cummins & Danesi, 1990; Turner, 1995.
32. Wilbur, 1987.
33. Lucas & Valli, 1992.
34. Lane & Battison, 1978.
35. Battison, 1978.
36. Lucas & Valli, 1990; Woodward & Markowicz, 1975.
37. Zimmer, 1989.
38. Gumperz quoted in Markowicz & Woodward, 1978.
39. Kannapell, 1989.
40. Quoted in Schein, 1989, p. 39.
41. Quoted in Padden & Humphries, 1988, p.63.
42. Quoted in Lane, 1984, p. 233.
43. Kannapell, 1989.
44. Hall, 1989.
45. Becker, 1980, p.65
46. Padden, 1980, p. 96.
47. Johnson, 1994.
48. Hall, 1989.
49. Supalla, 1992.
50. Mottez, 1985.
51. Mindess, 1990.

Chapter 4 Form and Function in ASL

1. Liddell & Johnson, 1989.
2. Fischer, 1982.
3. Battison, 1978.
4. Klima & Bellugi, 1979.
5. Bellugi & Fischer, 1972.
6. Aarons et al., 1992; Fischer, 1975; Padden, 1988.
7. Petitto & Bellugi, 1988.
8. Emmorey, Bellugi, Friederici & Horn, 1995.
9. Klima & Bellugi, 1979.
10. Supalla & Newport, 1978; Also see Padden & Perlmutter, 1987.
11. Shick, 1990; Supalla, 1986.
12. Emmorey & Corina, 1992.
13. Emmorey & Corina, 1992.
14. Emmorey & Corina, 1990.
15. Mayberry & Fischer, 1989; Mayberry & Eichen, 1991.
16. Newport, 1990.
17. Reilly, McIntire & Bellugi, 1994.
18. Wilbur, 1994.
19. Liddell, 1977.
20. Bahan, 1996; Baker, 1976; Baker & Padden, 1978.
21. Aarons, Bahan, Kegl & Neidle, 1992; Kegl, 1985.
22. Aarons, Bahan, Kegl & Neidle, 1992; Kegl, 1985; Lillo-Martin, 1992.
23. Bahan & Supalla, 1994.
24. Baker, 1976, 1977; Baker & Padden, 1978.
25. Clark & Clark, 1968.
26. Bellugi & Klima, 1976.
27. See Wilbur, 1987.
28. Bellugi & Siple, 1974.
29. Klima & Bellugi, 1979.
30. Mills & Weldon, 1983.
31. Poizner, Newkirk, Bellugi & Klima, 1981.
32. Mayberry & Fischer, 1989.
33. Hanson, 1986.
34. Hanson, Shankweiler & Fischer, 1983.
35. O'Grady, Van Hoek & Bellugi, 1990; Padden, 1991; Padden, 1995, personal communication.
36. Shand, 1982.
37. Hanson, 1989.
38. Hanson, 1986, 1989.
39. Hanson, Shankweiler & Fischer, 1983.
40. Geers & Moog, 1987; Moores & Sweet, 1990.
41. Hanson, 1982; Hanson, Shankweiler & Fischer, 1983; Padden, 1991.
42. Padden, 1991.

Chapter 4 Form and Function in ASL (cont.)

43. Hanson & Bellugi, 1982.
44. Jarvella, 1971.
45. Poizner, Klima & Bellugi, 1987.
46. Emmorey & Casey, 1995; Lane, 1986.
47. Emmorey, 1995; Emmorey & Casey, 1995.
48. Emmorey, 1995.
49. Liddell, 1990, disputes this analysis.
50. Emmorey, Corina & Bellugi, 1995.
51. Emmorey, 1995.
52. Bellugi, O'Grady, Lilo-Martin, O'Grady-Hynes, van Hoek & Corina, 1994; Conrad, 1979; Karchmer, Trybus & Paquin, 1978; Sisco & Anderson, 1980; Vernon, 1969a.
53. Bellugi, O'Grady, Lilo-Martin, O'Grady-Hynes, van Hoek & Corina, 1994; Bettger, 1992; Emmorey, 1993.
54. Siple, 1978.
55. Neville, 1988.
56. Bettger, 1992; Klima, Tzeng, Fok, Bellugi, Corina & Bettger, in press.
57. Discussion based on Klima & Bellugi, 1979.
58. Panara, 1987.
59. Description adapted from Kuntze, 1994.
60. The excerpt is reprinted from Padden & Humphries, 1988, p. 107, and the discussion is based on theirs.
61. Valli, 1995.
62. Excerpted from Valli, 1990. The analysis is based on a phonological theory of ASL by Liddell & Johnson, 1986.
63. Bienvenu, 1994.

Chapter 5 Deaf Culture

1. Van Cleve & Crouch, 1989, p. ix.
2. Van Cleve & Crouch, 1989.
3. Lane, 1984; Winzer, 1986.
4. Van Cleve & Crouch, 1989; Lane, 1984.
5. Britain: Van Cleve & Crouch, 1989; France: Lane, 1984. Also see Bullard, 1986.
6. Levesque, 1994.
7. Y. Andersson quoted in Christiansen & Barnartt, 1995, p. 37.
8. The description of the Gallaudet Revolution is based on Gannon, 1988. Also see Christiansen & Barnartt, 1995; Gannon, 1989.
9. For hearing people, 1995.
10. Stewart, 1991.
11. Gross, 1994.
12. Hall, 1991, p. 421.
13. Quotation from Foster, 1989.
14. Gannon, 1981.
15. Baker-Shenk, 1985.
16. Veditz, 1933.
17. Creighton, 1994.
18. Bernard, 1993; Karakostas, 1990.
19. Panara, 1987; Dr. Betty Miller, 1995, personal communication.
20. Mannes, 1987.
21. Willard, 1989.
22. Miller, 1994.
23. Painting description by L.K. Elion, with permission.
24. Baird, 1993.
25. Based on materials supplied by D. Bahl.
26. Silver, 1993; Sonnenstrahl, 1993.
27. Halverson, 1987.
28. Quoted in Baldwin, 1995, p. 21.
29. Baldwin, 1995.
30. Lentz, 1995.
31. Rutherford, 1995. Personal communication.
32. Banks & Bryan, 1993.
33. Bangs, 1987.
34. See the discussion in Bangs, 1994.
35. Bangs, 1994.
36. Neisser, 1983.
37. Schuchman, 1988.
38. Supalla, 1994a, b.
39. Padden, 1980.
40. Gannon, 1981.
41. Rutherford & Mocenigo, 1984.
42. Supalla, & Bahan, 1994.
43. Carlin, 1847.
44. Luczak, 1992.
45. Rutherford, 1989.
46. Bouchauveau, 1994.
47. Bienvenu, 1994; Coleman & Jankowski, 1994; Rutherford, 1989.
48. Jacobowitz, 1992.
49. Markowicz & Woodward, 1978.
50. Cohen, 1994a.
51. Wood & Holcomb, 1989.
52. Bournazian, 1993.
53. Aramburo, 1994; Woodward, 1976; Woodward & De Santis, 1977; Woodward & Erting, 1975b.
54. Hairston & Smith, 1983.
55. Aramburo, 1994; Higgins, 1980.
56. Anderson, 1994.
57. Anderson, 1992; Anderson & Grace, 1991; Dunn, 1989.
58. Emery & Slone, 1994.
59. Aramburo, 1989.

Chapter 5 Deaf Culture (cont.)

60. Hairston & Smith, 1983.
61. Farrell, 1989.
62. Rodriguez & Santiviago, 1991.
63. Cohen, 1993; Gerner de Garcia, 1993; Jackson-Maldonado, 1993.
64. Lopez, 1993.
65. Cheng, 1993.
66. Hammond & Meiners, 1993.
67. Kane, 1994.
68. Renteria, 1995.
69. Luczak, 1993, p. 15.
70. Smith et al., 1994; Wolf, 1987.
71. Wolf, 1987.
72. Chiccioli, 1994.
73. Reiman, Bullis, Davis & Cole, 1991.
74. Wolff & Harkins, 1986. See Lane, 1992, for a critique of teacher rating of Deaf student handicaps.
75. Allen, 1986a.
76. Hoffmeister, in press.
77. Preston, 1994.
78. Bahan, 1994; Padden, 1980; Preston, 1994; Sidransky, 1990; Walker, 1986.

Chapter 6 The World Deaf Scene

1. Woodward, 1978.
2. Lane, 1984.
3. Calvet, 1974.
4. Javal, 1887.
5. Karakostas, 1993a; Mottez, 1993.
6. Truffaut, 1994.
7. Colin, 1978, p. 13.
8. Mottez, 1993, p. 57.
9. Mottez & Markowicz, 1980.
10. Abbou, 1993; Brusque, 1993.
11. Bouchauveau, 1990.
12. Cuxac, 1983; Grémion, 1990; Moody, 1983.
13. Karakostas, 1990.
14. Belissen, 1993, p. 4.
15. Mottez, 1993.
16. Bouillon, 1993.
17. Cuxac, 1993.
18. Burgos, 1993.
19. Abbou, 1994; Bouchauveau, 1993; Karakostas, 1993b; Smith, 1994.
20. Truffaut, 1993.
21. This discussion of the French scene is based in part on Lane, 1993b.
22. Edenas, 1994.
23. Heiling, 1995, cited in Davies, 1990.
24. Mahshie, 1995.
25. Davies, 1990.
26. Wallin, 1994, pp. 320-321.
27. Wallin, 1995.
28. Andersson, 1994.
29. Wågström-Lundqvist, 1994.
30. Edmondson & Karlsson, 1990.
31. European Parliament, 1988.
32. Jones & Pullen, 1989.
33. Andersson, 1987.
34. Andersson, 1994a.
35. Joutselainen, 1991.
36. Commonwealth Secretariat, 1972.
37. UNESCO, 1985.
38. World Federation of the Deaf, 1993b.
39. Based on Bahan & Poole, 1995.
40. Respectively: Bahan & Poole, 1995; Groce, 1985. Johnson, 1994. Frishberg, 1987. Washbaugh, 1986; Woodward, 1978. Kakumasu, 1968; Farb, 1973.
41. Groce, 1985.
42. Attributed to T. Supalla, personal communication, in Bahan & Poole, 1995.
43. Johnson, 1994.
44. Moody, 1989.
45. Supalla & Webb, 1995.
46. Andersson, 1994.

Chapter 7 Disabling the DEAF-WORLD

1. Lane, 1984, pp. 15–16.

Chapter 8 Educational Placement and the Deaf Child

1. Luetke-Stahlman, 1988a, b.
2. Maxwell, Bernstein, & Matthews, 1990, 1991.
3. Woodward, 1990.
4. Moores, 1987.
5. Goppold, 1988.
6. Hoffmeister, 1982.
7. Moores, 1987.
8. Allen & Karchmer, 1990.
9. Moores, Weiss, & Goodwin, 1978.
10. Vincent, 1995.
11. Luterman, 1986.
12. Cited in Paul & Quigley, 1990. Also see Sabatino, 1982.
13. Hoffmeister, in press; Hoffmeister, 1993b; Lane, 1988.
14. Woodward, 1990.
15. Policy guidance issued October 30, 1992.

Chapter 8 Educational Placement and the Deaf Child (cont.)

See Baker-Hawkins & Esterbrooks, 1994.
16. DuBow, Geer & Strauss, 1992.
17. Moores, 1992.
18. Lane, 1992.
19. Woodward, 1990.
20. Nover, 1994.
21. Kluwin, Moores & Gonter-Gaustad, 1992.
22. Hallahan & Kaufman, 1995.
23. Allen, Rawlings & Schildroth, 1989; Craig & Garrity, 1994.
24. Stedt, 1992.
25. Patrie, 1994.
26. Dahl & Wilcox, 1990; Stedt, 1992.
27. Stedt, 1992.
28. Patrie, 1994.
29. Wilcox, Schroeder, & Martinez, 1990.
30. Schick & Williams, 1994.
31. Schick & Williams, 1994.
32. Wilcox, Schroeder, & Martinez, 1990.
33. Dahl, 1994; Dahl & Wilcox, 1990.
34. Wilcox, Schroeder, & Martinez, 1990.
35. Kluwin & Moores, 1985.
36. Wilcox, Schroeder, & Martinez, 1990.
37. Roy, 1992.
38. Roy, 1992.
39. Stedt, 1992.
40. Stedt, 1992.
41. Patrie, 1994.
42. Dahl, 1994.
43. Dahl & Wilcox, 1990; Patrie, 1994.
44. Patrie, 1994.
45. Hoffmeister, 1993a, 1994; Nover, 1993a, b, 1994. But see Wilcox, Schroeder, & Martinez, 1990.
46. Cokely, 1986.
47. Schick & Williams, 1994.
48. Lederberg, 1991; Vandell, Anderson, Ehrhardt, & Wilson, 1982.
49. Ramsey, 1993.

Chapter 9 Language and Literacy

1. Moores, 1987, p. 198.
2. Lane, 1984.
3. Israelite, Ewoldt & Hoffmeister, 1989.
4. Corson, 1973; Brasel & Quigley, 1975; Moores, Weiss & Goodwin, 1978. Also see: Moores, 1987; DeVillers, 1988.
5. Nover, 1993b.
6. Johnson, Liddell & Erting, 1989.
7. Allen & Karchmer, 1990.
8. Allen & Karchmer, 1990; Woodward, 1990.
9. Bornstein, Saulnier & Luczak, 1984.
10. Gustason, Pfeitzing & Zowolokow, 1992; Gustason, 1988
11. Anthony, 1971.
12. Allen, 1986.
13. Bickerton, 1982; Romaine, 1988; Singleton, 1989.
14. Andersen, 1983; Gee & Goodhart, 1988; Gee and Mounty, 1991.
15. Meier, 1990; Hoffmeister, 1990.
16. Cummins, 1984.
17. Cummins, 1984; Cummins & Swain, 1986; Cummins, 1988.
18. Cummins & Swain, 1986.
19. Pattison, 1982.
20. Marmor & Petitto, 1978; Wodlinger-Cohen, 1991; Gaustad, 1992.
21. Supalla, 1991; Wodlinger-Cohen, 1991; Hoffmeister, 1993a, 1995.
22. Erting, 1981, 1985; Williams & Capizzi-Snipper, 1990.
23. Smith, 1978; Wells, 1981.
24. Davey & King, 1990.
25. Dummet, 1981.
26. Davey, Lassaso & Cacready, 1983; Davey & King, 1990; Ewoldt, 1993; Marshall, 1970; Moores, 1970; Odom, Blanton, & Nunnally, 1967; Paul & Jackson, 1993.
27. Davey, Lassaso & Cacready, 1983; Davey & King, 1990; Marshall, 1970; Moores, 1970; Odom, Blanton, & Nunnally, 1967.
28. Fischler, 1983; Moores, 1970; Webster, 1987.
29. Davey & King, 1990; Sternberg, 1987.
30. Strassman et al., 1987.
31. Davey & King, 1990.
32. Davey & King, 1990; Nagy, Anderson & Herman, 1987.
33. Davey, 1987.
34. Davey & King, 1990.
35. Paul, 1994.
36. Bloom, 1984; Moores, 1987; Walberg, 1984.
37. Allen & Karchmer, 1990.
38. Ewoldt, 1985, 1993.
39. Mathews & Reich, 1993.
40. Erting, 1988; Mather, 1987.
41. Johnson & Griffith, 1986; Mather, 1987, 1993.
42. Johnson & Griffith, 1986; Mather, 1987, 1993; Mather & Matthews, 1993.
43. Hoffmeister, 1995.
44. Ewoldt, 1993.
45. Allen, 1986a.
46. Lane, 1984.

Chapter 10 Bilingual and Bicultural Education for Deaf Children

1. Kannapell, 1989; Mahshie, 1995.
2. Bilingual Education Act, PL 89-10. Civil Rights statutes: PL 88-352, Title VI, 1964; PL 93-380, 1974.
3. 20 USCS 3222
4. 500.4; 34 CFR Ch. V 7-1-87 edition.
5. 414 US at 566.
6. 20 USC sec 1703f 1976.
7. 480 F Supp at 22, E.D.N.Y., 1978; cf., 648 F.2d 989, 5th Cir., 1981.
8. Willig, 1985.
9. Mace-Matluck, Hoover & Calfee, 1984.
10. Swain & Lapkin, 1991.
11. Ramirez, Yuen & Ramey, 1991.
12. Cummins, 1986; Cummins & Swain, 1986.
13. Troikje, 1978; Obgu, 1978.
14. Hakuta, 1986.
15. Lambert, 1977.
16. Reynolds, 1991.
17. Haft, 1983.
18. Porter, 1990.
19. Crawford, 1992.
20. Commission on the Education of the Deaf, 1988.
21. Hakuta, 1986.
22. Erting, 1992.
23. Gee, 1990.
24. Sanders, 1994.
25. Supalla & Bahan, 1994.
26. Hoffmeister & Shettle, 1983; Hoffmeister,1985.
27. Greenberg, 1983.
28. Hoffmeister, 1982; 1985; Newport & Meier, 1985 for reviews, Singleton, 1989.
29. Akamatsu, 1987, 1989.
30. Goppold, 1988.
31. Snow et al., 1991.
32. Meadow, 1980.
33. Rodda & Grove, 1987.
34. Rodda & Grove, 1987; Greenberg, 1980.
35. Snow et. al, 1991.

Chapter 11 Evaluating Deaf People

1. Erdman, 1994.
2. Chorover, 1979.
3. Goddard, 1917; Chorover, 1979.
4. Herrnstein & Murray, 1994.
5. Foucault, 1980.
6. Scott, 1981, p. 103.
7. Rudner, 1978.
8. Quigley & Kretschmer, 1982.
9. Ragosta, 1987.
10. Conrad & Weiskrantz, 1981; Sisco & Anderson, 1980.
11. Braun, Ragosta & Kaplan, 1986.
12. Montgomery, 1978. One investigator estimates at least eighth-grade reading ability is required to take the MMPI: Smith, 1986.
13. Quigley & Kretschmer, 1982; Wolk & Allen, 1984.
14. Lane, 1988.
15. Lebuffe & Lebuffe, 1979, p. 299.
16. Hoyt, Siegelman & Schlesinger, 1981; Meadow, 1981.
17. Gerber & Goldberg, 1980; Meadow-Orlans, 1987, p. 124.
18. Schlesinger 1987, p. 11.
19. Freeman, Malkin & Hastings, 1975.
20. Rodda and & Grove, 1987.
21. Altshuler, Deming, Vollenweider, Rainer & Tendler, 1976.
22. Allen & Sligar, 1994.
23. Allen & Sligar, 1994.
24. Allen, 1986b.
25. Allen & Sligar, 1994.
26. Allen, 1986b.
27. Holt, 1994; Schildroth, 1990.
28. Ewoldt, 1987.
29. Moores, 1967; O'Neill, 1973.
30. Allen, Holt, Bloomquist & Starke, 1987.
31. Allen, 1986b.
32. Allen, 1986a.
33. Charrow & Fletcher, 1974.
34. Anderson & Sisco, 1977.
35. Blennerhassett, 1990.
36. Allen & Sligar, 1994.
37. Graham & Shapiro, 1953.
38. Moores & Sweet, 1990.
39. Brill, 1974; Conrad, 1979; Conrad & Weiskrantz, 1981; Karchmer Trybus & Paquin, 1978; Sisco & Anderson, 1980; Vernon, 1969a.
40. Vernon, 1969a.
41. Vernon, 1969a.
42. Brauer, 1994.
43. Evans & Elliott, 1987; Orr, De Mateo, Heller, Lee & Nguyen, 1987.
44. Moores & Sweet, 1990.
45. Quigley & Paul, 1984.
46. Moores & Sweet, 1990.
47. Engen & Engen, 1983.
48. Newport, 1990; Supalla et al., in press.
49. This test is not currently included in the battery.

Chapter 12 The Hearing Agenda I: To Mitigate a Disability

1. United Nations, 1994.
2. Department of Education and Science, 1978.
3. Nagase, 1995.
4. Foucault, 1980, p. 273.
5. Gregory & Hartley, 1991.
6. Abberley, 1987; Oliver, 1991.
7. Kaufman, 1986.
8. Driedger, 1989.
9. Hevey, 1993, p. 426.
10. DuBow, Geer & Strauss, 1992.
11. Bowe, 1994.
12. Bowe, 1994.
13. Schein & Delk, 1974.
14. Allen, Rawlings & Schildroth, 1989.
15. Schildroth, Rawlings & Allen, 1991.
16. Commission on the Education of the Deaf, 1988.
17. Watson, 1994.
18. Allen & Sligar, 1994.
19. Rawlings, Karchmer & DeCaro, 1988.
20. Schildroth, Rawlins & Allen, 1991.
21. Crammatte, 1987.
22. Craig & Garrity, 1994.
23. Vernon, 1991.
24. Better, Fine & Doss, 1980.
25. Equal Employment Opportunity Commission, 1991, p. I-34.
26. Chess & Fernandez, 1980.
27. Levine, 1981.
28. Schlesinger, 1985.
29. DuBow, Geer & Strauss, 1992.
30. Steinberg, 1991.
31. Loera, 1994.
32. Dickert, 1988.
33. Cf. Steinberg, 1991.
34. Based on Denmark, 1994.
35. Harvey, 1995.
36. Pollard, Gutman, DeMatteo & Stewart, 1991.
37. Spragins, Karchmer & Schildroth, 1981.
38. Pollard, 1995
39. Willigan & King, 1992.
40. Harvey, 1989.
41. Vernon, 1995.
42. Guthmann, Lybarger & Sandberg, 1995.
43. Based on the discussion in DuBow, Geer & Strauss, 1992.
44. Information provided by the Massachusetts Commission on the Deaf and Hard of Hearing; Irma Kale, interpreter coordinator.
45. DuBow, Geer & Strass, 1992.
46. Based on DuBow, Geer & Strauss, 1992.
47. Based on discussions in Baker-Shenk, 1985, 1988, 1992; McIntire & Sanderson, 1993; Moody, 1994.
48. Baker-Shenk, 1988.
49. Gagné & Tye-Murray, 1994.
50. Kewley-Port, 1994
51. Robards-Armstrong & Stone, 1994
52. Albrecht, 1992.
53. Albrecht, 1992.
54. Estes, 1994.
55. Geers, 1994.
56. McGarr & Harris, 1983; Wolk & Schildroth, 1986.
57. Boothroyd, 1989.
58. Brown & Gustafson, 1995.
59. Estimate from American Hearing Aid Society.
60. Based on discussion in Stone & Hurwitz, 1994.
61. Sandlin, 1994.
62. Boothroyd, 1989.
63. Reed, Durlach, Delhorne & Rabinowitz, 1989.
64. Berstein, 1989.

Chapter 13 The Future of the DEAF-WORLD

1. Jankowski, 1992.

Chapter 14 The Hearing Agenda II: Eradicating the DEAF-WORLD

1. Pride in a silent language, 1993.
2. Plann, 1993.
3. Lane, 1984.
4. Berthier, 1837.
5. Winzer, 1993.
6. Gallaudet, 1891. Cited in Winefield, 1987.
7. Lane, 1996.
8. Cited in Lane, 1984, p. 326.
9. Cited in Van Cleve, 1984, p. 209.
10. Cf. Lane, 1984.
11. Bruce, 1973, p. 393; Van Cleve, 1993.
12. Wisconsin Phonological Institute, 1894.
13. Van Cleve, 1993.
14. Johnson, 1918.
15. Bell, 1883, p. 216.
16. Bell, 1883, p. 216.
17. Lane, 1993a, p. 287.
18. Fay, 1898.
19. Ruben, 1991.
20. Biesold, 1993.

Chapter 14 The Hearing Agenda II: Eradicating the DEAF-WORLD (cont.)

21. Muhs, 1995.
22. Peter, 1934.
23. Higgins, 1993; Ruben, 1991.
24. BU Team, 1992; Gene that Causes, 1992.
25. Fraser, 1976.
26. Fraser, 1987.
27. National Institute on Deafness and Other Communication Disorders, 1992.
28. National Institute on Deafness and Other Communication Disorders, 1989.
29. Tye-Murray, 1992, p. 64.
30. Lane, 1992.
31. Dagron, 1994.
32. Tye-Murray, 1992.
33. Chronology based in part on Blume, 1993.
34. National Association of the Deaf, 1991.
35. Cited in Lane, 1994.
36. Cited in Lane, 1994.
37. Cited in Lane, 1994.
38. Cited in Lane, 1994.
39. Resolution of the XIIth World Congress of the World Federation of the Deaf, Vienna Austria, 1995.
40. Kohut, 1988.
41. National Institutes of Health, 1995
42. Letter dated 2/13/91 from the Vice-President, American Academy of Otolaryngology-Head and Neck Surgery, to the National Association of the Deaf.
43. Cohen, 1994a.
44. Laurenzi, 1993.
45. Lane, 1991, 1995a.
46. Allen, Rawlings & Remington, 1994; Schildroth & Hoto, 1993.
47. Osberger, Todd, Berry, Robbins & Miyamoto, 1991.
48. Staller, Beiter, Brimacombe, Mecklenburg & Arndt, 1991.
49. Somers, 1991.
50. Shea, Domico & Lupfer, 1994.
51. Osberger, Miyamoto, Zimmerman-Phillips et al., 1991.
52. Waltzman, Cohen, Gomolin, Shapiro, Ozdamar & Hoffman, 1994.
53. Fryauf-Bertschy, Tyler, Kelsay & Gantz, 1992.
54. Rose, 1994.
55. Blamey & Cowan, 1992.
56. Rabinowitz, Eddington, Delhorne & Cuneo, 1992.
57. Petitto & Marentette, 1991.
58. Neville, Schmidt & Kutas, 1983.
59. Neville, 1988.
60. Allen, Rawlings & Remington, 1994.
61. Lane, 1991.
62. Quoted in Lane, 1984.
63. Grodin & Glantz, 1994, p. 85.
64. Grodin & Glantz, 1994, p. 94.
65. Grodin & Glantz, 1994, p. 97.
66. Doomed Ghetto culture, 1993.
67. Cohen, 1994b, p. 19; Tyler, 1993.
68. Humphries, 1993, p. 6, 14.
69. Balkany & Hodges, 1994.

Chapter 15 The Deaf Agenda: Enriching the DEAF-WORLD

1. Chouard, 1978, p. 21.
2. Greg Hlibok, cited in this protest, 1988.
3. Abberley, 1987; Lane, 1995.
4. United Nations, 1994; Shapiro, 1993.
5. Shapiro, 1993, p. 144.
6. Schein, 1989.
7. Gusfield, 1989, p. 432.
8. Lane, 1995b; Morris, 1990; Scott, 1981.
9. cf. Barton, 1993.
10. Dowler & Hirsh, 1994.
11. Castle, 1990; Ross & Calvert 1967; Wilson, Ross & Calvert, 1974.
12. Open University, 1991.
13. Based on the discussion in Hawcroft, 1991.
14. Wright, 1994.
15. Kyle, 1990, 1991; Parratt & Tipping, 1991.
16. Fishman, 1982.
17. United Nations, 1994.
18. Kauppinen, 1994, p. 1.
19. Markowicz & Woodward, 1978.
20. Lane, 1992.
21. Johnson, Liddell & Erting, 1989.
22. World Federation of the Deaf, 1993a.
23. Mäkipää, 1993.
24. Finnish Association of the Deaf, 1994, p. 34.
25. Jacobwitz, 1995.
26. Address to the XII World Congress, World Federation of the Deaf, July 6, 1995.
27. World Federation of the Deaf, 1992, p. 38.
28. UNESCO, 1985.
29. European Parliament, 1988.
30. Joutselainen, 1991.
31. Mbewe, 1995.
32. United Nations, 1994, Rule 6, subsection 9.
33. Commission on the Education of the Deaf, 1988.
34. Kauppinen, 1994, p. 2.
35. Innes, 1994.

Chapter 15 The Deaf Agenda: Enriching the DEAF-WORLD (cont.)

36. UNESCO, 1994.
37. United Nations, 1994.
38. Woodward, Allen & Schildroth, 1985.
39. Innes, 1993.
40. Kauppinen, 1994.
41. National Association of the Deaf, 1994.
42. Commission on the Education of the Deaf, 1988.
43. Bergmann, 1994; Finnish Association of the Deaf, 1994.
44. Goodstein, 1994.
45. DuBow, Geer & Strauss, 1992.
46. National Captioning Institute, 1993a.
47. National Captioning Institute, 1993b.
48. WGBH Boston, 1993.
49. National Association of the Deaf, 1995.
50. Humphries, 1991, p. 209.
51. Kauppinen, 1994.
52. Crammatte, 1987.
53. Jacobowitz, 1995.
54. Hagemeyer, 1993.
55. Oliver, 1991.
56. Jordan, 1991.

References

Aarons, D., Bahan, B., Kegl, J., & Neidle, C. (1992). Clausal structure and a tier for grammatical marking in American Sign Language. *Nordic Journal of Linguistics, 15,* 103-142.

Abberley, P. (1987). The concept of oppression and the development of a social theory of disability. *Disability, Handicap & Society, 2,* 5-19.

Abbou, D. (1994). Hearing-Deaf relations. In C. Erting, R. E. Johnson, D. L. Smith & B. D. Snider (Eds.), *The Deaf Way: Perspectives from the International Conference on Deaf Culture* (pp. 674-676). Washington, DC: Gallaudet University Press.

Abbou, M. T. (1993). The uncertified deaf teacher in a bilingual class. In H. Lane (Ed.), *Parallel views: Education and access for Deaf people in France and the United States* (pp. 144-146). Washington, DC: Gallaudet University Press.

Akamatsu, C. T. (1987). *The role of instruction in text structure and metacognitive strategy instruction in deaf students' learning to read and write stories.* Paper presented at the meeting of the American Educational Research Association, Washington, DC.

Akamatsu, C. T., & Stewart, D. A. (1989). The role of fingerspelling in simultaneous communication. *Sign Language Studies, 65,* 361-374.

Albrecht, G. L. (1992). *The disability business: Rehabilitation in America.* Newbury Park, CA: Sage.

Allen, T. E. (1986a). Patterns of academic achievement among hearing-impaired students: 1974 and 1983. In A. N. Schildroth & M. A. Karchmer (Eds.), *Deaf children in America* (pp. 161-206). San Diego: College-Hill.

Allen, T. E. (1986b). *Understanding the scores: Hearing-impaired students and the Stanford Achievement Test* (7th ed.). Washington, DC: Center for Assessment and Demographic Studies, Gallaudet University.

Allen, T. E. (1992). Subgroup differences in educational placement for deaf and hard-of-hearing students. *American Annals of the Deaf, 137,* 381-388.

Allen, T. E., Holt, J. A., Bloomquist, C. A., & Starke, M. C. (1987). *Item analysis for the Stanford Achievement Test 7th edition 1983 standardization with hearing-impaired students.* Unpublished report, Center for Assessment and Demographic Studies, Gallaudet University, Washington, DC.

Allen, T. E., & Karchmer, M. (1990). Communication in classrooms for deaf students: Student, teacher, and program characteristics. In H. Bornstein (Ed.), *Manual communication: Implications for education* (pp. 45-66). Washington, DC: Gallaudet University Press.

Allen, T. E., Rawlings, B. W., & Remington, E. (1994). Demographic and audiologic profiles of deaf children in Texas with cochlear implants. *American Annals of the Deaf, 138,* 260-266.

Allen, T. E., Rawlings, B. W., & Schildroth, A. N. (1989). *Deaf students and the school to work transition.* Baltimore, MD: Brooks.

Allen, T. E., & Sligar, S. R. (1994). The assessment of deaf individuals in the context of rehabilitation. In R. C. Nowell & L. E. Marshak (Eds.), *Understanding deafness and the rehabilitation process* (pp. 113-141). Boston: Allyn & Bacon.

Altshuler, K., Deming, W. E., Vollenweider, J., Rainer, J. D., & Tendler, R. (1976). Impulsivity and profound early deafness: A cross-cultural inquiry. *American Annals of the Deaf, 121*, 331-345.

Andersen, R. (1983). A language acquisition interpretation of pidginization and creolization. In R. Anderson (Ed.), *Pidginization and creolization as language acquisition*. Rowley, MA: Newbury House.

Anderson, G. B., & Grace, C. (1991). Black deaf adolescents: A diverse and underserved population. *Volta Review, 93*, 73-86.

Anderson, G. B. (1994). Tools for a wiser, healthier, Black Deaf community. *Deaf American Monographs, 44*, 1-4.

Anderson, H. (1992). Perspectives on discrimination and barriers encountered by Black deaf Americans. In G. B. Anderson & D. Watson (Eds.), *The Black deaf experience: Excellence and equity. Proceedings of a national conference March 12-14, 1992* (pp. 49-51). Little Rock, AR: University of Arkansas.

Anderson, R. J., & Sisco, F. H. (1977). *Standardization of the WISC-R performance scale for deaf children.* Unpublished report, Center for Assessment and Demographic Studies, Washington, DC.: Gallaudet University.

Andersson, Y. (1987). World Federation of the Deaf. In J. V. Van Cleve (Ed.), *Gallaudet encyclopedia of deaf people and deafness* (pp. 344-347). New York: McGraw-Hill.

Andersson, Y. (1994a). A survey of selected national organizations of the Deaf: Preliminary findings. *Deaf American Monographs, 44*, 5-7.

Andersson, Y. (1994b). The Stockholm deaf club: A case study. In C. Erting, R. E. Johnson, D. L. Smith & B. D. Snider (Eds.), *The Deaf Way: Perspectives from the International Conference on Deaf Culture* (pp. 516-521). Washington, DC: Gallaudet University Press.

Anthony, D. (1971). *Seeing Essential English manual (books 1 and 2)*. Anaheim, CA: Anaheim Union High School District.

Aramburo, A. (1994). Sociolinguistic aspects of the Black deaf community. In C. Erting, R. E. Johnson, D. L. Smith & B. D. Snider (Eds.), *The Deaf Way: Perspectives from the International Conference on Deaf Culture* (pp. 474-482). Washington, DC: Gallaudet University Press.

Aramburo, A. J. (1989). *Sociolinguistic aspects of the Black Deaf community*. In C. Lucas (Ed.), The sociolinguistics of the Deaf community (pp. 103-119). New York: Academic Press.

Bahan, B. (1994). Comment on Turner. *Sign Language Studies, 84*, 241-249.

Bahan, B. (1996). *Non-manual realization of agreement in American Sign Language*. Unpublished doctoral dissertation, Boston University, Boston.

Bahan, B., & Poole-Nash, J. (1995, April). *Formation of signing communities: Perspective from Martha's Vineyard.* Paper presented at the Deaf Studies IV Conference, Woburn, MA.

Baird, C. (1993). *Chuck Baird: 35 Plates. Text and introduction by L.K. Elion*. San Diego:DawnSignPress.

Baker, C. (1976). What's not on the other hand in American Sign Language. In S. Mufwene, C. Walker & S. Steever (Eds.), *Papers from the Twelfth Regional Meeting, Chicago Linguistics Society*. Chicago: University of Chicago Press.

Baker, C., & Padden, C. (1978). Focusing on the nonmanual components of American Sign Language. In P. Siple (Ed.), *Understanding language through sign language research* (pp. 27-58). New York: Academic Press.

Baker-Hawkins, S., & Esterbrooks, S. (Eds.) (1994). *Deaf and hard-of-hearing students: Educational service guidelines*. Alexandria, VA: National Association of State Directors of Special Education.

Baker-Shenk, C. (1985). Liberation theology and the deaf community: The Claggett Statement. *Sojourners*, 30-32.

Baker-Shenk, C. (1988). *Dialogue on interpreter roles, varying perspectives.* Unpublished paper.

Baker-Shenk, C. (1992). The interpreter: machine, advocate or ally. In J. Plant-Moeller (Ed.), *Expanding horizons: Proceedings of the 12th National Congress of Registries of Interpreters for the Deaf. Aug. 6-11, 1991* (pp. 120-140).

References

Baldwin, S. (1995). *Pictures in the air: The story of the National Theatre of the Deaf*. Washington, DC: Gallaudet University Press.

Balkany, T. (1994, January 28). A brief perspective on cochlear implants. *New England Journal of Medicine, 328*, 281-282.

Balkany, T., & Hodges, A. (1994). Misleading the deaf community about cochlear implantation in children. *Annals of Otology, Rhinology & Laryngology, 103*, 148-149.

Bangs, D. (1987). Television and motion pictures: Deaf cultural programming. In J. V. Van Cleve (Ed.), *Gallaudet encyclopedia of deaf people and deafness* (pp. 273-275). New York: McGraw-Hill.

Bangs, D. (1994). What is a deaf performing arts experience? In C. Erting, R. E. Johnson, D. L. Smith & B. D. Snider (Eds.), *The Deaf Way: Perspectives from the International Conference on Deaf Culture* (pp. 751-761). Washington, DC: Gallaudet University Press.

Banks, M., & Bryan, A. M. (1993). African-American Deaf women in performing arts: Theater and film. In College for Continuing Education (Ed.), *Deaf studies III: Bridging cultures in the 21st century*. Proceedings of a conference April 22-25, 1993 (pp. 75-79). Washington, DC: Gallaudet University Press.

Barton, L. (1993). The struggle for citizenship: the case of disabled people. *Disability, Handicap & Society, 8*, 235-248.

Battison, R. (1978). *Lexical borrowing in American Sign Language*. Silver Spring, MD: Linstok Press.

Becker, G. (1980). *Growing old in silence*. Berkeley: University of California Press.

Belissen, P. (1993). The language and culture of the deaf community. In H. Lane (Ed.), *Parallel views: Education and access for Deaf people in France and the United States* (pp. 95-97). Washington, DC: Gallaudet University Press.

Bell, A. G. (1883). *Memoir upon the formation of a deaf variety of the human race*. Reprinted, 1969. Washington, DC: Volta Bureau.

Bellugi, U., & Fischer, S. (1972). A comparison of sign language and spoken language. *Cognition, 1*, 173-200.

Bellugi, U., & Klima, E. (1976). Two faces of sign: Iconic and abstract. In S. Harnad, H. Steklis & J. Lancaster (Eds.), *Origins and evolution of language and speech*. New York: New York Academy of Sciences.

Bellugi, U., O'Grady, L., Lillo-Martin, D., O'Grady-Hynes, M., van Hoek, K., & Corina, D. (1994). Enhancement of spatial cognition in deaf children. In V. Volterra & C. Erting (Eds.), *From gesture to language in hearing and deaf children* (pp. 278-298). Berlin: Springer Verlag.

Bellugi, U., & Siple, P. (1974). Remembering with and without words. In F. Bresson (Ed.), *Current problems in psycho-linguistics*. Paris: CNRS.

Bergmann, R. (1994). Teaching sign language as the mother tongue in the education of deaf children in Denmark. In I. Ahlgren & K. Hyltenstam (Eds.), *Bilingualism in deaf education* (pp. 84-90). Hamburg: Signum.

Bernard, Y. (1993). Silent artists. In R. Fischer & H. Lane (Eds.), *Looking back: A reader on the history of deaf communities and their sign languages* (pp. 75-87). Hamburg: Signum.

Bernstein, L. (1989). Computer-based speech training for profoundly hearing-impaired children: some design considerations. *Volta Review, 91*, 19-28.

Berthier, F. (1837). Lettre sur les difficultés au marriage des sourds-mutes. *Le sourd-muet et l'aveugle, 1*, 190-195.

Better, S. R., Fine, P. R., & Doss, G. H. (1980). Overcoming disincentives to the rehabilitation of SSI and SSDI beneficiaries. *International Journal of Rehabilitation Research, 3*, 62-64.

Bettger, J. (1992). *The effects of experience on spatial cognition: Deafness and knowledge of ASL*. Unpublished doctoral dissertation, University of Illinois, Urbana-Champaign.

Bickerton, D., (1982). *Roots of language*. Ann Arbor, MI: Karoma Press.

Bienvenu, M. J. (1994). Reflections of Deaf culture in Deaf humor. In C. Erting, R. E. Johnson, D. L. Smith & B. D. Snider (Eds.), *The Deaf Way: Perspectives from the International Conference on Deaf Culture* (pp. 16-23). Washington, DC: Gallaudet University Press.

Biesold, H. (1993). The fate of the Israelite Asylum for the Deaf and Dumb in Berlin. In R. Fischer & H. Lane (Eds.), *Looking back: A reader on the history of deaf communities and their sign languages* (pp. 157-170). Hamburg: Signum.

Blamey, P. J., & Cowan, R. S. C. (1992). The potential benefit and cost effectiveness of tactile devices in comparison with cochlear implants. In I. R. Summers (Ed.), *Tactile aids for the hearing impaired* (pp. 187-217). London: Whurr.

Blennerhassett, L. (1990). Intellectual assessment. In D. F. Moores & K. Meadow-Orlans (Eds.), *Educational and developmental aspects of deafness* (pp. 255-280). Washington, DC: Gallaudet University Press.

Bloom, B. (1984). The 2 sigma problem: The search for methods of group instruction as effective as one-to-one tutoring. *Educational Researcher, 13*, 4-16.

Blume, S. (1993). Cochlear implantation and the politics of deafness: Britain and the Netherlands compared. Paper presented at a meeting of the Deaf Studies Research Unit, University of Durham.

Bonvillian, J. D., Orlansky, M. D., & Folven, R. J. (1994). Early sign language acquisition: implications for theories of language acquisition. In V. Volterra & C. Erting (Eds.), *From gesture to language in hearing and deaf children* (pp. 219-232). Berlin: Springer Verlag.

Boothroyd, A. (1989). Developing and evaluating a tactile speechreading aid. *Volta Review, 91*, 101-112.

Bornstein, H. & Saulnier, K., & Luczak, K. (1984). *The Signed English starter*. Washington, DC: Gallaudet College Press.

Bouchauveau, G. (1990). La Langue des Signes Française de 1978 à nos jours. In: A. Karakostas (Ed.), *Le Pouvoir des signes* (pp. 208-214). Paris: Institut National de Jeunes Sourds.

Bouchauveau, G. (1993). Access to culture in France. In H. Lane (Ed.), *Parallel views: Education and access for Deaf people in France and the United States* (pp. 215-219). Washington, DC: Gallaudet University Press.

Bouchauveau, G. (1994). Deaf humor and culture. In C. Erting, R. E. Johnson, D. L. Smith & B. D. Snider (Eds.), *The Deaf Way: Perspectives from the International Conference on Deaf Culture* (pp. 24-30). Washington, DC: Gallaudet University Press.

Bouillon, J.P. (1993). Regulations affecting social access for the deaf in France. In H. Lane (Ed.), *Parallel views: Education and access for Deaf people in France and the United States* (pp. 190-193). Washington, DC: Gallaudet University Press.

Bournazian, A. (1993). *Gender roles in the American Deaf community*. Unpublished manuscript, Northeastern University.

Bowe, F. G. (1994). Accessibility: Legal issues. In R. C. Nowell & L. E. Marshak (Eds.), *Understanding deafness and the rehabilitation process* (pp. 223-237). Boston: Allyn & Bacon.

Brauer, B. (1994). Adequacy of a translation of the MMPI into American Sign Language for use with deaf individuals: Linguistic equivalency issues. *Rehabilitation Psychology, 38*, 247-260.

Brasel, K.E. (1975). *The influence of early language and communication environments on the development of language in Deaf children.* Unpublished doctoral dissertation, University of Illinois, Urbana-Champaign.

Brasel, K.E. & Quigley, S.E. (1977). Influence of certain language and communication environments in early childhood on development of language in deaf individuals. *Journal of Speech and Hearing Research, 20*, 95-107.

Braun, H., Ragosta, M., & Kaplan, B. (1986). *The predictive validity of the Scholastic Aptitude Test for disabled students.* Princeton, NJ: Educational Testing Service.

Brill, R. G. (1974). The superior IQs of deaf children of deaf parents. In P. J. Fine (Ed.), *Deafness in infancy and early childhood* (pp. 151-161). New York: Medcom.

References

Brown, P. M., & Gustafson, M. S. (1995). Showing sensitivity to deaf culture. ASHA, 37, 46-47.

Bruce, R. V. (1973). *Bell. Alexander Graham Bell and the conquest of solitude*. Boston: Little Brown.

Brusque, M. (1993). Experimental bilingual classes in France. In H. Lane (Ed.), *Parallel views: Education and access for Deaf people in France and the United States* (pp. 140-143). Washington, DC: Gallaudet University Press.

BU Team (1992, March). BU team finds genetic cause of Waardenburg Syndrome. *Deaf Community News*, March.

Bullard, D. (1986). *Islay*. Silver Spring, MD: TJ Publishers.

Burgos, J. (1993). Postsecondary education in France. In H. Lane (Ed.), *Parallel views: Education and access for Deaf people in France and the United States* (pp. 164-169). Washington, DC: Gallaudet University Press.

Calvet, L.J. (1974). *Linguistique et colonialisme*. Paris. Payot.

Carlin, J. (1847). The mute's lament. *American Annals of the Deaf, 1*, 15-16.

Castle, D. (1990). Employment bridges cultures. *Deaf American, 40*, 19-21.

Charrow, V., & Fletcher, J. D. (1974). English as the second language of deaf children. *Developmental Psychology, 10*, 436-470.

Cheng, L. L. (1993). Deafness: An Asian/Pacific Island perspective. In K. M. Christensen & G. L. Delgado(Eds.), *Multicultural issues in deafness* (pp. 113-126). White Plains, NY: Longman.

Chess, S., & Fernandez, P. (1980). Do deaf children have a typical personality? *Journal of the American Academy of Child Psychiatry, 19*, 654-664.

Chiccioli, T., Harrison, S., Kesner, B., Lejeune, J., Stender, A., Tunison, W., Herrada-Benites, R., & Levine, F. (1994). We have Usher Syndrome. *Silent News, 26*, 3.

Chorover, S. (1979). *From Genesis to genocide*. Cambridge, MA: MIT Press.

Chouard, C.-H. (1978). *Entendre sans oreille*. Paris: Laffont.

Christiansen, J. B., & Barnartt, S. N. (1995). *Deaf President Now! The 1988 revolution at Gallaudet University*. Washington, DC: Gallaudet University Press.

Clark, H., & Clark, E. (1968). Semantic distinctions and memory for complex sentences. *Quarterly Journal of Experimental Psychology, 20*, 129-138.

Cohen, N. (1994a). The ethics of cochlear implants in young children. *American Journal of Otology, 15*, 1-2.

Cohen, N. (1994b). cochlear implants in young children: Ethical considerations. *Annals of Otology, Rhinology & Laryngology, 103*, 17-19.

Cohen, O. P. (1991). At-risk deaf adolescents. *Volta Review, 93*, 57-72.

Cohen, O. P. (1993). Educational needs of African-American and Hispanic deaf children and youth. In K. M. Christensen & G. L. Delgado (Eds.), *Multicultural issues in deafness* (pp. 45-68). White Plains, NY: Longman.

Cokely, D. (1986). The effects of lag time on interpreter errors. *Sign Language Studies, 53*, 341-375.

Coleman, L., & Jankowski, K. (1994). Empowering Deaf people through folklore and storytelling. In C. Erting, R. E. Johnson, D. L. Smith & B. D. Snider (Eds.), *The Deaf Way: Perspectives from the International Conference on Deaf Culture* (pp. 55-60). Washington, DC: Gallaudet University Press.

Colin, D. (1978). *Psychologie de l'enfant sourd*. Paris: Masson.

Commission on the Education of the Deaf (1988). *Toward equality: Education of the deaf. A report to the President and the Congress of the United States*. Washington, DC: U.S. Government Printing Office.

Commonwealth Secretariat (1972). Special education in the developing countries of the Commonwealth. *Education in the Commonwealth, 5*, 27-51.

Congress on Deaf - International - First (1879). *Compte-rendu . . . Congrès universel pour l'amelioration du sort des aveugles et des sourds-muets*. Paris: Imprimerie Nationale.

Conrad, R. (1979). *The deaf schoolchild.* London: Harper Row.

Conrad, R., & Weiskrantz, B. C. (1981). On the cognitive ability of deaf children with deaf parents. *American Annals of the Deaf, 126*, 995-1003.

Corson, H. (1973). *Comparing deaf children of oral deaf parents and deaf children using manual communication with deaf children of hearing parents on academic, social, and communicative functioning.* Unpublished doctoral dissertation, University of Cincinnati.

Craig, H., & Garrity, R. P. (1994). The post-secondary transition: From school to independent living. In R. C. Nowell & L. E. Marshak (Eds.), *Understanding deafness and the rehabilitation process* (pp. 83-112). Boston: Allyn & Bacon.

Crammatte, A. B. (1987). *Meeting the challenge: Hearing-impaired professionals in the workplace.* Washington, DC: Gallaudet University Press.

Crawford, J. *Hold your tongue: Bilingualism and the politics of "English Only."* Reading, MA: Addison-Wesley.

Creighton, N. (1994). Maureen Amy Yates, Miss Deaf America. *National Association of the Deaf Broadcaster, 16* (11), 1-2, 39-40.

Cummins, J. (1986). Empowering minority students: a framework for intervention. *Harvard Educational Review, 56,* 18-36.

Cummins, J., & Danesi, M. (1990). *Heritage languages: The development and denial of Canada's linguistic resources.* Toronto: Garamond.

Cummins, J., & Swain, M. (1986). *Bilingualism in education.* New York: Longman.

Cuxac, C. (1983). *Le langage des sourds.* Paris: Payot.

Cuxac, C. (1993). La langue des signes: Construction d'un objet scientifique. *Psychoanalyses, 46-47,* 97-113.

Dagron, J. (1994). *Implant cochléaire: problèmes éthiques.* Paris: Presses d'Aujourd'hui.

Dahl, C. (1994). Another Certificate? *Registry of Interpreters for the Deaf Views, 11*, 2, 18.

Dahl, C. & Wilcox, S. (1990). Preparing the educational interpreter: A survey of sign language interpreter training programs. *American Annals of the Deaf, 135*, 4.

Davey, B. (1987). Relations between word knowledge and comprehension: Generalization across tasks and readers. *Journal of Educational Research, 80,* 179-183.

Davey, B. and King, S. (1990). Acquisition of word meanings from context by deaf readers. *American Annals of the Deaf, 135*, 227-234.

Davey, B. LaSasso, C. & Macready, G. (1983). A comparison of reading comprehension task performance for deaf and hearing subjects. *Journal of Speech and Hearing Research, 26*, 622-628.

Davies, S. (1990a). *Bilingual education of deaf children in Sweden and Denmark: Strategies for transition and implementation.* Washington, DC: Gallaudet Research Institute.

Davies, S. (1990b). *Two languages for deaf children in Sweden and Denmark.* Ideas Portfolio II. New York: Rehabilitation International and the World Institute on Disabilities.

Denmark, J. (1994). *Deafness and mental health.* London: Kingsley.

Department of Education and Science (1978). *Special educational needs: Report of the committee of inquiry into the education of handicapped children and young people.* Warnock report. London: Her Majesty's Stationery Office.

De Villiers, J. (1988). *A longitudinal study of the language development in young oral deaf children.* Unpublished manuscript.

Dickert, J. (1988). Examination of bias in mental health evaluation of deaf patients. *Social Work*, 273-274.

Doomed ghetto culture (Letters to the editor of the Atlantic Monthly reprinted). *Deaf Life,* December, 1993, 33.

Dowler, D. L., & Hirsh, A. (1994). Accommodations in the workplace for people who are deaf or hard-of-hearing. *Technology and Disability, 3,* 15-25.

Driedger, D. (1989). *The last civil rights movement.* London Hurst.

DuBow, S. (1987). Legal services. In J. V. Van Cleve (Ed.), *Gallaudet encyclopedia of deaf people and deafness* (pp. 158-161). New York: McGraw-Hill.

DuBow, S., Geer, S. & Strauss, K. P. (Eds.) (1992). *Legal rights: The guide for deaf and hard of hearing people.* Washington, DC: Gallaudet University Press.

Dummett, M. (1981). *Frege: Philosophy of language.* Cambridge, MA: Harvard University Press.

Dunn, L. (1989). Setting the pace in Black deaf America. In G. Olsen (Ed.), *A kaleidoscope of deaf America* (pp. 22-23). Silver Spring, MD: National Association of the Deaf.

Edenas, C. (1994). Improving sign language skills of hearing teachers: A Swedish experiment. In C. Erting, R. E. Johnson, D. L. Smith & B. D. Snider (Eds.), *The Deaf Way: Perspectives from the International Conference on Deaf Culture* (pp. 615-620). Washington, DC: Gallaudet University Press.

Edmondson, W. H., & Karlsson, F. (1990). SLR'87: *Papers from the Fourth International Symposium on Sign Language Research,* 1987. Hamburg: Signum.

Emery, S., & Slone, J. (1994). How long must we wait? In C. Erting, R. E. Johnson, D. L. Smith & B. D. Snider (Eds.), *The Deaf Way: Perspectives from the International Conference on Deaf Culture* (pp. 470-473). Washington, DC: Gallaudet University Press.

Emmorey, K. (1993). Processing a dynamic visual-spatial language: Psycholinguistic studies of American Sign Language. *Journal of Psycholinguistic Research, 22,* 153-187.

Emmorey, K. (1995). The confluence of space and language in signed languages. In P. Bloom, M. Peterson, L. Nadel & M. Garrett (Eds.), *Language and space.* Cambridge, MA: MIT Press.

Emmorey, K., Bellugi, U., Friederici, A., & Horn, P. (1995). Effects of age of acquisition on grammatical sensitivity: evidence from on-line and off-line tasks. *Applied Psycholinguistics, 16,* 1-23.

Emmorey, K., & Casey, S. (1995). A comparison of spatial language in English and American Sign Language. *Sign Language Studies, 88,* 255-288.

Emmorey, K., & Corina, D. (1990). Lexical recognition in sign language: Effects of phonetic structure and morphology. *Perceptual and Motor Skills, 71,* 1227-1252.

Emmorey, K., & Corina, D. (1992). *Differential sensitivity to classifier morphology in ASL signers.* Paper presented at the meeting of the Linguistic Society of America, Chicago, IL.

Emmorey, K., Corina, D., & Bellugi, U. (1995). Differential processing of topographic and referential functions of space. In K. Emmorey & J. Reilly (Eds.), *Language, gesture and space* (pp. 43-62). Hillsdale, NJ: Lawrence Erlbaum Associates.

Emmorey, K., Kosslyn, S.M., & Bellugi, U. (1993). Visual imagery and visual-spatial language: Enhanced imagery abilities in deaf and hearing ASL signers. *Cognition, 46,* 139-181.

Engen, E., & Engen, T. (1983). *Rhode Island Test of Language Structure.* Austin, TX: Pro-Ed.

Equal Employment Opportunity Commission (1991). *Americans with Disabilities Act handbook.* Washington, DC: U.S. Government Printing Office.

Erdman, S. (1994). Self-assessment: From research focus to research tool. In J. P. Gagné & N. Tye-Murray (Eds.), *Research in audiological rehabilitation* (pp. 66-90). Cedar Falls, IA: American Academy of Rehabilitative Audiology.

Erting, C.J. (1981). An anthropological approach to the study of the communicative competence of deaf children. *Sign Language Studies, 32,* 221-238.

Erting, C.J. (1985). Sociocultural dimensions of deaf education: Belief systems and communicative interaction. *Sign Language Studies, 47,* 111-126.

Erting, C.J. (1988). Acquiring linguistic and social identity: Interactions of deaf children with a hearing teacher and a deaf adult. In M. Strong (Ed.), *Language Learning and Deafness.* Cambridge: Cambridge University Press.

Erting, C.J. (1992). Deafness and literacy: Why can't Sam read? *Sign Language Studies, 75,* 97-112.

Estes, C. (1994). Technical aids for deaf Americans. In H. Lane (Ed.), *Parallel views: Education and access for deaf people in France and the United States* (pp. 223-227). Washington, DC: Gallaudet University Press.

European Parliament (1988, July 18). *Official Gazette of the European Community* (Doc. A2-302/87).

Evans, J. W., & Elliott, H. (1987). The mental status examination. In H. Elliott, L. Glass & J. W. Evans (Eds.), *Mental health assessment of deaf clients: A practical manual* (pp. 83-92). San Diego: College-Hill.

Ewoldt, C. (1985). A descriptive study of the developing literacy of young hearing-impaired children. *Volta Review, 87*, 109-126.

Ewoldt, C. (1987). Reading tests and the deaf reader. Can we measure how well deaf students read? *Perspectives for teachers of the hearing-impaired, 5*, 21-24.

Ewoldt, C. (1993) Whole language. *American Annals of the Deaf, 138*, 10-12.

Farb, P. (1973). *Word play: What happens when people talk?* New York: Alfred Knopf.

Farrell, C. (1989). Students who are Black and deaf say they face dual discrimination. *Black Issues in Higher Education*, 14-15.

Fay, E. A. (1898). *Marriages of the deaf in America*. Washington, DC: Volta Bureau.

Finnish Association of the Deaf (1994). An educational policy program for the Deaf. *Deaf American Monographs, 44*, 33-40.

Fischer, S. (1975). Influences on word order change in ASL. In C. Li (Ed.), *Word order and word order change* (pp. 1-25). Austin, TX: University of Texas Press.

Fischer, S. (1978). Sign language and creoles. In P. Siple (Ed.), *Understanding language through sign language research* (pp. 309-332). New York: Academic Press.

Fischer, S. (1982). Sign language and manual communication. In D. G. Sims & G. G. Walter (Eds.), *Deafness and communication: Assessment and training*. Baltimore, MD: Williams & Wilkins.

Fischler, I. (1983). Contextual constraint and comprehension of written sentences by deaf college students. *American Annals of the Deaf, 128*, 418-424.

Fishman, J. (1982). A critique of six papers on the socialization of the deaf child. In J. B. Christiansen (Ed.), *Conference highlights: National research conference on the social aspects of deafness* (pp. 6-20). Washington, DC: Gallaudet College.

For hearing people only. (1995). *Deaf Life, 8* (3), 6-7.

Foster, S. (1989). Social alienation and peer identification: A study of the social construction of deafness. *Human Organization, 48*, 226-235.

Foucault, M. (1980). *Power/Knowledge: Selected interviews and other writings, 1972-1977*. Brighton: Harvester Press.

Fraser, G. R. (1976). *The causes of profound deafness in childhood*. Baltimore: Johns Hopkins.

Fraser, G. R. (1987). Hearing loss: Genetic causes. In J. V. Van Cleve (Ed.), *Gallaudet encyclopedia of deaf people and deafness* (pp. 20-23). New York: McGraw-Hill.

Freeman, R. D., Boese, R., & Carbin, R., (1975). *Can't your child hear?* Baltimore, MD: University Park Press.

Freeman, R. D., Malkin, S. F., & Hastings, J. O. (1975). Psychosocial problems of deaf children and their families: a comparative study. *American Annals of the Deaf, 121*, 391-405.

Frishberg, N. (1975). Arbitrariness and iconicity: Historical change in American Sign Language. *Language, 51*, 676-710.

Frishberg, N. (1987). Sign languages: Ghanaian. In J. V. Van Cleve (Ed.), *Gallaudet encyclopedia of deaf people and deafness* (pp. 78-79). New York: McGraw-Hill.

Fryauf-Bertschy, H., Tyler, R. S., Kelsay, D., & Gantz, B. J. (1992). Performance over time of congenitally and postlingually deafened children using a multi-channel cochlear implant. *Journal of Speech and Hearing Research, 35*, 913-920.

References

Gagné, J. P., & Tye-Murray, N. (Eds.). (1994). *Research in audiological rehabilitation: Current trends and future directions*. Cedar Falls, IA: American Academy of Rehabilitative Audiology.

Gannon, J. (1981). *Deaf heritage*. Silver Spring: National Association of the Deaf.

Gannon, J. (1988). The week the world heard Gallaudet. *Gallaudet Alumni Newsletter, 22*, 1-3.

Gannon, J. (1989). *The week the world heard Gallaudet*. Washington, DC: Gallaudet University Press.

Gaustad, M. (1992). Long-term effects of manual codes on English skills. *Applied Psycholinguistics, 7*, 101-128.

Gee, J. P. (1990). *Social linguistics and literacies*. Philadelphia: Taylor & Francis Falmer Press.

Gee, J. P. & Goodhart, W. (1988). American Sign Language and the human biological capacity for language. In M. Strong (Ed.), *Language learning and deafness*. Cambridge: Cambridge University Press.

Gee, J. P., & Mounty, J. L. (1991). Nativization, variability, and style shifting in the sign language development of deaf children of hearing parents. In P. Siple & S. Fischer (Eds.), *Theoretical issues in sign language research Vol. 2* (pp. 65-84). Chicago IL: University of Chicago Press.

Geers, A. E. (1994). Closing comments on the decision to implant a deaf child. *Annals of Otology, Rhinology & Laryngology, 103*, 20-21.

Geers, A. E., & Moog, J. S. (1987). *Factors predictive of the development of reading and writing skills in the congenitally deaf: report of the oral sample*. Rockville, MD: National Institute on Deafness and other Communication Disorders.

Geers, A. E. & Schick, B. (1988). Acquisition of spoken and signed English by hearing-impaired children of hearing-impaired or hearing parents. *Journal of Speech and Hearing Disorders, 53*, 136-143.

Gene that causes (1992, Feburary 18). *Gene that causes Waardenburg's Syndrome. New York Times, 141*, B7,C2.

Gerber, B. M., & Goldberg, H. K. (1980). Psychiatric consultation in a school program for multiply handicapped deaf children. *American Annals of the Deaf, 125*, 579-585.

Gerner de Garcia, B. (1993). Addressing the needs of Hispanic deaf children. In K. M. Christensen & G. L. Delgado (Eds.), *Multicultural issues in deafness* (pp. 69-90). White Plains, NY: Longman.

Gilman, L., Davis, J. & Raffin, M. (1980). Use of common morphemes by hearing-impaired children exposed to a system of manual English. *Journal of Auditory Research, 20*, 57-69.

Gjerdingen, D. (1987). Summation. *American Annals of the Deaf, 132*, 350.

Goddard, H. (1917). Mental tests and the immigrant. *Journal of Delinquency, 2*, 243-277.

Goldin-Meadow, S. (1985). Language development under atypical learning conditions. *Children's Language, 5*, 197-245.

Goldin-Meadow, S., & Mylander, C. (1984). The development of morphology without a conventional language model. *Chicago Linguistic Society, 20*, 119-135.

Goldin-Meadow, S. & Mylander, C. (1990a). The role of parental input in the development of a morphological system. *Journal of Child Language, 17*, 527-563.

Goldin-Meadow, S., & Mylander,C. (1990b). Beyond the input given: The child's role in the acquisition of language. *Journal of the Linguistic Society of America, 66*, 323-355.

Goodstein, H. (1994). Information superhighway. *National Association of the Deaf Broadcaster, 16*, 5, 7.

Goppold, L. (1988). Early intervention for preschool deaf children: The longitudinal academic effects relative to program methodology. *American Annals of the Deaf, 133*, 285-288.

Graham, E., & Shapiro, E. (1953). Use of the performance scale of the WISC with the deaf child. *Journal of Consulting Psychology, 17*, 396-398.

Greenberg, M. T. (1980). Hearing families with deaf children: stress and functioning as related to communication method. *American Annals of the Deaf, 125*, 1063-1071.

Greenberg, M. T. (1983). Family stress and child competence: The effects of early intervention for families with deaf infants. *American Annals of the Deaf, 128*, 407-417.

Gregory, S. (1976). *The deaf child and his family*. London: George Allen.

Gregory, S. & Hartley, G. M. (Eds.). (1991). *Constructing deafness*. London: Pinter.

Grémion, J. (1990). *La Planète des sourds*. Paris: Messinger.

Groce, N. (1985). *Everyone here spoke sign language*. Cambridge, MA: Harvard University Press.

Grodin, M. A., & Glantz, L. H. (1994). *Children as research subjects*. New York: Oxford University Press.

Grosjean, F. (1982). *Life with two languages*. Cambridge, MA: Harvard University Press.

Gross, B. (1994). Mainstreaming—A new concept for recreation and leisure in the deaf community. In C. Erting, R. E. Johnson, D. L. Smith & B. D. Snider (Eds.), *The Deaf Way: Perspectives from the International Conference on Deaf Culture* (pp. 545-547). Washington, DC: Gallaudet University Press.

Gusfield, J. (1989). Constructing the ownership of social problems: fun and profit in the welfare state. *Social Problems, 36,* 431-441.

Gustason, G. (1988) Why Signing Exact English was developed. In G. Gustason, (Ed.), *Signing Exact English: Exact or not?* A collection of articles. Los Alamitos, CA: Modern Signs Press, Inc.

Gustason, G., Pfetzing, D., Zawolkow,E. (1992). *Signing Exact English*. Los Angeles, CA: Modern Signs Press.

Guthmann, D. G., Lybarger, R., & Sandberg, K. A. (1995). *Chemical dependency treatment: Specialized approaches for deaf and hard-of-hearing clients*. Minneapolis, MN: Minnesota Chemical Dependency Program.

Haft, J. (1983). Assuring equal educational opportunity for language-minority students: Bilingual education and the Equal Educational Opportunity Act of 1974. *Columbia Journal of Law and Social Problems, 18*, 209-293.

Hagemeyer, A. L. (1993). Looking to the future: A librarian's perspective. *Deaf American, 43*, 33-38.

Hairston, E., & Smith, L. (1983). *Black and deaf in America*. Silver Spring, MD: TJ Publishers.

Hakuta, K. (1986). *Mirror of Language: The Debate on Bilingualism*. New York: Basic Books.

Hall, S. (1989). Train-Gone-Sorry: The etiquette of social conversation in American Sign Language. In S. Wilcox (Ed.), *American Deaf Culture* (pp. 89-102). Silver Spring, MD: Linstok Press.

Hall, S. (1991). Door into American Deaf culture: Folklore in an American Deaf social club. *Sign Language Studies, 73*, 421-429.

Hallahan, D., & Kaufman, J. (1994). *Exceptional children: Introduction to special education*. Boston, MA: Allyn & Bacon.

Halverson, B. (1987). Theater, college. In J. V. Van Cleve (Ed.), *Gallaudet encyclopedia of deaf people and deafness* (pp. 284-287). New York: McGraw-Hill.

Hammond, S. A., & Meiners, L. H. (1993). American Indian deaf children and youth. In K. M. Christensen & G. L. Delgado (Eds.), *Multicultural issues in deafness* (pp. 143-166). White Plains, NY: Longman.

Hansen, B., & Kjaer-Sorensen, R. (1976). *The sign language of deaf children in Denmark*. Copenhagen Denmark: The School for the Deaf.

Hanson, V. L. (1982). Use of orthographic structure by deaf adults: Recognition of fingerspelled words. *Applied Psycholinguistics, 3*, 343-356.

Hanson, V. L. (1986). Access to spoken language and the acquisition of orthographic structure: evidence from deaf readers. *Quarterly Journal of Experimental Psychology A: Human Experimental Psychology, 38*, 193-212.

Hanson, V. L. (1989). Phonology and reading: Evidence from profoundly deaf readers. In D. Shankweiler & I. Y. Liberman (Eds.), *Phonology and reading disability: Solving the reading puzzle*. Ann Arbor: University Michigan Press.

Hanson, V. L., & Bellugi, U. (1982). On the role of sign order and morphological structure in memory for American Sign Language. *Journal of Verbal Learning and Verbal Behavior, 21*, 621-633.

References

Hanson, V. L., Shankweiler, D., & Fischer, F. W. (1983). Determinants of spelling ability in deaf and hearing adults: access to linguistic structure. *Cognition, 14*, 323-44.

Harris, R. (1978). Impulse control in deaf children. Research and clinical issues. In L. S. Liben (Ed.), *Deaf children: Developmental perspectives*. New York: Academic Press.

Harvey, M(1989). *Psychotherapy with deaf and hard-of-hearing persons*. Hillsdale: Lawrence Erlbaum Associates.

Harvey, M. (1995). Utilization of traumatic transference by a hearing therapist. In M. Harvey & N. Glickman (Eds.), *Culturally-sensitive psychotherapy with Deaf persons*. Hillsdale, NJ: Lawrence Erlbaum Associates.

Hawcroft, L. (1991). *D251: Deaf people in hearing worlds. Unit 7. Whose welfare?* Milton Keynes: Open University.

Hawkins, L. & Baker-Hawkins, S. (1991). Perspectives on deafness: Hearing parents of deaf children. In M. Garretson (Ed.), *Perspectives on Deafness: A Deaf American Monograph* (pp. 63-66). Silver Spring, MD: National Association of the Deaf.

Heiling, K. (1995). Education of the deaf in Sweden. In A. W. Brejle (Ed.), *A worldwide summary of education of the deaf*. Portland, OR: Lewis and Clark College.

Herrnstein, R., & Murray, C. (1994). *The bell curve*. New York: Free Press.

Hevey, D. (1993). From self-love to the picket line: strategies for change in disability representation. *Disability, Handicap & Society, 8*, 423-430.

Higgins, P. C. (1980). *Outsiders in a hearing world*. Beverly Hills, CA: Sage.

Higgins, W. (Ed.) (1993). La parole des sourds. *Psychoanalystes, 46-47*, 1-216.

Holt, J. (1994). Classroom attributes and achievement test scores for deaf and hard-of-hearing students. *American Annals of the Deaf, 139*, 430-437.

Hoffmeister, R. (1982). The acquisition of language abilities by deaf children. In H. Hoeman & R. Wilbur (Eds.), *Communication in two societies, monographs in social aspects of deafness*. Washington, DC: Gallaudet University Press.

Hoffmeister, R. (1985). Families with deaf parents: A functional perspective. In K. Thurman, (Ed.), *Children with handicapped parents: Research and perspectives*. Academic Press, New York.

Hoffmeister, R. (1990). ASL and its implications for education. In H. Bornstein (Ed.), *Manual communication in America*. Washington, DC: Gallaudet University Press.

Hoffmeister, R. (1993a). *The problem of manually coded English in deaf children*. Paper presented at the Annual Convention of American Instructors of the Deaf, Baltimore, MD.

Hoffmeister, R. (1993b). *Can bilingual/bicultural education of the deaf survive special education?* Paper presented at the Annual Convention of American Instructors of the Deaf, Baltimore, MD.

Hoffmeister, R. (1994). Metalinguistic skills in deaf children. In College for Continuing Education (Ed.), *Post Milan ASL and English literacy: Issues, trends and research. Conference proceedings, October 20-22, 1993*. Washington, DC: Gallaudet University.

Hoffmeister, R. (1995, April). *What deaf kids know about ASL even though they 'see' MCE!* Paper presented at the Deaf Studies IV Conference, Woburn, MA.

Hoffmeister, R. (in press). Cross cultural misinformation: What special education says about the Deaf. *Disability & Society*.

Hoffmeister, R. & Shettle, C. (1983). Adaptations in communication made by deaf signers to different audience types. *Discourse Processes, 6*, 258-274.

Hoffmeister, H. & Wilbur, R. (1980). The acquisition of American Sign Language: Review. In H. Lane & F. Grosjean (Eds.), *Recent perspectives on American Sign Language*. Hillsdale, NJ: Lawrence Erlbaum Associates.

Hoyt, M. F., Siegelman, E. Y., & Schlesinger, H. S. (1981). Special issues regarding psychotherapy with the deaf. *American Journal of Psychiatry, 138*, 807-811.

Humphries, T. (1991). An introduction to the culture of deaf people in the United States: Content notes and reference materials for teachers. *Sign Language Studies, 72*, 209-240.

Humphries, T. (1993). Multicultural issues in deafness. In K. M. Christensen & G. L. Delgado (Eds.), *Multicultural issues in deafness*. White Plains, NY: Longman.

Innes, J. (1993). Education section. *National Association of the Deaf Broadcaster, 15* (4), 18.

Innes, J. (1994). National Association of the Deaf comments on IDEA. *National Association of the Deaf Broadcaster, 16* (12), 1-2.

Israelite, N., Ewoldt, C., & Hoffmeister, R. (1989). *Bilingual/bicultural education for deaf and hard-of-hearing students: A review of the literature on effective use of native sign language on the acquisition of a majority language by hearing-impaired students*. Ontario: Ministry of Education.

Jackson-Maldo, D. (1993). Mexico and the United States: A cross-cultural perspective on the education of deaf children. In K. M. Christensen & G. L. Delgado (Eds.), *Multicultural issues in deafness* (pp. 91-112). White Plains, NY: Longman.

Jacobowitz, E. L. (1992). Humor and wit in the Deaf community. In College for Continuing Education (Ed.), Deaf studies: *What's up? Proceedings of a conference October 24, 1991* (pp. 187-192). Washington, DC: Gallaudet University.

Jacobowitz, L. (1995). Legislative recognition of ASL as a foreign language. *National Association of the Deaf Broadcaster, 17* (12), 12-13.

Jankowski, K. A. (1992). The battle of ideologies: A struggle for ownership in the Deaf community. Unpublished doctoral dissertation. University of Maryland, College Park. Jarvella, R. (1971). Syntactic processing of connected speech. *Journal of Verbal Learning and Verbal Behavior, 10*, 409-416.

Javal, E. (1887). Adieu aux professeurs sourds. *Revue Internationale de l'Enseignement des Sourds-Muets, 3*, 285-287.

Jodoin, J. & Hoffmeister, R. (1994). *Views of the deaf in speech and hearing texts*. Working Paper #30. Center for the Study of Communication and Deafness, Boston University, Boston, MA.

Johnson, H., & Griffith, P., (1986). The instructional pattern of two fourth-grade spelling classes: A mainstream issue. *American Annals of the Deaf, 121*, 4, 331-338.

Johnson, R. E. (1994). Sign language and the concept of deafness in a traditional Yucatec Mayan village. In C. Erting, R. E. Johnson, D. L. Smith & B. D. Snider (Eds.), *The Deaf Way: Perspectives from the International Conference on Deaf Culture* (pp. 103-109). Washington, DC: Gallaudet University Press.

Johnson, R. E., Liddell, S. K., & Erting, C.J. (1989). *Unlocking the curriculum: principles for achieving access in deaf education*. Washington, DC: Gallaudet University, Gallaudet Research Institute.

Johnson, R. H. (1918). The marriage of the deaf. *Jewish Deaf*, 5-6.

Jones, L., & Pullen, G. (1989). 'Inside we are all equal': A European social policy survey of people who are deaf. In L. Barton (Ed.), *Disability and dependency* (pp. 127-137). Bristol, PA: Taylor & Francis Falmer Press.

Jordan, K. (1991). Ethical issues in the genetic study of deafness. *Annals of the New York Academy of Sciences, 630*, 236-239.

Joutselainen, M. (1991). *WFD Survey of deaf people in the developing world*. Helsinki: World Federation of the Deaf.

Kakumasu, J. (1968). Urubu Sign Language. *International Journal of American Linguistics, 34*, 275-281.

Kane, T. P. (1994). Deaf Gay men's culture. In C. Erting, R. E.Johnson, D. L. Smith & B. D. Snider (Eds.), *The Deaf Way: Perspectives from the International Conference on Deaf Culture* (pp. 483-485). Washington, DC: Gallaudet University Press.

Kannapell, B. (1989). Inside the deaf community. In S. Wilcox (Ed.), *American Deaf culture* (pp. 21-28). Silver Spring, MD: Linstok Press.

Karakostas, A. (Ed.) (1990). *Le Pouvoir des signes*. Paris: Institut National de Jeunes Sourds.

References

Karakostas, A. (1993a). Fragments of glottophagia: Ferdinand Berthier and the birth of the deaf movement in France. In R. Fischer & H. Lane (Eds.), *Look back: A reader on the history of Deaf communities and their sign languages* (pp. 133-142). Hamburg: Signum.

Karakostas, A. (1993b). Access to mental health care in France. In H. Lane (Ed.), *Parallel views: Education and access for Deaf people in France and the United States* (pp. 202-207). Washington, DC: Gallaudet University Press.

Karchmer, M. A., Trybus, R. J., & Paquin, M. M. (1978). *Early manual communication, parental hearing status, and the academic achievement of deaf students*. Paper presented at the meeting of the American Educational Research Association, Toronto.

Kaufman, C. (1986). Role obligations and health status in chronic disease: The experience of men and women with arthritis. *Disability, Handicap & Society, 1*, 261-271.

Kauppinen, L. (1994). *The standard rules*. Helsinki: World Federation of the Deaf, Secretariat.

Kegl, J. (1985). *Locative relations in American Sign Language word formation, syntax and discourse* Unpublished doctoral dissertation, Massachusetts Institute of Technology, Cambridge, MA.

Kewley-Port, D. (1994). Speech technology and speech training for the hearing impaired. In J. P. Gagné & N. Tye-Murray (Eds.), *Research in audiological rehabilitation* (pp. 251-265). Cedar Falls, IA: American Academy of Rehabilitative Audiology.

Klima, E., & Bellugi, U. (1979). On the creation of new lexical items by compounding. In E. S. Klima & U. Bellugi (Eds.), *The signs of language*. (3rd ed., pp. 272-315). Cambridge, MA: Harvard University Press.

Klima, E., Tzeng, O. J. L., Fok, Y. Y. A., Bellugi, U., Corina, D., & Bettger, J. (in press). From sign to script: Effects of linguistic experience on perceptual categorization. *Journal of Chinese Linguistics: Special issue on brain bases of language*.

Kluwin, T. & Moores, D. (1985). The effects on the mathematics achievement of hearing-impaired adolescents. *Exceptional Children, 52*, 153-160.

Kluwin, T., Moores, D., & Gonter-Gaustad, M. (Eds.), (1992). *Toward effective public school programs for deaf students: context, process & outcomes*. New York Teachers College Press

Kohut, R. I. (Ed.). (1988). Cochlear implants. *National Institutes of Health Consensus Development Conference Statement, 7*, 1-25.

Kourbetis, V. (1987). *Deaf children of deaf parents and deaf children of hearing parents in Greece: a comparative study*. Unpublished doctoral dissertation, Boston University, Boston.

Kuntze, M. (1994). Developing students' literary skills in ASL. In College for Continuing Education (Ed.), *Post Milan ASL and English literacy: Issues, trends and research. Conference proceedings, October 20-22, 1993* (pp. 267-281). Washington, DC: Gallaudet University.

Kyle, J. (1990). The Deaf community: Culture, custom and tradition. In S. Prillwitz & T. Vollhaber (Eds.), *Sign language research and application* (pp. 175-185). Hamburg: Signum.

Kyle, J. (1991). Deaf people and minority groups in the U.K. In S. Gregory & G. M. Hartley (Eds.), *Constructing deafness* (pp. 272-277). London: Pinter.

Lambert, W. (1977). Culture and language as factors in education. In F. Eckman (Ed.), *Current themes in linguistics: Bilingualism, experimental linguistics, and language typologies*. Washington, DC: Hemisphere Publishing.

Lane, H. (1984). *When the mind hears: A history of the deaf*. New York: Random House.

Lane, H. (1986). On language, power, and the deaf. In M. McIntire (Ed.), *Interpreting: The art of cross-cultural mediation*. Silver Spring, MD: Registry of Interpreters for the Deaf.

Lane, H. (1988). Is there a "psychology of the deaf?" *Exceptional Children, 55*, 7-19.

Lane, H. (1991). Cultural and disability models of Deaf Americans. *Journal of the American Academy of Rehabilitative Audiology, 1991, 23*, 11-26.

Lane, H. (1992). *The mask of benevolence: Disabling the Deaf community*. New York: Alfred Knopf.

Lane, H. (1993a). Cochlear implants: Their cultural and historical meaning. In J. Van Cleve (Ed.), *Deaf history unveiled*. Washington, DC: Gallaudet University Press.

Lane, H. (1993b). Constructing deafness in France and the United States. In H. Lane (Ed.), *Parallel views: Education and access for Deaf people in France and the United States* (pp. 3-22). Washington, DC: Gallaudet University Press.

Lane, H. (1994). The cochlear implant controversy. *World Federation of the Deaf News, (2-3)*, 22-28.

Lane, H. (1995a). Acquisition of speech perception ability in prelingually deaf children with a multi-channel cochlear implant. Letter to the Editor. *American Journal of Otology, 16*, 393-399.

Lane, H. (1995b). Constructions of deafness. *Disability and Society, 10*, 171-189.

Lane, H. (1996). Who are hearing people? In N. Glickman and M. Harvey (Eds.), *Culturally affirmative psychotherapy with Deaf persons*. Hillsdale, NJ: Lawrence Erlbaum Associates.

Lane, H., & Battison, R. (1978). The role of oral language in the evolution of manual language. In D. Gerver & W. Sinaiko (Eds.), *Language interpretation and communication*. New York: Plenum.

Laurenzi, C. (1993). The bionic ear and the mythology of cochlear implants. *British Journal of Audiology, 27*, 1-5.

Lebuffe, F. P., & Lebuffe, L. A. (1979). Psychiatric aspects of deafness. *Primary Care, 6*, 295-310.

Lederberg, A. (1991). Social interactions among deaf preschoolers: The effects of language ability and age. *American Annals of the Deaf, 136*, 53-59.

Lenneberg, E. (1967). *Biological foundations of language*. New York: Wiley.

Lentz, E. (1995). *The Treasure: Poems by Ella Mae Lentz* (videotape). Berkeley, CA: In Motion Press.

Levesque, J. (1992). My mother's last words. *DCARA News, 13*, 2.

Levesque, J. (1994). Its a Deaf Deaf Deaf world. *DCARA News, 15*, 2.

Levine, E. (1981). *Ecology of early deafness*. New York: Columbia University Press.

Liddell, S. K. (1977). *An investigation into the syntactic structure of American Sign Language*. Unpublished doctoral dissertation, University of California, San Diego.

Liddell, S. K. (1990). Four functions of a locus: Reexamining the structure of space in ASL. In C. Lucas (Ed.), *Sign language research: Theoretical issues Vol. 2* (pp. 176-200). Washington, DC: Gallaudet University Press.

Liddell, S. K., & Johnson, R. E. (1989). American Sign Language: The phonological base. *Sign Language Studies, 64*, 195-277.

Liddell, S. K., & Johnson, R. E. (1986). American Sign Language compound formation processes, lexicalization, and phonological remnants. *Natural Language and Linguistic Theory, 4*, 445-513.

Lillo-Martin, D. (1992, August). *The point of view predicate in American Sign Language*. Paper presented at the Conference on Theoretical Issues in Sign Language Research, San Diego.

Livingston, S. (1983). Levels of development in the language of deaf children. *Sign Language Studies, 40*, 193-286.

Loera, P. A. (1994). The use and application of cognitive- behavioral psychotherapy with Deaf persons. In R. C. Nowell & L. E. Marshak (Eds.), *Understanding deafness and the rehabilitation process* (pp. 155-187). Boston: Allyn & Bacon.

Lopez, J. R. (1993). Transforming leadership for the 21st century. *Deaf American, 43*, 83-92.

Lucas, C., & Valli, C. (1990). ASL, English and contact signing. In C. Lucas (Ed.), *Sign language research: Theoretical issues* (pp. 288-307). Washington, DC: Gallaudet University Press.

Lucas, C., & Valli, C. (1992). *Language contact in the American deaf community*. New York: Academic Press.

Luczak, R. (1992). Learning to speak I. In J. Jepson (Ed.), *No walls of stone: An anthology of literature by deaf and hard-of-hearing writers* (p. 78). Washington, DC: Gallaudet University Press.

Luczak, R. (1993). *Eyes of desire: A Deaf Gay and Lesbian reader*. Boston: Alyson.

Luetke-Stahlman, B., (1988a). Documenting syntactically and semantically incomplete bimodal input to hearing-impaired subjects. *American Annals of the Deaf, 133*, 230-234.

Luetke-Stahlman, B. (1988b). SEE-2 in the classroom: How well is English represented? In G. Gustason (Ed.), *Signing English in total communication*. Los Lalamitos, CA: Modern Sign Press.

Luterman, D. (Ed.) (1986). *Deafness in perspective*. New York: Taylor & Francis.

Mace-Matluck, B. J., Hoover, W. A., & Calfee, R. C. (1984). *Teaching reading to bilingual children*. Austin, TX: Southwest Educational Development Laboratory.

Mahshie, S. N. (1995). *Educating deaf children bilingually: With insights and applications from Sweden and Denmark*. Washington, DC: Gallaudet University.

Mäkipää, A. (1993, February). Focus on the human rights dimension of deafness. *World Federation of the Deaf News*, 13-14.

Mannes, J. P. (1987). Broderson, Morris. In J. V. Van Cleve (Ed.), *Gallaudet encyclopedia of deaf people and deafness* (pp. 159-160). New York: McGraw-Hill.

Markowicz, H., & Woodward, J. (1978). Language and the maintenance of ethnic boundaries in the Deaf community. *Communication and Cognition, 11*, 29-38.

Marlowe, J. (1987). Early identification and the hearing-impaired child's right to become. *American Annals of the Deaf, 132*, 337-339.

Marmor, G. & Petitto, L. (1979). Simultaneous communication in the classroom: How well is English grammar represented? *Sign Language Studies, 23*, 99-136.

Martin, F. (1994). *Introduction to audiology*. Fifth ed. Englewood Cliffs, NJ: Prentice Hall.

Marshall, W. (1970). *Quantitative and qualitative analysis of the language of deaf children*. Unpublished doctoral dissertation, University of Illinois, Urbana Champaign, IL.

Mather, S. (1987). Eye gaze and communication in a deaf classroom. *Sign Language Studies, 54* 11-30.

Mather, S. (1993). Adult/Deaf-toddler discourse. In College of Continuing Education (Ed.), *Post Milan ASL and English literacy: Issues, trends and research. Conference proceedings, October 20-22, 1993* (pp. 283-298). Washington, DC: Gallaudet University.

Mather, S. & Mitchell, R. (1993). Communication abuse: A sociolinguistic perspective. In College of Continuing Education (Ed.) *Post Milan ASL and English literacy: Issues, trends and research. Conference proceedings, October 20-22, 1993* (pp. 117-134). Washington, DC: Gallaudet University Press.

Matthews, T. & Reich, C. (1993). Constraints on communication in classrooms for the deaf. *American Annals of the Deaf, 138*, 14-18.

Mayberry, R., & Eichen, E. (1991). The long-lasting advantage of learning sign language in childhood: another look at the critical period for language acquisition. *Journal of Memory and Language, 30*, 486-512.

Mayberry, R., & Fischer, S. (1989). Looking through phonological shape to lexical meaning: the bottleneck of non-native sign language processing. *Memory and Cognition, 17*, 740-754.

Maxwell, M., Bernstein, M., & Matthews, K. (1990). Bimodal & bilingual communication in schools for the deaf. *Sign Language Studies, 47*, 127-140.

Maxwell, M. & Bernstein, M., & Matthews, K. (1991). Bimodal language production. In P. Siple & S. Fischer (Eds.), *Theoretical issues in sign language research Vol. 2* (pp. 171-190). Chicago, IL: University of Chicago Press.

Mbewe, E. (1995, January). Give Deaf women a chance to contribute! *World Federation of the Deaf News*, 26-28.

McGarr, N. S., & Harris, K. S. (1983). Articulatory control in a deaf speaker. In I. Hochberg, H. Levitt & M. J. Osberger (Eds.), *Speech of the hearing-impaired* (pp. 75-95). Baltimore, MD: University Park Press.

McIntire, M. (1977). The acquisition of American Sign Language hand configurations. *Sign Language Studies, 16*, 247-266.

McIntire, M., & Sanderson, G. (1993). *Bye-bye Bi-Bi. Questions of empowerment and role.* Paper presented at the Convention of the Registry of Interpreters for the Deaf, Evansville, IN.

Meadow, K. P. (1968). Early manual communication in relation to the deaf child's intellectual, social and communicative functioning. *American Annals of the Deaf, 113*, 29-41.

Meadow, K. P. (1980). *Deafness and child development.* Berkeley, CA: University of California Press.

Meadow, K. P. (1981). Studies of behavior problems of deaf children. In L. K. Stein, E. D. Mindel & T. Jabaley (Eds.), *Deafness and mental health* (pp. 3-22). New York: Grune & Stratton.

Meadow-Orlans, K. P. (1987). Psychosocial intervention with deaf children. In B. W. Heller, L. M. Flohr & L. S. Zegans (Eds.), *Psychosocial interventions with sensorially disabled persons* (pp. 115-130). Orlando, FL: Grune & Stratton.

Meier, R. P. (1990). Personal deixis in American Sign Language. In S. Fischer & P. Siple (Eds.), *Theoretical issues in sign language research Vol. 1.* Chicago IL: University of Chicago Press.

Meier, R. P., & Newport, E. L. (1990). Out of the hands of babes: On a possible sign advantage in language acquisition. *Language, 66*, 1-23.

Meyer, M. (1994). Access in California: A case study. In H. Lane (Ed.), *Parallel views: Education and access for Deaf people in France and the United States* (pp. 194-201). Washington, DC: Gallaudet University Press.

Miller, B. (1994). De'VIA (Deaf View/Image Art). In C. Erting, R. E. Johnson, D. L. Smith & B. D. Snider (Eds.), *The Deaf Way: Perspectives from the International Conference on Deaf Culture* (pp. 770-772). Washington, DC: Gallaudet University Press.

Mills, C., & Weldon, L. (1983). Effects of semantic and cheremic context on acquisition of manual signs. *Memory and Cognition, 11*, 93-100.

Mindel, E. & Vernon, M. (1971). *They grow in silence.* Silver Spring, MD: National Association of the Deaf.

Mindess, A. (1990). What name signs can tell us about deaf culture. *Sign Language Studies, 66*, 1-24.

Montgomery, G. (Ed.) (1978). *Of sound and mind: Deafness, personality, and mental health.* Edinburgh: Scottish Workshop Publications.

Moody, W. (1983). *Introduction à l'histoire et à la grammaire de la langue des signes.* Paris: International Visual Theatre.

Moody, W. (1987). Desloges, Pierre. In J. V. Van Cleve (Ed.), *Gallaudet encyclopedia of deaf people and deafness* (pp. 301-302). New York: McGraw-Hill.

Moody, W. (1989). La communication internationale chez les sourds. *Rééducation orthophonique, 17*, 213-224.

Moody, W. (1994). Interpreting for Deaf and hearing people in the United States. In H. Lane (Ed.), *Parallel views: Education and access for Deaf people in France and the United States* (pp. 63-75). Washington, DC: Gallaudet University Press.

Moores, D. (1967). *Applications of "cloze" procedures to the assessment of psycholinguistic abilities of the deaf.* Unpublished doctoral dissertation, University of Illinois, Urbana-Champaign, IL.

Moores, D. (1970). Investigation of psycholinguistic abilities of deaf adolescents. *Exceptional Children, 36*, 645-654.

Moores, D. (1987). *Educating the deaf: Psychology, principles, and practices.* Hougton Mifflin: Boston, MA.

Moores, D. (1992). What did we know and when did we know it. In M. Walworth, D. Moores, & T. O'Rourke (Eds.), *A freehand: Enfranchising the education of Deaf children* (pp. 67-68). Silver Spring, MD: T. J. Publishers.

Moores, D., & Meadow-Orlans, K. P., (Eds.) (1990). *Educational and developmental aspects of deafness.* Washington, DC: Gallaudet University Press.

Moores, D., & Sweet, C. (1990). Factors predictive of achievement. In D. F. Moores & K. Meadow-Orlans (Eds.), *Educational and developmental aspects of deafness* (pp. 154-201). Washington, DC: Gallaudet University Press.

Moores, D., Weiss, K., Goodwin, M., (1978). Early intervention programs for hearing impaired children: a longitudinal assessment. *American Annals of the Deaf, 123*, 925-936.

Morris, J. (1990). *Pride against prejudice*. London: Women's Press. Mottez, B. (1985). Aspects de la culture sourde. Santé Mentale, 85, 13-16.

Mottez, B. (1993). Aspects of a French-American comparison. In H. Lane (Ed.), *Parallel views: Education and access for Deaf people in France and the United States* (pp. 55-59). Washington, DC: Gallaudet University Press.

Mottez, B. (1993). The deaf-mute banquets and the birth of the deaf movement. In R. Fischer & H. Lane (Eds.), *Look back: A reader on the history of Deaf communities and their sign languages* (pp. 143-155). Hamburg: Signum.

Mottez, B. & Markowicz, H. (1980). The social movement for the acceptance of French Sign Language. In C. Baker and R. Battison (Eds.), *Sign language and the deaf community. Essays in honor of William Stokoe* (221-232). Silver Spring, MD: National Association of the Deaf.

Muhs, J. (1995). *Followers and outcasts. The history of Berlin's Deaf community under National Socialism* (1933-1945). Unpublished manuscript, Berlin Deaf Club.

Nagase, O. (1995, October). *Disabled persons' fundamental law in Japan*. Paper presented at the Disability Rights Symposium of European Regions, Southampton.

Nagy, W., Anderson, R., & Herman, P. (1987). Learning word meanings from context during normal reading. *American Educational Research Journal, 24*, 237-270.

National Association of the Deaf (1991). Report of the Task Force on Childhood Cochlear Implants. *National Association of the Deaf Broadcaster, 13*, 1.

National Association of the Deaf (1994). ASL position paper approved by National Association of the Deaf. *National Association of the Deaf Broadcaster, 16*, 39.

National Association of the Deaf (1995). State association presidents' interpreting concerns. *National Association of the Deaf Broadcaster, 17*, 28.

National Captioning Institute (1993a). *Nearly 100 million Americans can benefit from watching captioned TV*. Falls Church VA: NCI.

National Captioning Institute (1993b). *Backgrounder: A brief history of captioned television*. Falls Church VA: NCI.

National Institutes of Health (1995). NIH Consensus Development Conference: Cochlear implants in adults and children. *Journal of the American Medical Association, 274*, 1955-1961.

Neisser, A. (1983). *The other side of silence: Sign language and the deaf community in America*. New York: Alfred Knopf.

Neville, H. (1988). Cerebral organization for spatial attention. In J. Stiles-Davis, M. Kritchevsky & U. Bellugi (Eds.), *Spatial cognition: Brain bases and development* (pp. 327-341). Hillsdale, NJ: Lawrence Erlbaum Associates.

Neville, H., Schmidt, A., & Kutas, M. (1983). Altered visual evoked potentials in congenitally deaf adults. *Brain Research, 266*, 127-132.

Newport, E. (1988). Constraints on learning and their role in language acquisition: Studies of the acquisition of American Sign Language. *Language Sciences, 10*, 147-172.

Newport, E. (1990). Maturational constraints on language learning. *Cognitive Science, 14*, 11-28.

Newport, E. & Gleitman, L. (1977). Maternal self-repetition and the child's acquisition of language. *Papers and Reports on Child Language Development, 13*, 46-55.

Newport, E., & Meier, R. (1985). Acquisition of American Sign Language. In D. I. Slobin (Ed.), *The Cross-linguistic study of language acquisition* (pp. 881 938). Hillsdale, NJ: Lawrence Erlbaum Associates.

National Institute on Deafness and other Communication Disorders (1989). *National research plan.* Bethesda, MD: National Institutes of Health.

National Institute on Deafness and other Communication Disorders (1992). *National strategic research plan for hearing and hearing impairment and voice and voice disorders. NIH pub. 93- 3443.* Bethesda, MD: National Institutes of Health.

Nover, S. (1993a). Who will shape the future of Deaf education. *Deaf American, 43,* 117-123.

Nover, S. (1993b, June). *Our voices, our vision: Politics of deaf education.* Paper presented at the Convention of American Instructors of the Deaf, Baltimore, MD.

Nover, S. (1994, October). *Full inclusion for deaf students: an ethnographic perspective.* Paper presented at the Conference on Inclusion—Defining Quality Education for Deaf and Hard-of-Hearing Students, Washington, DC.

Odom P., Blanton, R.L., & Nunnally, J. (1967). Some "cloze" technique studies of language capability in the deaf. *Journal of Speech And Hearing Research, 10,* 816-827.

Ogbu, J. (1978). *Minority education and caste.* New York: Academic Press.

O'Grady, L., Van Hoek, K., & Bellugi, U. (1990). The intersection of signing, spelling and script. In W. H. Edmondson & F. Karlsson (Eds.), *SLR '87: Papers from the Fourth International Symposium on Sign language Research* (pp. 224-234). Hamburg: Signum.

Oliver, M. (1991). Multispecialist and multidisciplinary — a recipe for confusion? 'Too many cooks spoil the broth'. *Disability, Handicap & Society, 6,* 65-68.

O'Neil, M. (1973). *The receptive language competence of deaf children in the use of the base structure rules of transformational generative grammar.* Unpublished doctoral dissertation, University of Pittsburgh, PA.

Open University (1991). *D251: Deaf people in hearing worlds.* Milton Keynes: Open University.

Orr, F. C., De Matteo, A., Heller, B., Lee, M., & Nguyen, M. (1987). Psychological assessment. In H. Elliott, L. Glass & J. W. Evans (Eds.), *Mental health assessment of deaf clients: a practical manual* (pp. 93-106). San Diego: College-Hill.

Osberger, M. J., Miyamoto, R. T., Zimmerman-Phillips, S., Kemink, J. L., Stroer, B., Firszt, J. B., & Novak, M. A. (1991). Independent evaluations of the speech perception abilities of children with the Nucleus 22-channel cochlear implant system. *Ear and Hearing 12* (4) (Suppl. 66S-80S).

Osberger, M. J., Todd, S. L., Berry, S. W., Robbins, A. M., & Miyamoto, R. T. (1991). Effect of age of onset of deafness on children's speech perception abilities with a cochlear implant. *Annals of Otology, Rhinology, and Laryngology, 100,* 883-888.

Padden, C. (1980). The deaf community and the culture of deaf people. In C. Baker & R. Battison (Eds.), *Sign language and the deaf community: Essays in honor of William C. Stokoe* (pp. 89-103). Silver Spring, MD: National Association of the Deaf.

Padden, C. (1988). *Interaction of morphology and syntax in American Sign language.* New York: Garland. University of California, San Diego.

Padden, C. (1991). The acquisition of fingerspelling in deaf children. In P. Siple & S. Fischer (Eds.), *Theoretical issues in sign language research* (Vol. 2, pp. 191-210). Chicago: University of Chicago Press.

Padden, C., & Humphries, T. (1988). *Deaf in America: Voices from a culture.* Cambridge, MA: Harvard University Press.

Padden, C., & Perlmutter, D. (1987). American Sign Language and the architecture of phonological theory. *Natural Language and Linguistic Theory, 5,* 335-375.

Panara, R. (1987a). Cultural programs. In J. V. Van Cleve (Ed.), *Gallaudet encyclopedia of deaf people and deafness* (pp. 216-222). New York: McGraw-Hill.

Panara, R. (1987b). Performing arts. In J. V. Van Cleve (Ed.), *Gallaudet encyclopedia of deaf people and deafness* (pp. 274-276). New York: McGraw-Hill.

Parratt, D. & Tipping, B. (1991). The state, social work and deafness. In S. Gregory & G. M. Hartley (Eds.), *Constructing deafness* (pp. 247-252). London: Pinter.

Patrie, C. (1994). Educational interpreting: Who leads the way? *Registry of Interpreters for the Deaf Views, 11 (2)*, 1,19-20.

Pattison, R. (1982). *On literacy*. New York: Oxford University Press.

Paul, P. (1994). *Toward an understanding of deafness and second-language literacy*. Paper presented at the Annual Conference of Teachers of English and Language Arts: Convention of American Instructors of the Deaf. Youngstown, OH.

Paul, P. & Jackson, D. (1993). *Toward a psychology of deafness*. Boston, MA: Allyn & Bacon.

Paul, P. & Quigley, S. (1990). *Education and deafness*. New York, Longman.

Peter, W. W. (1934). Germany's sterilization program. *American Journal of Public Health, 24 (3)*, 187-191.

Petitto, L. A. (1993). On the ontogenetic requirements for early language acquisition. In B. de Boysson-Bardies, S. de Schonen, P. Jusczyk & J. Morton (Eds.), *Developmental neurocognition: speech and face processing in the first year of life* (pp. 365-383). New York: Kuwer Academic Press.

Petitto, L. A., & Bellugi, U. (1988). Spatial cognition and brain organization: Clues from the acquisition of a language in space. In J. Stiles-Davis, M. Kritchevsky & U. Bellugi (Eds.), *Spatial cognition: Brain bases and development* (pp. 299-327). Hillsdale, NJ: Lawrence Erlbaum Associates.

Petitto, L. A., & Marentette, P. F. (1991). Babbling in the manual mode: Evidence for the ontogeny of language. *Science, 251*, 1493-1496.

Pizzuto, E. (1994). The early development of deixis in American Sign Language: What is the point? In V. Volterra & C. Erting (Eds.), *From gesture to language in hearing and Deaf children* (pp. 142-152). Washington, DC: Gallaudet University Press.

Plann, S. (1993). Pedro Ponce de Leon: Myth and reality. In J. Van Cleve (Ed.), *Deaf history unveiled* (pp. 1-12). Washington, DC: Gallaudet University Press.

Poizner, H., Klima, E., & Bellugi, U. (1987). *What the hands reveal about the brain*. Cambridge, MA: Massachusetts Institute of Technology Press.

Poizner, H., Newkirk, D., Bellugi, U., & Klima, E. (1981). Representation of inflected signs from American Sign Language in short-term memory. *Memory and Cognition, 9*, 121-131.

Pollard, R. Q., Gutman, V. A., DeMatteo, A. D., & Stewart, L. (1991). *Training in deafness and mental health: Studies and issues*. Paper presented at the meeting of the American Psychological Association, San Francisco.

Pollard, R. Q. (1995). Public mental health service and diagnostic trends regarding individuals who are deaf or hard of hearing. *Rehabilitation Psychology, 39*, 147-160.

Porter, R. P. (1990). *Forked tongue: The politics of bilingual education*. New York: Basic Books.

Preston, P. (1994). *Mother father deaf: Living between sound and silence*. Cambridge, MA: Harvard University Press.

Pride in a silent language (1993, May 16). *New York Times*, 22.

Quigley, S., & Kretschmer, R. (1982). *The education of deaf children*. Baltimore, MD: University Park Press.

Quigley, S., & Paul, P. (1984). *Language and deafness*. San Diego: College Hill Press.

Rabinowitz, W. M., Eddington, D. K., Delhorne, L. A., & Cuneo, P. A. (1992). Relations among different measures of speech reception in subjects using a cochlear implant. *Journal of the Acoustical Society of America, 92*, 1869-1881.

Ragosta, M. (1987). *Students with disabilities. Four years of data from special test administrations of the Scholastic Aptitude Test 1980-1983*. (Report 87-2). New York: College Board.

Ramirez, J. D., Yuen, S. D., & Ramey, D. R. (1991). *Final report: Longitudinal study of structured immersion strategy, early-exit and late-exit transitional bilingual education programs for language-minority children*. San Mateo, CA: Aguirre International.

Ramsey, C. (1993). *A description of classroom discourse an literacy learning among deaf elementary students in a mainstream program.* Unpublished doctoral dissertation, University of California, Berkeley, CA.

Rawlings, B., Karchmer, M., & DeCaro, J. J. (Eds.). (1988). *College and career programs for deaf students.* Washington, DC: Gallaudet University.

Reed, C. M., Durlach, N. I., Delhorne, L. A., Rabinowitz, W. M., & Grant, K. W. (1989). Research on tactual communication of speech: Ideas, issues, and findings. *Volta Review, 91*, 65-78.

Reilly, J. S., McIntire, M. L., & Bellugi, U. (1994). Faces: The relationship between language and affect. In V. Volterra & C. Erting (Eds.), *From gesture to language in hearing and Deaf children* (pp. 128-141). Washington, DC: Gallaudet University Press.

Reiman, J., Bullis, M., Davis, C., & Cole, A. (1991). "Lower- achieving" deaf people: Overview and case study. *Volta Review, 93*, 99-120.

Renteria, D. (1995, March). Deaf Gay and Lesbian coalition. *DCARA News.*

Reynolds, A. G. (1991). The cognitive consequences of bilingualism. In A. G. Reynolds (Ed.), *Bilingualism, multiculturalism, and second language learning* (pp. 145-182). Hillsdale, NJ: Lawrence Erlbaum Associates.

Robards-Armstrong, C., & Stone, H. E. (1994). Research in audiological rehabilitation: Current trends and future directions; The consumer's perspective. In J. P. Gagné & N. Tye-Murray (Eds.), *Research in audiological rehabilitation* (pp. 25-44). Cedar Falls, IA: American Academy of Rehabilitative Audiology.

Rodda, M., & Grove, C. (1987). *Language, cognition and deafness.* Hillsdale, NJ: Lawrence Erlbaum Associates.

Rodriguez, O., & Santiviago, M. (1991). Hispanic deaf adolescents: A multicultural minority. *Volta Review, 93*, 89-97.

Romaine, S. (1988). *Pidgin & creole languages.* New York: Longman.

Rose, D. E. (1994). Cochlear implants in children with prelingual deafness: Another side of the coin. *American Journal of Audiology, 3, 6.*

Ross, M. (Ed.), (1990). *Hearing-impaired children in the mainstream.* Parkton, MD: York Press.

Ross, M., & Calvert, D. R. (1967). Semantics of deafness. *Volta Review, 69*, 644-649.

Roy, C. (1992). A sociolinguistic analysis of the interpreter's role in simultaneous talk in a face-to-face interpreted dialogue. *Sign Language Studies, 74*, 21-61.

Ruben, R. J. (1991). The history of genetics of hearing impairment. *Annals of the New York Academy of Sciences, 630*, 6-15.

Rudner, L. (1978). Using standard tests with the hearing-impaired. *Volta Review, 80*, 31-40.

Rutherford, S. (1989). Funny in Deaf—not in hearing. In S. Wilcox (Ed.), *American Deaf Culture* (pp. 65-82). Silver Spring, MD: Linstok Press.

Rutherford, S., & Mocenigo, R. (1984). *American culture: The Deaf perspective. Vol. 2 Deaf folklore. Vol. 3 Deaf literature* (Videotapes). San Francisco, CA: San Francisco Public Library.

Sabatino, D. (1982). Preparing individual educational programs (IEPs). In D. Sabatino & L. Mann (Eds.), *A handbook of diagnostic and prescriptive teaching* (pp. 19-70). Rockville, MD: Aspen.

Sanders, B. (1994). *A is for ox.* New York: Pantheon Books.

Sandlin, R. E. (1994). *Understanding digitally programmable hearing aids.* Boston: Allyn & Bacon.

Schein, J. D. (1989). *At home among strangers.* Washington, DC: Gallaudet University Press.

Schein, J. D., & Delk, M. T. (1974). The deaf population of the United States. Silver Spring, MD: National Association of the Deaf.

Schick, B. (1990). Classifier predicates in American Sign Language. *International Journal of Sign Linguistics, 1*, 15-40.

Schick, B., & Williams, K. (1994). Evaluating educational interpreters using classroom performance. *Registry of Interpreters for the Deaf Views, 11*, 15.

Schildroth, A. (1990). *Achievement testing of deaf students: the 8th edition Stanford Achievement Test.* Washington, DC: Center for Assessment and Demographic Studies, Gallaudet University.

Schildroth, A., & Hoto, S. (1991). Annual survey of hearing-impaired children and youth: 1989-90 school year. *American Annals of the Deaf, 136*, 155-164.

Schildroth, A., & Hotto, S. (1993). Annual survey of hearing-impaired children and youth. *American Annals of the Deaf, 138*, 163-171.

Schildroth, A., Rawlings, B., & Allen, T. E. (1991). Deaf students in transition: Education and employment issues for deaf adolescents. *Volta Review, 93*, 41-53.

Schlesinger, H. S. (1972). Meaning and enjoyment: Language acquisition of deaf children. In T. O'Rourke (Ed.), *Psycholinguistics and Total Communication: The state of the art.* Silver Spring, MD: National Association of the Deaf.

Schlesinger, H. S. (1985). Deafness, mental health, and language. In F. Powell, T. Finitzo-Hieber, S. Friel-Patti & D. Henderson (Eds.), *Education of the hearing-impaired child* (pp. 103-119). San Diego: College-Hill.

Schlesinger, H. S. (1987). Effects of powerlessness on dialog and development: Disability, poverty and the human condition. In B. W. Heller, L. M. Flohr & L. S. Zegans (Eds.), *Psychosocial interventions with sensorially disabled persons* (pp. 1-28). Orlando, FL: Grune & Stratton.

Schlesinger, H. S. & Meadow, K. (1972). *Sound and sign: Childhood deafness and mental health.* Berkeley, CA: University of California Press.

Schuchman, J. S. (1988). *Hollywood speaks: Deafness and the film entertainment industry*. Urbana: University of Illinois Press.

Scott, R. A. (1981). *The making of blind men*. New Brunswick, NJ: Transaction.

Shand, M. (1982). Sign-based short-term coding of American Sign Language signs and printed English words by congenitally deaf signers. *Cognitive Psychology, 14*, 1-12.

Shapiro, J. P. (1993). *No pity: People with disabilities forging a new civil rights movement.* New York: Times Books.

Shea, J. J., Domico, E. H., & Lupfer, M. (1994). Speech perception after multichannel cochlear implantation in the pediatric patient. *American Journal of Otology, 15*, 66-70.

Shroyer, E. H., & Shroyer, S. P. (1984). *Signs across America.* Washington, DC: Gallaudet University Press.

Sidransky, R. (1990). *In silence: Growing up hearing in a deaf world.* New York: St. Martin's Press.

Silver, A. (1993). Reframing Deaf art/De'VIA for the 21st century. In College for Continuing Education (Ed.), *Deaf studies III: Bridging cultures in the 21st century. Proceedings of a conference April 22-25, 1993* (pp. 67-74). Washington, DC: Gallaudet University.

Singleton, J. (1989). *Restructuring of language from Impoverished input: Evidence for linguistic compensation.* Unpublished Doctoral Dissertation, University of Illinois, Urbana-Champaign, IL.

Siple, P. (1978). Visual constraints and the forms of signs. *Sign Language Studies, 19*, 95-110.

Sisco, F. H., & Anderson, R. J. (1980). Deaf children's performance on the WISC-R relative to hearing status of parents and child-rearing experiences. *American Annals of the Deaf, 125*, 923-930.

Smith, D. (1986). Mental health research enters realm of linguistics. *Research at Gallaudet*, 3-5.

Smith, F. (1978). *Understanding reading*. New York: Holt, Rinehart & Winston.

Smith, P. (1994). *A professional deaf educator in spite of the system.* In C. Erting, R. E. Johnson, D. L.

Smith & B. D. Snider (Eds.). *The Deaf Way: Perspectives from the International Conference on Deaf Culture* (pp. 669-673). Washington, DC: Gallaudet University Press.

Smith, R. H., Berlin, C. I., Hejmancik, J. F., Keats, B. J. B., Kimberling, E. J., Lewis, R. A., Moller, C. G., Peliias, M. Z., & Trenebjarg, L.(1994). Clinical diagnosis of the Usher Syndromes. *American Journal of Medical Genetics, 50*, 32-38.

Snow, C., Barnes, W., Chandler, J., Goodman, I., & Hemphill, L. (1991). *Unfulfilled expectations: Home and school influences on literacy*. Cambridge, MA: Harvard University Press.

Somers, M. N. (1991). Speech perception abilities in children with cochlear implants or hearing aids. *American Journal of Otology, 12*, 174-178.

Sonnenstrahl, D. (1993). Visual arts in Deaf studies: Historical perspectives on Deaf artists. In College for Continuing Education (Ed.), *Deaf studies III: Bridging cultures in the 21st century. Proceedings of a conference April 22-25, 1993* (pp. 19-24). Washington, DC: Gallaudet University.

Spradley, T. S., & Spradley, J. P. (1978). *Deaf like me*. New York: Random House.

Spragins, A. B., Karchmer, M. B., & Schildroth, A. N. (1981). Profile of psychological services providers to hearing-impaired students. *American Annals of the Deaf, 126*, 94-105.

Stedt, J. (1992). Issues of education interpreting. In Kluwin, T., Moores, D., & Gonter-Gaustad, M. (Eds.), *Toward effective public school programs for deaf students: context, process, and outcomes* (pp. 83-99). New York: Teachers College Press.

Steinberg, A. (1991). Issues in providing mental health services to hearing impaired persons. *Hospital and Community Psychiatry, 42*, 380-389.

Sternberg, R. J. (1987). Most vocabulary is learned from context. In M. G. McKeown & M. E. Curtis (Eds.), *The nature of vocabulary acquisition* (pp. 89-105). Hillsdale, NJ: Lawrence Erlbaum Associates.

Stewart, D. A. (1991). *Deaf sport: The impact of sports within the Deaf community*. Washington, DC: Gallaudet University Press.

Stone, H. E., & Hurwitz, T. A. (1994). Accessibility to the hearing world: Assistive devices and specialized support. In R. C. Nowell & L. E. Marshak (Eds.), *Understanding deafness and the rehabilitation process* (pp. 239-268). Boston: Allyn & Bacon.

Strassler, B. (1995, August). Eugene Hairston. *Silent News, 27*, 37.

Strassman, B., Kretchmer, R., & Bilsky, L. (1987). The Instantiation of general terms by deaf adolescents/adults. *Journal of Communication Disorders, 20*, 1-13.

Supalla, S. (1986). *The modality question in Signed English development*. Unpublished master's thesis, University of Illinois.

Supalla, S. (1990). *Segmentation of manually coded English: Problems in the mapping of English in the visual/gestural mode*. Unpublished doctoral dissertation, University of Illinois, Urbana-Champaign.

Supalla, S. (1991). Manually coded English: The modality question in signed language development. In P. Siple & S. Fischer (Eds.), *Theoretical issues in sign language research* (Vol. 2, pp. 85-109). Chicago, IL: University of Chicago Press.

Supalla, S. (1992). *The book of name signs: Naming in American Sign Language*. San Diego: DawnSignPress.

Supalla, S. & Bahan, B. (1994). *ASL literature series: "Bird of a different feather" and "For a decent living." (1) Teachers videotape (2) Teachers guide (3) Student workbook (4) Student videotape*. San Diego: DawnSignPress.

Supalla, T. (1986). The classifier system in American Sign Language. In C. Craig (Ed.), *Noun classes and categorization* (pp. 181-214). Philadelphia: Benjamins.

Supalla, T. (1994a). *Charles Krauel: A profile of a deaf filmmaker*. San Diego: DawnSignPress.

Supalla, T. (1994b). Deaf folklife film collection project. In C. Erting, R. E. Johnson, D. L. Smith & B. D. Snider (Eds.), *The Deaf Way: Perspectives from the International Conference on Deaf Culture* (pp. 285-290). Washington, DC: Gallaudet University Press.

Supalla, T., & Newport, E. (1978). How many seats in a chair? The derivation of nouns and verbs in ASL. In P. Siple (Ed.) *Understanding language through sign language research* (pp. 91-132). New York: Academic Press.

Supalla, T., Newport, E., Singleton, J., Supalla, S., Metlay, D., & Coulter, G. (in press). *Test battery of American Sign Language morphology and syntax*. San Diego: DawnSignPress.

Supalla, T., & Webb, R. (1995). *Structure of an international sign language pidgin.* Unpublished paper, University of Rochester, Rochester, NY.

Swain, M., & Lapkin, S. (1991). Additive bilingualism and French immersion education: Roles of language proficiency and literacy. In A. G. Reynolds (Ed.), *Bilingualism, multiculturalism, and second language learning* (pp. 203-216). Hillsdale, NJ: Lawrence Erlbaum Associates.

Swisher, V. (1983). Characteristics of hearing mothers' manually coded English. In W. Stokoe & V. Volterra (Eds.), *SLR '83: Proceedings of the International Symposium on Sign Language Research* (pp. 38-47). Silver Spring, MD: Linstok Press.

Swisher, V. (1984). Signed input of hearing mothers to deaf children. *Language learning, 34* 69-86.

Swisher, V. & Thompson, M. (1985). Mothers learning simultaneous communication: The dimensions of the task. *American Annals of the Deaf, 130*, 212-217.

This protest helped us find pride—and hope. (1988, March 15). *USA Today*, p. 11a.

Troike, R. C. (1978). Research evidence for the effectiveness of bilingual education. *NABE Journal, 3*, 13-24.

Tronick, E., Als, H., Adamson, L., Wise, S., Brazelton, T. (1978). The infant's response to entrapment between two contradictory messages in face-to-face interaction. *Journal of the American Academy of Child Psychiatry, 27*, 74-77.

Truffaut, B. (1993). Etienne de Fay and the history of the deaf. In H. Lane & R. Fischer (Eds.), *Looking back: A reader on the history of deaf communities and their sign languages* (pp. 13-24). Hamburg: Signum.

Truffaut, B. (1994). The French deaf movement after the Milan Congress. In C. Erting, R. E. Johnson, D. L. Smith & B. D. Snider (Eds.), *The Deaf Way: Perspectives from the International Conference on Deaf Culture* (pp. 172-175). Washington, DC: Gallaudet University Press.

Tucker, I., & Nolan, M. (1984). Educational audiology. London: Croom Helm.

Turner, G. (1995). *Signing in the twilight zone.* Unpublished manuscript, Dept. of Educational Studies, University of Central Lancashire, Preston, England.

Tye-Murray, N. (1992). *Cochlear implants and children: a handbook for parents, teachers and speech professionals.* Washington, DC: Alexander Graham Bell Association.

Tyler, R. (1993). Cochlear implants and the deaf culture. *American Journal of Audiology, 2*, 26-32.

United Nations (1994). *The standard rules on the equalization of opportunities for persons with disabilities.* New York: United Nations.

UNESCO (1985). *Consultation on alternative approaches for the education of the deaf ED-84/ws/102.* Paris: UNESCO.

UNESCO (1994). *The Salamanca statement and framework for action on special needs education ED-94/ws/18.* Paris: UNESCO.

Valentine, V. (1996). Listening to deaf Blacks, *Emerge*, Janurary, 56-61.

Valli, C. (1990). The nature of a line in ASL poetry. In W. H. Edmondson & F. Karlsson (Eds.), *SLR'87: Papers from the Fourth International Symposium on Sign Language Research,* 1987 (pp. 171-182). Hamburg: Signum.

Valli, C. (1995). *ASL poetry, selected works of Clayton Valli* [Videotape and workbook]. San Diego: DawnSignPress.

Van Cleve, J. V. (1993). The academic integration of deaf children: a historical perspective. In R. Fischer & H. Lane (Eds.), *Looking back: A reader on the history of deaf communities and their sign languages* (pp. 333-348). Hamburg: Signum.

Van Cleve, J. V. (1984). Nebraska's oral law of 1911 and the deaf community. *Nebraska History, 65*, 195-220.

Van Cleve, J. V., & Crouch, B. (1989). *A place of their own: Creating the deaf community in America.* Washington, DC: Gallaudet University Press.

Vandell, D., Anderson, L., Ehrhardt, G., & Wilson, K. (1982). Integrating hearing and deaf preschoolers: An attempt to enhance hearing children's interactions with deaf peers. *Child Development, 53*, 1354-1363.

Veditz, G. (1933, June 1). The genesis of the National Association. *Deaf-Mutes Journal, 62* (22), 1.

Vernon, M. (1969a). *Multiply-handicapped deaf children: medical, educational, and psychological considerations.* Washington, DC: Council for Exceptional Children.

Vernon, M. (1969b). Sociological and psychological factors associated with hearing loss. *Journal of Speech and Hearing Research, 12*, 541-563.

Vernon, M. (1991). At the crossroads: the future workplace and implications for rehabilitation. In D. Watson & M. Taff- Watson (Eds.), *At the crossroads: A celebration of diversity. Proceedings of the Twelfth Biennial Conference of American Deafness and Rehabilitation Association* (pp. 3-10). Little Rock, AR: American Deafness and Rehabilitation Association.

Vernon, M. (1995, March). Psychology and deafness: Past and prologue. *Gallaudet Today, 25*, 12-17.

Vincent, N. (1995). *Parent-infant programming*. Paper presented at the Deaf Studies IV Conference, Woburn, MA.

Wagstrom-Lundqvist, G. (1994). The challenge to deaf people in the arts today. In C. Erting, R. E. Johnson, D. L. Smith & B. D. Snider (Eds.), *The Deaf Way: Perspectives from the International Conference on Deaf Culture* (pp. 726-730). Washington, DC: Gallaudet University Press.

Walberg, H. (1984). Improving the productivity of America's schools. *Educational Leadership, 41*, 19-30.

Walker, L. A. (1986). *A loss for words*. New York: Harper Row.

Wallin, L. (1994). The study of sign language in society: Part two. In C. Erting, R. E. Johnson, D. L. Smith & B. D. Snider (Eds.), *The Deaf Way: Perspectives from the International Conference on Deaf Culture* (pp. 318-330). Washington, DC: Gallaudet University Press.

Wallin, L. (1995). *One culture, two languages*. Paper presented at the Deaf Studies IV Conference, Woburn MA.

Waltzman, S. B., Cohen, N. L., Gomolin, R. H., Shapiro, W. H., Ozdamar, S. R., & Hoffman, R. A. (1994). Long-term results of early cochlear implantation in congenitally and prelingually deafened children. *American Journal of Otology, 15 (suppl.)*, 9-13.

Walworth, M. (1992) ESL/ASL: Unanswered questions, unquestioned answers. In M. Walworth, D. Moores, & T. O'Rourke (Eds.), *A freehand: Enfranchising the education of Deaf children* (pp. 119-139). Silver Spring, MD: T. J. Publishers.

Washabaugh, W. (1986). *Five fingers for survival.* Ann Arbor MI: Karoma Publishers.

Watson, D. (1994). Education and jobs in the United States. In H. Lane (Ed.), *Parallel views: Education and access for Deaf people in France and the United States* (pp. 149-163). Washington, DC: Gallaudet University Press.

Webster, A. (1987). Reading and writing in severely hearing-impaired children. *International Journal of Rehabilitation Research, 10*, 227-229.

Weisel, A., & Reichstein, J. (1987). Parental hearing status, reading comprehension skills, and social-emotional adjustment. In R. Ojala (Ed.), *Proceedings of the Tenth World Congress of the World Federation of the Deaf.* Helsinki: Finnish Association of the Deaf.

Wells, G. (1981). *Learning through language: The study of language development Vol. 1.* Cambridge: Cambridge University Press.

WGBH (1993). *Line 21 Closed captions: History and description.* Boston, MA: WGBH.

Wilbur, R. B. (1987). *American Sign Language* (2nd ed.). Boston: Little-Brown.

Wilbur, R. B. (1994). Eyeblinks and ASL phrase structure. *Sign Language Studies, 84*, 221-240.

Wilcox, P., Schroeder, F., & Martinez, T. (1990). A commitment to professionalism: Educational interpreting standards within a large public school system. *Sign Language Studies, 68*, 277-286.

Willard, T. (1989). Shining a spotlight on America's Deaf visual artists. In G. Olsen (Ed.), *A kaleidoscope of Deaf America* (p. 27). Silver Spring, MD: National Association of the Deaf.

Williams, J. & Capizzi-Snipper, G. (1990). *Literacy and bilingualism.* White Plains, NY: Longman.

Willig, A. (1985). A meta-analysis of selected studies on the effectiveness of bilingual education. *Review of Educational Research, 55*, 269-318.

Willigan, B. A., & King, S. J. (Eds.) (1992). *Mental health services for deaf people*. Washington, DC: Gallaudet Research Institute.

Wilson, G. B., Ross, M., & Calvert, D. R. (1974). An experimental study of the semantics of deafness. *Volta Review, 76*, 408-414.

Winefield, R. (1987). *Never the twain shall meet: The communications debate*. Washington, DC: Gallaudet University Press.

Winzer, M. A. (1993). Education, urbanization and the deaf community: A case study of Toronto, 1870-1900. In J. Van Cleve (Ed.), *Deaf history unveiled* (pp. 127-145). Washington, DC: Gallaudet University Press.

Winzer, M. A. (1986). Deaf-Mutia: Responses to alienation by the deaf in the mid-nineteenth century. *American Annals of the Deaf, 131*, 29-32.

Wisconsin Phonological Institute (1894). *Improvement of the Wisconsin system of education for deaf-mutes*. Milwaukee: WPI.

Wodlinger-Cohen, R. (1991). The manual representation of speech by Deaf children, their mothers and their teachers. In P. Siple & S. Fischer (Eds.), *Theoretical issues in sign language research Vol. 2* (pp. 149-170). Chicago, IL: University of Chicago Press.

Wolf, E. G. (1987). Deafblindness. In J. V. Van Cleve (Ed.), *Gallaudet encyclopedia of deaf people and deafness* (pp. 226-250). New York: McGraw-Hill.

Wolff, A. B., & Harkins, J. E. (1986). Multihandicapped students. In A. N. Schildroth & M. A. Karchmer (Eds.), *Deaf children in America* (pp. 55-82). San Diego: College-Hill.

Wolk, S., & Allen, T. E. (1984). A five-year follow-up of reading comprehension achievement of hearing-impaired students in special education programs. *Journal of Special Education, 18*, 161-176.

Wolk, S., & Schildroth, A. N. (1986). Deaf children and speech intelligibility: A national study. In A. N. Schildroth & M. A. Karchmer (Eds.), *Deaf children in America* (pp. 139-160). San Diego: College-Hill.

Wood, S., & Holcomb, M. (1989). Deaf women at vanguard of history. In G. Olsen (Ed.), *A kaleidoscope of Deaf America* (pp. 20-21). Silver Spring, MD: National Association of the Deaf.

Woodward, J. (1973). Interrule implication in American Sign Language. *Sign Language Studies, 3*, 47-56.

Woodward, J. (1974). Implicational variation in American Sign Language: Negative incorporation. *Sign Language Studies, 5*, 20-30.

Woodward, J. (1976). Black southern signing. *Language in Society, 5*, 211-218.

Woodward, J. (1978a). Attitudes toward deaf people on Providence Island, Colombia. *American Anthropologist, 63*, 49-68.

Woodward, J. (1978b). Historical bases of American Sign Language. In P. Siple (Ed.), *Understanding language through sign language research*. New York: Academic Press.

Woodward, J. (1990). Sign English in the education of deaf students. In H. Bornstein (Ed.), *Manual communication in America* (pp. 67-80). Washington, DC: Gallaudet University Press.

Woodward, J., Allen, T. E., & Schildroth, A. (1985). Teachers and deaf students: An ethnography of classroom communication. In S. DeLancey & R. Tomlin (Eds.), *Proceedings of the First Annual Pacific Linguistics Conference* (pp. 479-493). Eugene, OR: University of Oregon Press.

Woodward, J., & De Santis, S. (1977). Two to one it happens: Dynamic phonology in two sign languages. *Sign Language Studies, 17*, 329-346.

Woodward, J., & Markowicz, H. (1975). *Some handy new ideas on pidgins and creoles: Pidgin sign languages*. Paper presented at the Conference on Pidgin and Creole Languages, Honolulu, Hawaii.

Woodward, J. C., & Erting, C. (1975). Synchronic variation and historical change in American Sign Language. *Language Science, 37*, 9-12.

World Federation of the Deaf (1992). *Proceedings of the XIth World Congress of the World Federation of the Deaf, Tokyo, July 2-11, 1991*. Tokyo: World Federation of the Deaf.

World Federation of the Deaf (1993a). Violations of human rights. *World Federation of the Deaf News*, 14.

World Federation of the Deaf (1993b). Sign languages oppressed; Deaf community not satisfied. *World Federation of the Deaf News*, 20-21.

World Health Organization (1980). *International classification of impairments, disabilities, and handicaps*. Geneva: World Health Organization.

Wright, L. (1994, July 25). Annals of politics: One drop of blood. *The New Yorker*, 46-55.

Zimmer, J. (1989). Toward a description of register variation in American Sign Language. In C. Lucas (Ed.), *The sociolinguistics of the Deaf community* (pp. 253-272). New York: Academic Press.

Zweibel, A. (1987). More on the effects of early manual communication on the cognitive development of deaf children. *American Annals of the Deaf, 132*, 16-20.

Index

A

C

D

E

F

G

H

I

M

N

O

P

S

T

U

V

W

About the Authors

❦

HARLAN LANE is a recipient of the prestigious MacArthur Fellowship and of the World Federation of the Deaf International Social Merit Award. He is Matthews University Distinguished Professor at Northeastern University, Research Affiliate at the Massachusetts Institute of Technology. His Deaf history, *When the Mind Hears*, and contemporary commentary, *The Mask of Benevolence: Disabling the Deaf Community*, have won the Literary Achievement Award of the National Association of the Deaf.

ROBERT HOFFMEISTER is Associate Professor of Education at Boston University, where he directs the oldest Deaf Studies program in the U.S.; programs for education of the Deaf and ASL; and the Center for the Study of Communication and Deafness. He is a prolific writer and advocate for the DEAF–WORLD, in which he grew up as the hearing son of Deaf parents.

BEN BAHAN is Associate Professor of Deaf Studies at Gallaudet University. He is a noted Deaf scholar in ASL linguistics, a lecturer on history, culture and education of the Deaf, and a celebrated ASL storyteller in the DEAF–WORLD.

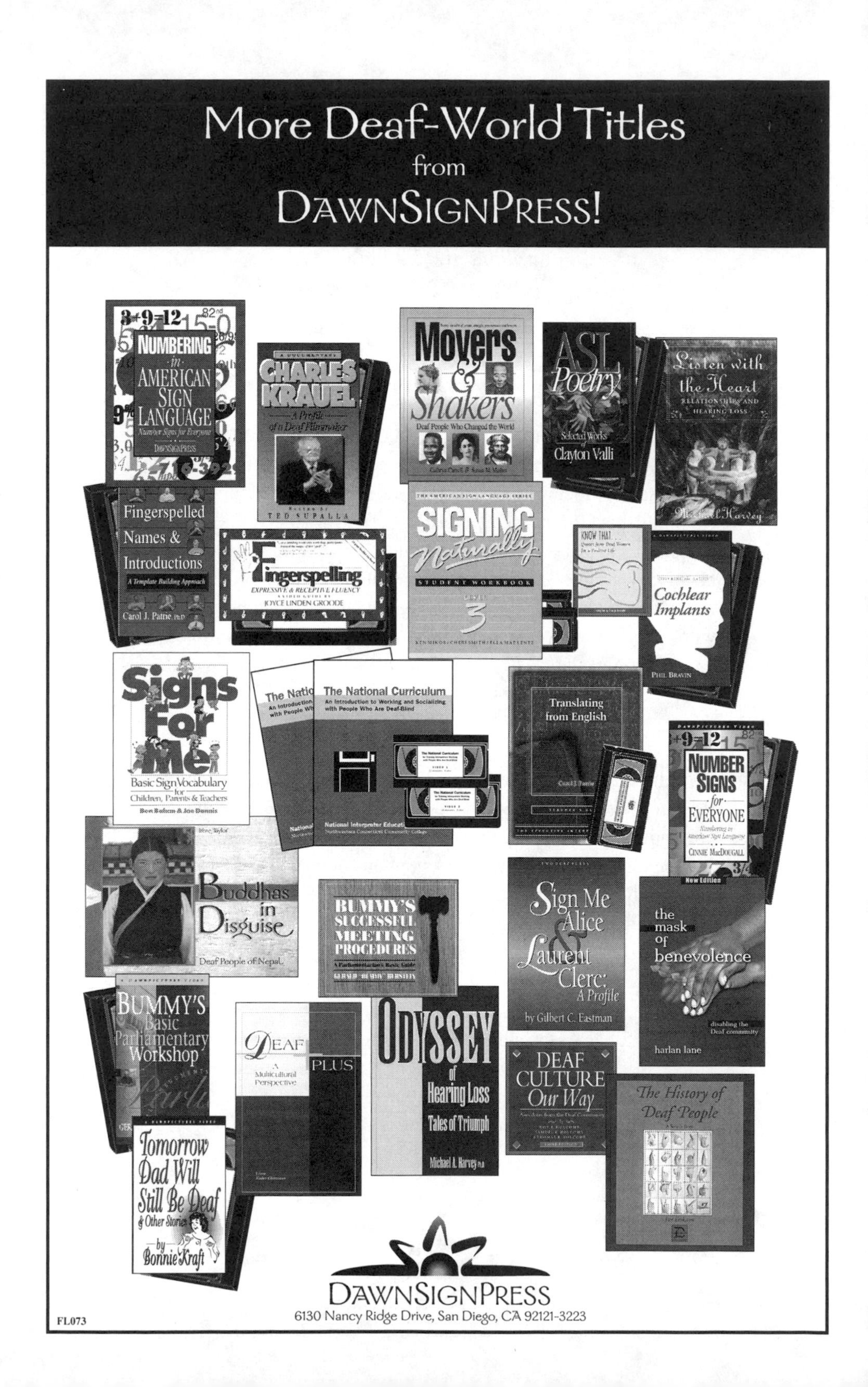